Phonology

as Human Behavior

Sound

and Meaning

The Roman Jakobson Series

in Linguistics and Poetics

C. H. van Schooneveld,

Series Editor

Phonology as Human Behavior

Theoretical Implications and Clinical Applications

Yishai Tobin

Duke
University Press
Durham & London
1997

Printed in the United States of America on acid-free paper ∞

Typeset in Times with Futura display by Tseng Information Systems, Inc.

Library of Congress Cataloging-in-Publication Data appear on the last printed page of this book.

In memory of

Professor William Diver

As this book was going to press, I was informed

of Professor Diver's untimely passing. It is with

great sadness, regret, respect, and affection

that I dedicate this volume

to his memory

In the study of isolated sounds, to note the position of the vocal organs is sufficient, . . . as for articulation, the speaker has unlimited freedom. But when we come to the pronunciation of two sounds that are joined, the problem is not so simple; and we must bear in mind the possible discrepancy between the effect desired and the effect produced. We do not always have the ability to pronounce what we intend. Freedom in linking phonological species is checked by the possibility of linking articulatory movements. . . . The importance of combinatory phonology in general linguistics is obvious. Whereas traditional phonology generally gives rules for articulating all sounds—variable and accidental elements of language—and stops there, combinatory phonology limits the possibilities and defines the constant relations of interdependent phonemes.
—Ferdinand de Saussure ([1916] 1966: 50–51)

I will try to promote an approach to phonology that I think will do for the field what Buddhism promises to do for the soul: to permit it to escape the endless agonizing cycle of birth and death of trendy theories, schools, frameworks, etc. and achieve oneness with the spirit and principles that guide all scientific endeavor, be it physics, chemistry, physiology, psychology, or linguistics.
—J. J. Ohala (1987: 207)

Contents

List of Figures and Tables xiii
Preface xvii

I Phonetics and Phonology *A Historical Overview* 1

1 Phonetics versus Phonology: The Prague School and Beyond 3

Theoretical and Methodological Assumptions . 3 The Historical Development of Phonetics versus Phonology . 8 Defining Language Synergetically . 18 Summary and Conclusions . 23

2 Phonology as Human Behavior 25

The Columbia School . 25 Phonetics and Phonology in the Columbia School . 27 The Identification of Unobservable Units . 28 The Statement of the Problem . 30 The Fundamental Analytic Position . 32 The Analysis . 33 Summary and Conclusions . 46

II Phonology as Human Behavior across Languages 51

3 The Italian and Latin Connections 53

Combinatory Phonology . 53 The Study . 56 The Analysis . 59 Summary and Conclusions . 86

4 The Hebrew and Yiddish Connections 88

Theoretical and Methodological Background . 88 The Triconsonantal (CCC) Root System . 89 Consonant Clusters in Hebrew . 106 Consonant Clusters in Yiddish . 112 Summary and Conclusions . 119

III Phonology as Human Behavior *Panchronic, Pedagogical, and Textual Applications* 123

5 Panchronic Applications in Hebrew Phonology 125

The Stop/Spirant Alternation in Hebrew . 125 Summary and Conclusions . 144

6 Pedagogical and Textual Applications 145
Teaching Phonetics as Human Behavior . 145 A Text Analysis: "Jabberwocky" . 150 The Analysis . 152 Summary and Conclusions . 169

IV Phonology as Human Behavior
Developmental and Clinical Applications 171

7 Developmental Phonology and Functional Clinical Applications 173
Language Acquisition and Phonology as Human Behavior . 173 The Role of Roman Jakobson and Developmental Phonology . 174 Jakobson's Claims and Phonology as Human Behavior . 178 Post-1968 Claims and Phonology as Human Behavior . 182 Phonological Processes and Phonology as Human Behavior . 184 Functional Processes in Hebrew-Speaking Children . 191 Functional Processes in a Hearing Child of Deaf Parents . 194 Functional Clinical Applications . 195 Defining Language Disorders . 196 The Aims of Clinical Linguistics . 200 Phonology as Human Behavior and Functional Clinical Applications . 201 Description versus Explanation in the Clinic . 206 Summary and Conclusions . 209

8 Clinical Applications to Organic Disorders 210
Phonological Theory and the Speech Clinic . 210 Phonology as Human Behavior and the Speech Clinic . 211 Clinical Applications to Organic Disorders . 215 Summary and Conclusions . 250

V Phonology as Human Behavior
Audiology and Aphasia 253

9 Audiology, Hearing Impairment, and Cochlear Implants 255
Audiology and Hearing Impairment . 255 The Speech of the Hearing Impaired from a Traditional Point of View . 257 The Speech of the Hearing Impaired and Functional Processes . 260 The Speech of the Hearing Impaired and Phonology as Human Behavior . 262 Audiology and Phonology as Human Behavior . 270 Cochlear Implants and Phonology as Human Behavior . 279 Summary and Conclusions . 283

10 Aphasia 284
Aphasia: Definition and Classification . 284 Linguistics, Phonology, and Aphasia . 285 The Language of Apraxia and Aphasia and Phonology as Human Behavior . 290 Aphasia and Phonology as Human Behavior . 292 Summary and Conclusions . 303

Appendices 307
Notes 311
References 337
Index 375

List of Figures and Tables

Figures

1.1 The Structuralist Paradigm 6
1.2 Phonetics versus Phonology 7
1.3 The Synergetic Relation between the Encoder and the Decoder 22
2.1 The linguistic Sign 26

Tables

1.1 Trubetzkoy's Classes of Vowels and Consonants 14
2.1 Frequency Distributions for Occurrence of *l* and *r* in Initial Clusters in English 34
3.1 Phonemic Inventory of Italian (Hypothesized) 58
3.2 Phonetic Characterization by Stricture and Airflow 60
3.3 Frequencies of Phonemes of Constriction by Class 62
3.4 Phonemes Characterized by Articulators, Aperture, and Airflow 70
3.5 Frequencies of Initial Latin Phonemes of Constriction, by Class 73
3.6 Proportions of Stems from Sources Other than Classical Latin, from a Random Sample 74
3.7 Class II Phonemes Evaluated for Factors A, Q, V, E, and T 76
3.8 Distribution of Clusters of Classes II and III 78
3.9 Distribution of Clusters of Classes II and III, by Class III Phoneme 79
3.10 Stable and Mobile Coordination 81
4.1 The Hebrew Consonant System: Active Articulators 91
4.2 The Disfavoring of Additional Articulators in Adjacent Phonetic Environments 95
4.3 The Favoring of Phonemes with Complete Constriction in Root-Initial and Root-Final Positions 96
4.4 The Disfavoring of the Same Articulators in Adjacent Phonetic Environments 99

4.5 The Disfavoring of the Same Phoneme in Adjacent Phonetic Environments 102
4.6 The Favoring of the Apex in the Phonemic Inventory of Hebrew 103
4.7 The Favoring of the Apex in C-I Position 104
4.8 The Favoring of the Apex in C-II Position 104
4.9 The Favoring of the Apex in C-III Position 105
4.10 The Favoring of Visible Phonemes in C-I = C-II Position 106
4.11 Frequency Distributions for Occurrences of *l* and *r* in Initial Clusters in Hebrew 107
4.12 Frequency Distributions for Occurrences of *l* and *r* in Initial Clusters in Yiddish 112
5.1 Rule Opacity 130
5.2 Opacity of Phonetic Motivation 132
5.3 Opacity by Parasites 135
6.1 Number of Syllables per Word (General Corpus) 153
6.2 Number of Syllables per Word (Neologisms) 153
6.3 Stressed Syllables (General Corpus) 155
6.4 Stressed Syllables (Neologisms) 155
6.5 Voicing in Word-Initial Position (General Corpus) 157
6.6 Voicing in Word-Initial Position (Neologisms) 157
6.7 Distribution of Active Articulators in Word-Initial Position (General Corpus) 158
6.8 Distribution of Active Articulators in Word-Initial Position (Neologisms) 159
6.9 The Favoring of Visible Phonemes in Word-Initial Position (General Corpus) 160
6.10 The Favoring of Explosive Phonemes in Word-Initial Position (General Corpus) 161
6.11 The Favoring of Explosive Phonemes in Word-Initial Position (Neologisms) 161
6.12 The Favoring of Apical Phonemes in Word-Final Position (General Corpus) 162
6.13 Percentage of Active Articulators in Word-Initial and Word-Final Position (General Corpus) 162
6.14 The Favoring of Apical Phonemes in Word-Final Position (Neologisms) 163
6.15 Percentage of Active Articulators in Word-Initial and Word-Final Position (Neologisms) 163

6.16 The Disfavoring of Additional Articulators in Adjacent Phonetic Environments (General Corpus) 164
6.17 The Disfavoring of Additional Articulators in Adjacent Phonetic Environments (Neologisms) 165
6.18 The Distribution of the Same Articulators in Adjacent Phonetic Environments (General Corpus) 167
6.19 The Distribution of the Same Articulators in Adjacent Phonetic Environments (Neologisms) 168
8.1 Deaffrication in a Mentally Retarded Child 244
8.2 Consonant Cluster Reduction in a Mentally Retarded Child 245
8.3 Deletion of Velar Fricatives in a Mentally Retarded Child 246
8.4 Deletion of Unstressed Initial Syllables in a Mentally Retarded Child 248
9.1 Functional Processes in the Speech of Deaf Children 262

Preface

> The ultimate task of phonology is to discover the causes of the behavior of speech sounds. To do this phonologists must refer to the way speech is created and used by humans, including how it is stored in the brain, retrieved, executed and perceived, and used to facilitate social interaction among humans. —John J. Ohala (1983b: 189)

> Phonology, then, is for us an attempt to understand the non-random distribution within the signal, and grammar is the attempt to understand the non-random distribution of the signals themselves.
> —William Diver (1975: 13)

> It must be repeated yet again that it is not up to language to conform to the edicts of linguists, it is up to linguists to adapt their methods if they do not do full justice to the language being studied.
> —André Martinet (1955: 125–26)

> Let the language tell you how to analyze it. —C. H. van Schooneveld

The purpose of this book is to present the theory of phonology as human behavior, introduced by William Diver of the Columbia school of form-content analysis. This theory takes into account the communication and human orientations inherent in the definition of language as a system of signs used by human beings to communicate. The goal of this theory is to explain how the paradigmatic systems of phonemes and the nonrandom syntagmatic patterns of their distribution directly reflect the axiom that language represents a constant search for maximum communication with minimal effort.

Following the adage that the proof of the pudding is in the eating, I will show how the theory of phonology as human behavior may be applied to language in general via a series of language-specific and cross-linguistic analyses of English, Italian, Latin, Hebrew, and Yiddish. I will then show how the theory may be appealed to in order to explain a particularly thorny diachronic problem in Hebrew phonemics, one that has far-reaching socio-linguistic synchronic implications, and applied to the teaching of phonetics and the analysis of two poems by Lewis Carroll. Finally, I will apply the theory to language acquisition and use it to explain various functional and organic speech disorders in the speech and hearing clinic, including the language of aphasia.

The theory of phonology as human behavior may be viewed as part of the historical development of a larger twentieth-century structural, functional, and cognitive linguistics. The first basic theoretical and methodological principle of invariance versus variation was introduced by Ferdinand de Saussure. This fundamental concept was further developed within the teleological communication-oriented framework of Nikolai Trubetzkoy and Roman Jakobson of the Prague school in the form of markedness and distinctive feature theory. The human factor in the guise of a therapeutic–human economy orientation was outlined by André Martinet of the functional school of phonology. The synergetic combination of the communication and human factors as a means to explain the nonrandom distribution of sounds in language is what underlies and distinguishes the theory of phonology as human behavior developed by William Diver and his students.

This volume will begin with a historical discussion of the theoretical and methodological connection between phonetics and phonology. This discussion will highlight the need to establish a unit (or units) of analysis that will describe and explain the sounds of language and their synchronic distribution and diachronic development. More specifically, first I will attempt to justify the phoneme as the basic unit of this analysis. Then I will replace some of the formal distinctive features traditionally and neotraditionally associated with the phoneme (e.g., place and manner of articulation, voicing, nasality) with others that may more accurately reflect both the human and the communication factors (e.g., active articulators vs. passive receptors, stabile vs. mobile articulations, the number of sets of articulators to be controlled, and degrees of stricture and airflow). These new theoretical and methodological concepts will be applied to the realm of phonotactics or combinatory phonology in data taken from various languages and the clinic.

This volume represents the joint efforts of the author, a linguist who has spent almost two decades teaching phonetics and phonology, and his graduate and undergraduate students of linguistics, behavioral sciences, speech therapy, and audiology. During the last decade, we have attempted to apply the theory of phonology as human behavior to all aspects of the speech clinic. We are not attempting to sell the theory of phonology as human behavior as the best or the ultimate theory of phonology, nor do we view it as a panacea for all linguists and speech and hearing clinicians. This volume merely documents our attempts to apply a specific approach to language in general and to phonology in particular to both language and languages as well as to another area of linguistic research—clinical phonology and audiology.

At this initial stage of our research, we basically view both the theory and its clinical applications as being reasonably well founded empirically and potentially promising. Like all students of language and linguistics who optimistically attempt to apply linguistic theories to the clinic, we have a long way to go. The answers—if they ever come—will come only when we know more about the complexities of the human brain, human development and cognition, and human behavior. We view our research as a tenuous first step in achieving a better understanding of these mysteries.

We would like to acknowledge the Department of Communication Disorders, Speech, Language and Hearing of the School of Health Professions in the Sackler Faculty of Medicine of Tel-Aviv University at Tel-Hashomer, which provided the clinical framework for this study both in a graduate seminar on phonology and in several master's theses.

This research was also supported by a grant from the Faculty of Humanities and Social Sciences of the Ben-Gurion University of the Negev, and most of the material in this volume was presented as part of a workshop in the cognitive and developmental psychology and anthropology tracks in the Department of Behavioral Sciences of this faculty as well as in graduate and undergraduate seminars in linguistics, semiotics, and phonology in the Departments of Foreign Literatures and Linguistics and English Language and Literature at the Ben-Gurion University of the Negev and Haifa University.

We would also like to thank all our colleagues and friends—fellow faculty, students, and clinicians—for their interest, useful input, and constructive criticism. A particular expression of professional gratitude must be made to Professor Lawrence J. Raphael, whose constructive criticism, trenchant comments, and specific suggestions undoubtedly have made this a better book. A special personal *toda raba, dank je wel,* and thank you go to my family and friends in Israel, the Netherlands, and the United States, who have supported me throughout this entire endeavor.

The theory of phonology as human behavior is gaining recognition in Israel and has been the theme of a special issue of *Dibur u-Shmiya* (Speech and hearing disorders) (vol. 18, 1995), the journal of the Israeli Speech, Hearing and Language Association. I would like to thank Dr. Yael Frank, the editorial board, and the contributors to this special issue on phonology, which I guest edited.

In closing, we find it especially fitting that this volume appears in a series dedicated to Roman Jakobson, the first linguist to show the connection between and apply the then new science of phonology to first language acquisition and aphasia. We view our work as a modest step in the continuation of this tradition, and we wish to thank Professor C. H. van Schooneveld for inviting us to contribute this volume to this series. We hope to show how viewing phonology as an instance of human communicative behavior reflects the connections and interrelations among the phylogeny, ontogeny, and pathology of the development of sound systems in language. For this reason, we hope that our work will be seen as part of the legacy left by Roman Jakobson and Nikolai Trubetzkoy that is still upheld and advanced by such linguists as C. H. van Schooneveld, André Martinet, and Anatoly Liberman. This volume, however, primarily reflects the work of William Diver, his students, and their students who continue to analyze all aspects of language both as a system of communication and as an instance of human behavior, particularly—as I shall attempt to show here—in phonology.

1

Phonetics and Phonology

A Historical Overview

Sounds are too volatile and subtle for legal restraints;
to enchain syllables and to lash the wind,
are equally the undertakings of pride,
unwilling to measure its desires by its strength.
—Dr. Johnson

"Did you say *pig* or *fig?*" said the Cat.
"I said *pig,*" replied Alice; "and I wish you wouldn't
keep appearing and vanishing so suddenly:
you make one quite giddy."
—Lewis Carroll ([1865] 1961: 56)

Art is a form of speech. Speech must be based
on human needs, not abstract theories of grammar.
Or anything but the spoken word.
The real word.
—John Fowles (1974: 50)

Take care of the sense,
and the sounds will take care of themselves.
—Lewis Carroll ([1865] 1961: 75)

1 Phonetics versus Phonology

The Prague School and Beyond

The autonomy of linguistics and the use of the comparative method were suited to the task of describing and cataloguing the units and patterns in language. But in the 20th century linguists have started to ask *why* these units and patterns exist, i.e., they seek explanations for, not just descriptions of linguistic structure. We have reached the point where the continued re-working of the patterns in language no longer gives us answers to our questions.—J. J. Ohala (1983c: 232)

Linguists have for many decades recognized that not all possible sequences of types of sounds occur in the morphemes of any single language. These restrictions were called "phonotactic" or "distributional" constraints by the classical structuralists and "morpheme structure" rules or conditions by generative phonologists. Although these constraints may originally have been conceived as merely descriptive statements one could make about the sound pattern of the language, there is sufficient evidence now that native speakers are also aware of them, that is, that many of the constraints noted by linguists are psychologically real.
—J. J. Ohala and M. Ohala (1986: 239)

Theoretical and Methodological Assumptions

In this chapter, I will briefly examine the historical development of the distinction between phonetics and phonology as presented by the structuralist forerunners of the theory of phonology as human behavior: Ferdinand de Saussure; the Prague school communication-oriented approach; and André Martinet and the functional school approach. In particular, I will focus on how each approach specifically deals with phonetics and phonology from the point of view of the interaction between the communication (i.e., the establishment of oppositions) and the human (i.e., the cognition, perception, and behavior of human beings) factors underlying its definition of language. I have selected these particular Saussurian, sign-oriented, or semiotic approaches to compare and contrast because they all share a similar definition of language within a general European structuralist framework.[1]

Most of post-Saussurian twentieth-century humanistic thought (notably including semiotics and linguistics) as well as the social, behavioral, or cognitive sciences (e.g., sociology, psychology, and anthropology) ultimately can be defined and described as belonging to this larger structuralist paradigm. Yet, within this general structuralist framework as originally outlined in Saussure ([1916] 1966: 16), where linguistics was to be part of a larger science of semiology (later to be known as semiotics), linguistics (as opposed to semiotics) has often been considered to be the better-defined discipline and has even been viewed as the most developed branch within the larger structuralist paradigm. For example, in his brilliant and provocative introduction to Propp (1984: xx) (reviewed by Tobin and Simms 1988), Anatoly Liberman states: "In all discussions of structuralism, linguistics occupies a prominent place. Literary scholars, sociologists, and anthropologists constantly accuse their opponents of underestimating or overestimating the achievements of modern linguistics. Such arguments create the impression that linguistic structuralism is something well-defined, which is wrong. Practically all European and American linguistics after World War I has been structuralist."

The underlying assumption of my research is that every linguistic theory is the direct result of a specific set of theoretical axioms that is related to how the linguist defines language, defines a linguistic problem, determines the source, kind, and amount of data to be selected and analyzed, chooses a methodology to select and analyze the data, and compares and contrasts the analyses in light of all the above. These five criteria basically serve to describe how and what a particular linguist or school of linguistics views as the goals of linguistic research.

From a Saussurian, sign-oriented, or semiotic point of view, language may be defined as a system of systems that is composed of various subsystems (revolving around the notion of the linguistic sign) that are organized internally and systematically related to each other and that is used by human beings to communicate. *Theoretically,* this semiotic definition of language implies the dichotomy between *langue* and *parole, langue* being an abstract code composed of signals and meanings and their paradigmatic, or associative, and syntagmatic relations, a complex code that is shared by a community of speakers, and *parole* being the concrete and seemingly chaotic realization of this complex abstract code—exploited by individual speakers—to communicate specific discourse messages in different linguistic and situational contexts. The primary task of the linguist is to postulate the abstract code or system of systems of a language in order to explain the nonrandom distribution of the linguistic forms of that language in linguistic and situational discourse contexts. *Methodologically,* this definition of language implies a respect for and reliance on actual or real (as opposed to contrived or solely introspective) data culled from discourse and a commitment to deal with the human factor (i.e., the cognitive, perceptual linguistic and nonlinguistic behavior of human beings) as it is relevant to communication in different linguistic and situational contexts.

Many diverse models of linguistic analysis, both quantitative and qualitative, have been developed to describe, interpret, and explain concrete, individual linguistic phenomena (*parole*) according to general, communal, and abstract theoretical tenets (*langue*) in various structuralist guises and under quite different names.[2] The notion of a general structuralist model (following a basic semiotic orientation) may be viewed as being a theoretical and methodological bridge between the abstract and the concrete levels of human linguistic phenomena.

Indeed, one may safely say that a model has been established (a model basically derived from phonology within linguistics) that has then been extended to all of what Culler (1976: 10–11) defines as the "fundamental problems of what the French call the 'human sciences': the disciplines that deal with the world of meaningful objects and actions (as opposed to physical objects and events themselves) . . . based on the sign and on sign-systems [that] pave the way for a general study of the ways in which human experience is organized. In other words: a search for an underlying meaningful system to explain what may appear to be disparate, and even chaotic, superficial phenomena through the use of *meaningful signs.*"

The structuralist model for linguistics is illustrated schematically in figure 1.1. Very often, this methodological model has presupposed an analogy between the model itself and the phenomena it purports to explain. This is not surprising when we consider the fact that it is the analyst's definition of language that determines which linguistic phenomena are chosen as being important and relevant to the theory and the analysis. Therefore, the model is predetermined by the theoretical units found in the analyst's definition of language.

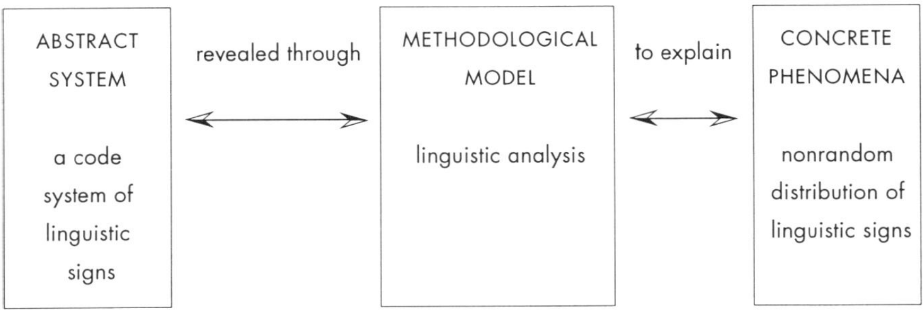

Figure 1.1 The structuralist paradigm.

Ferdinand de Saussure ([1916] 1966: 8) first maintained that one of the chief tasks of linguistics was to define itself. He further claimed that the objects of study in language are not given in advance, as are the objects of study in other sciences. In short, for linguistics, it is the definition of language espoused by a theory that actually creates the object of study.[3]

The structural model for linguistics that was later extended to other fields and disciplines was originally based on the sound systems of language, namely, the dichotomy between the abstract systems of hypothetical sound units postulated by the linguist and the concrete sounds of language produced and perceived by members of a speech community, which traditionally has been studied under the rubrics of phonology and phonetics, respectively.

More specifically, one may view the differences between phonetics and phonology in the following way. Phonetics is the description of what sounds occur where and which features (acoustic and articulatory) they are composed of (i.e., how they are articulated and perceived)—the "what," "how," and "where" of the realized sound system of (a) language:

what + how + where = description.

Phonology is a postulation and classification of the abstract units of the sound system of (a) language (e.g., the notions of phonemes and/or distinctive features etc.) as well as an explanation of the phonotactic distribution of sounds (both on the paradigmatic level, within different classes, and on the syntagmatic level)—"why" different sounds occur and do not occur in specific phonetic environments and/or in collocations with other sounds:

why = explanation.

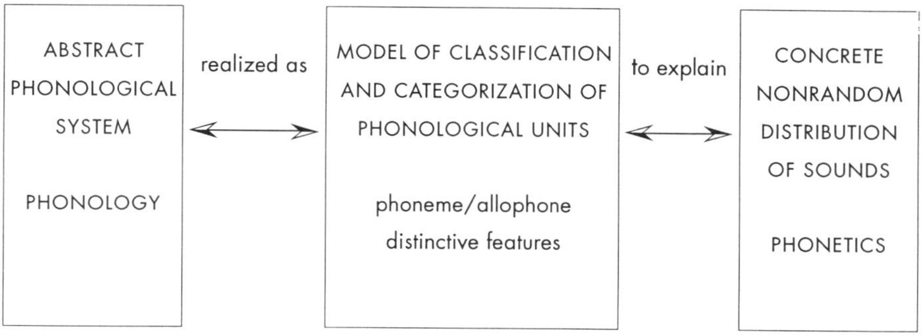

Figure 1.2 Phonetics versus phonology.

Schematically, one may place phonetics and phonology within the structuralist framework as illustrated in figure 1.2.

The theoretical and methodological distinctions between (a possibly autonomous?) phonetics and (a possibly autonomous?) phonology or the extent to which phonetics may or may not contribute to phonology (or possibly vice versa?) has not always been clearly defined in linguistics and may even be a point of contention between different linguistic approaches.[4] This chapter is based on four fundamental theoretical and methodological tenets:

1. The concept of the phoneme composed of distinctive articulatory and acoustic features—sounds that make communicative oppositions—reflects the abstract level of paradigmatic sound systems in *langue* and underlies the communication factor.

2. The concept of allophones composed of secondary or nondistinctive features—sounds that do not make communicative oppositions—reflects the concrete nonrandom syntagmatic distribution of the variations within a single and specific phoneme and may be related to the human factor.

3. In order to explain why the abstract phonemes of (a) language may also distribute—like allophones—in a nonrandom manner, we must appeal directly to the human factor in addition to merely classifying the phonemes and their distinctive features that underlie the communication factor.[5]

4. It is only through the incorporation of the human factor as a means to explain the nonrandom distributions of sounds (beyond the traditional communicative notions of phonemes/allophones and distinctive and secondary features) that a structural analysis can achieve both abstraction (via the postulated units of analysis) and explanatory generality (the ability to explain why these different sound units function and distribute as they do in realized speech on the largest scope possible).[6]

Therefore, in this chapter, I will trace the development of the interaction between the communication-oriented approach of Ferdinand de Saussure and the Prague school and the potential (and often unrealized role) of the human factor as found in the work of André Martinet and William Diver as a means to better understand the differences between phonetics and phonology.

The Historical Development of Phonetics versus Phonology

Ferdinand de Saussure: The Notion of System

In their usually accepted senses today, the terms *phonetics* and *phonology* were basically reversed by Saussure. What today is generally called *phonetics* (i.e., the physiological and acoustic features of sounds and their classification according to those features) was referred to as *phonology* by Saussure. On the other hand, Saussure viewed phonetics as a historical science, a study of the diachronic development or evolution of sounds, that is, analyzing speech events and changes over time. Therefore, what he labeled *phonetics* (and not phonology) belonged to his definition of linguistics as the scientific study of language. Saussure's notion of phonology, however, as consisting of the study of the articulatory mechanism and various perceptual implications of the various speech sounds, *all of which do not change,* was, therefore, viewed merely as an auxiliary discipline belonging exclusively to the realm of speaking. Despite the auxiliary nature of phonology, however, Saussure noted that it served as a necessary tool for dealing with the written forms of language. Linguistic evidence furnished by written forms is valid only when interpreted, thus requiring an understanding of the phonological system of each language, that is, a description of its sounds. Each language, of course, according to Saussure, operates with a fixed number of well-differentiated phonemes.[7]

Saussure laid the foundation for the distinction between phonology and phonetics (as established by his successors in the Prague school) by establishing the fundamental structuralist dichotomy of the abstract level of *langue* and the concrete level of *parole.* Furthermore, he laid the groundwork for the teleological, functional communication orientation in phonology as well as linking this teleological, functional communication approach to the role of the human factor. For Saussure, the description of sounds is directly linked with the articulatory act. The articulatory act is based on two elements that are constant, necessary, and sufficient for the production of sound: expiration and oral articulation (augmented by superimposed vibrations of the larynx and/or nasal resonances). Thus, Saussurian phonology consisted of the classification of sounds according to their oral articulation and degree of aperture and the organs involved in producing them:

1. occlusives (labials, dentals, gutterals);
2. fricatives or spirants (labiodentals, dentals, palatals, gutterals);
3. nasals;
4. liquids (lateral articulations [l], vibrant articulations [r]); and
5. vowels (subclassified by degree of opening).

Saussure also recognized the role of the distribution of sounds and the need to study sounds as part of a spoken chain taking the reciprocal relations of sounds into account as part of the study of phonology.

Despite the fact that Saussure predated the sound spectrograph by approximately four decades (and hence the Jakobsonian notion of acoustic distinctive features), his delimitation of sounds within the spoken chain is implicitly based on auditory impressions. The phoneme, for Saussure, was inherently the sum of the auditory impressions as well as the articulatory movements and mechanisms. If the Saussurian sign was the invariable pairing of signal and meaning, the Saussurian phoneme was the fundamental pairing of the acoustic and the articulatory aspects of the signal. Furthermore, for Saussure, oppositions were everything. Therefore, the importance of analyzing phonemes was for the oppositions that they created in speech and not only the process through which these oppositions were obtained. Thus, we may view Prague school phonology as a natural extension of Saussurian phonology.[8]

The Prague School: The Teleological-Functional-Communication Approach

The Prague school firmly distinguished phonology from phonetics. This distinction implied a theoretical model based on the dichotomy between *langue* and *parole* and a questioning of the Saussurian dichotomy between synchrony and diachrony on the sound level. Furthermore, it brought the teleological-functional notion of communication to the forefront of phonological analysis, making it the raison d'être of phonology.

Le Roy (1967: 64–65) sums up the role of the Prague school in distinguishing the difference between phonetics and phonology in the following way:

Phonetics which was formerly a science of observation—the ancient Indians achieved astonishing results in this field—and which studies the sounds of human speech from the articulatory and acoustic points of view, has been much improved since experimental methods were first applied to it at the end of the last century. From 1926 onwards a group of linguists from the Linguistic Circle of Prague, arguing from the fact that phonetics, since it started using apparatus and to be studied in the laboratories, has made enormous progress but at the same time has moved further and further away from linguistics, devised a completely different method for studying the sounds of language. At the first International Conference of Linguists at the Hague in 1928, R. Jakobson, S. Karcevskij and N. S. Trubetzkoy presented their famous *Proposition 22* which marks the birth of the new discipline of *phonology*. The proposition dealt with the "significant differences" that characterize the elements of every phonological system and of the "phonological correlations" that are constituted by series of binary oppositions.

Starting from the principle that any science, to be valid, must be general, the members of this school wished to reintegrate phonetics into the framework of linguistics by rescuing it from the examination of the purely individual facts of *parole* and applying it to the more general study of *langue*, with particular emphasis on the relationship between the sound (or the complex of sounds) and its meaning. One might also say that phonetics studies what is actually pronounced, something that varies from one individual to another and even within the usage of one individual, whilst phonology studies what one is conscious of pronouncing or of hearing pronounced, and this is a constant within a given linguistic community.[9]

Both Trubetzkoy and Jakobson recognize their intellectual debt to Saussure for the notions of system, *langue*, and *parole* and their emphasis on the functional communicative role of the phoneme and the phonological system. As Trubetzkoy ([1939] 1969: 3) says of the place of phonology in linguistic analysis:

Since *langue* consists of rules or norms, it is a system, or better, several partial systems, which *parole* is not. The grammatical categories form grammatical systems, the semantic categories various semantic systems. All these systems are properly balanced, so that all parts lend support to one another, and are related to one another. It is only for this reason that it is possible to relate the infinite variety of concepts and ideas that appear in the act of speech to the components of the subsystems of the language system. This is also true of the signifier aspect. The sound flow of the concrete speech event is an interrupted, seemingly unordered sequence of sound movements merging into each other. The units of the signifier aspect of the language system, on the other hand, form an ordered system. And due to the fact that the individual elements or movements of the sound flow realized in the speech event can be related to individual units of that system, the sound flow is ordered.

Trubetzkoy ([1939] 1969: 6) goes on to discuss Saussure, *langue,* and *parole:* "Ferdinand de Saussure, who recognized and clearly formulated the importance of the difference between *langue* and *parole,* also recognized, as he expressed it, the intangible nature of the signifier pertaining to *langue.* Nevertheless, he did not expressly insist on the necessity of distinguishing between the study of sound pertaining to the act of speech (*parole*) and that pertaining to the system of language (*langue*). In his *Cours de linguistique générale* this thought is merely hinted at. It seems that the founder of the Geneva school considered the distinction between the study of sound pertaining to *parole* and the study of sound pertaining to *langue* as being less important than the distinction between the descriptive and historical study of sound." Trubetzkoy ([1939] 1969: 10) then clearly defines the purpose or the function of the language system of phonology, relating it directly to communication: "It is the task of phonology to study which differences in sound are related to differences in meaning in a given language, in which way the discriminative elements . . . are related to each other, and the rules according to which they may be combined into words and sentences. It is clear that these objectives cannot be attained by the methods of the natural sciences. Rather phonology must use the same methods as are used in the study of the grammatical systems of language."

Along similar Saussurian functional lines, Jakobson describes the difference between phonetics and phonology in the following way:

> And in spite of the numerous contradictions in the teachings of Saussure, it is to him and his school that we owe the second idea crucial for the functional study of sounds, the idea of the *phonological system.* Once the point of departure for the study of the relation between sounds and meaning has been indicated . . . it was a matter of drawing out all the implications of this and actually developing the new discipline, the systematic study of the sounds of a language from the point of view of their linguistic functions. (Jakobson 1978: 42)

It is true that the phonetic substance of language has been studied thoroughly, and that such studies, especially over the last fifty years, have produced an abundance of illuminating results. But for the most part the phenomena under consideration have been investigated in abstraction from their function. In these circumstances it has been impossible to classify, or even understand, these phenomena. In the same way, it would be impossible to understand and classify machines or other instruments so long as attention was focussed exclusively on the materials with which they are made, or on their external form, with no consideration of what they are used for. In order to be able to interpret and classify the diverse actions of our phonatory organs it is essential that we take into account the acoustic phenomena that these actions aim at producing, *for we speak in order to be heard;* and in order to be able to interpret, classify and define the diverse sounds of our language we must take into account the meaning, *for it is in order to be understood that we speak to be heard.* (Jakobson 1978: 24–25)

Theoretically and methodologically, the distinction between phonology and phonetics as perceived by Jakobson and Trubetzkoy is a typically Praguian holistic one that can best be understood by examining the metaphoric way in which both have chosen to describe it:

Phonetics falls outside linguistics just as the chemistry of colours strictly speaking falls outside the theory of painting. On the other hand, the study of the use of sounds in language, (in other words, of sounds considered as verbal signs) is an integral part of linguistics just as the study of the use of colours considered as pictorial signs is part of the theory of figurative art and in particular of the theory of painting. This linguistic study of sounds, the study of sounds in the light of the work they perform in language, has come to be called phonology. (Jakobson 1978: 45)

The phonology of expression may thus be compared to the study of costumes in folklore. The difference between fat and skinny or between tall and small people is very important to the tailor, whose job is to make a particular costume. But from the point of view of folklore these differences are quite insignificant: only the conventionally specified form of the costume is important. The clothing of a sloppy person is dirty and rumpled. Absentminded persons do not always have all their buttons fastened. All of these characteristics are of no significance for the study of costumes in folklore. Folklore is interested in every characteristic, however minute, by which in accordance with prevailing custom the dress of a married woman is distinguished from that of a single girl, etc. People belonging to groups customarily characterized by ethnologically relevant differences in dress are also often distinguished by linguistic ("glottic") characteristics and especially by peculiarities pertaining to the "phonology of expression." Compare, for example, sex and age groups, social classes or occupational groups, educational classes, city dwellers and peasants, and regional groups. (Trubetzkoy [1939] 1969: 17)

As a result of this systematic study of sounds—phonology—within the teleological, functional communicative framework, the notion of the phoneme (signifying distinctiveness or "mere otherness") (Sangster 1982: 4) became the postulated abstract theoretical unit of *langue*. The mutual distinctiveness between the phonemic units themselves was then subsequently developed both by Trubetzkoy and by Jakobson (as well as by subsequent phonological theorists) into binary and hierarchical articulatory and acoustic distinctive features. Distinctive features allowed for the functional and theoretical distinctions between the phonemic or abstract sound units themselves. These distinctive features—along with the secondary nondistinctive features of allophones—are realized during the speech act of *parole*, but only distinctive features are postulated as part of the abstract code of *langue*.[10]

The development of distinctive feature theory is perhaps the best-known theoretical phonological construct that had its roots in the intellectual heritage of Prague school phonology. It, too, like the phoneme and most structural concepts, may be viewed as an attempt to postulate abstract categories that will describe and explain as large and general an amount of concrete linguistic data as possible. Both Trubetzkoy (1931) and Jakobson (Jakobson, Fant, and Halle 1952; Jakobson and Halle 1956) developed sets of "natural" articulatory and acoustic distinctive features as part of the functionally oriented theory and methodology of Prague school phonology.

Trubetzkoy (1931) postulated three natural classes for vowels and four for consonants, classes based on the oppositions developed by distinctive feature theory within the framework of Prague school phonology (see table 1.1). With the advent of the sound spectrograph and the subsequent advances made in the field of acoustics, Jakobson, Fant, and Halle (1952) and Jakobson and Halle (1956) extended the theory of distinctive features to include the acoustic correlates of speech sounds. From the phonological point of view, these features have been reduced to a stock of twelve binary oppositions that they believed to be sufficient to analyze all languages and that were thus presented as theoretical linguistic universals. The first nine oppositions represent features of sonority (similar to the features of quantity and force

Table 1.1 Trubetzkoy's Classes of Vowels and Consonants

Vowels	*Consonants*
Oppositions of quality:	Oppositions of localization:[a]
Aperture (sonority)	Oppositions of manner of articulation:
Timbre	Voice correlation
Rounding correlation	Correlation based on type of expiration:
Palatovelar correlation (front/back)	Aspirated/unaspirated
Oppositions of resonance:	Glottalized/nonglottalized
Nasalized/nonnasalized	Constriction correlation
Squeezed vowels/pure vowels	Oppositions of timbre:
Pharyngeal sounds/nonpharyngeal sounds	Palatalized/nonpalatalized
Oppositions of prosody:	Rounded/unrounded
Intensity:	Emphatic palatalization/nonemphatic palatalization
Dynamic	Emphatic velarization/nonemphatic velarization
Accented/unaccented	Retroflex/dental
Weak/strong	Oppositions of intensity:
Quantity:	Dynamic:
Long/short	Fortis/lenis
Melody (pitch):	Squeezed/nonsqueezed (*gedrängt/locker*)
Tone movement	Strong/weak
Register	Quantity:
Oppositions of close contact	Long/short
	Geminated/nongeminated

Source: Baltaxe (1978: 72–75).

[a]Oppositions based on point of articulation.

that are related to the amount and concentration of energy in the acoustic spectrum). The twelve binary oppositions or universal distinctive features (as presented in Jakobson and Halle 1956) are

1. vocalic versus nonvocalic,
2. consonantal versus nonconsonantal,

3. compact versus diffuse,
4. tense versus lax,
5. voiced versus voiceless,
6. nasal versus oral,
7. discontinuous (or interrupted) versus continuant,
8. strident versus mellow,
9. checked versus unchecked,
10. grave versus acute,
11. flat versus plain, and
12. sharp versus plain.

The Prague school distinction between the study of sounds on the level of *parole* and the study of sounds on the level of *langue,* that is, the distinction between phonetics and phonology, was a revolutionary advance in linguistic theory. It provided a more holistic and systematic approach to linguistic analysis at the expense of the distinction between synchrony and diachrony (at least in the field of phonology). It introduced the abstract notion of the distinctive phoneme to systematic phonological analysis, thus placing the teleological, functional communication aspect of the sound system of language at the very forefront of linguistic analysis. It further paved the way for the development of distinctive feature theory as a more abstract, general, and therefore scientific method of distinguishing between sounds or phonemes. We may thus view Prague school phonology as the first example of a teleological, functional communication-oriented structuralist approach to linguistics. The Prague school, however, presents a functionalist framework that does not necessarily make the *human factor* the most central element in the explanation of the ordering of the sounds of the language system. It is this theoretical and methodological need to include the human factor as a crucial and necessary element in an explanation of the nonrandom distribution of different sounds and classes of sounds in human language that motivates the work of André Martinet of the functionalist school and William Diver of the Columbia or form-content school in their work in phonology.

André Martinet: The Therapeutic View of Sound Change

Martinet took the essentially Praguian notion of the so-called therapeutic view of sound change and developed it into an explicit and sophisticated linguistic theory. According to Sampson (1980: 112), the therapeutic theory of sound change involves "the notion that sound changes were to be explained as a result of a striving towards a sort of ideal balance or resolution of various conflicting pressures; for instance the need for speech to be comprehensible [the communication factor] despite inevitably inexact pronunciation [the human factor]." This functional notion of therapeutic change (the striving for a balance or an equilibrium within the sound system of a language over time as a result of the conflict between the communication and the human factors) is rather at odds with the traditional Saussurian synchrony/diachrony dichotomy since it implies that there is an underlying system in diachrony as well as in synchrony. Jakobson (1929) had already noticed the systematic aspects of diachrony with regard to phonology.

The clearest explication of the concept of therapeutic change is found, of course, in Martinet's (1955) seminal *Économie des changements phonétiques.* It is precisely here that the role of the human factor in the nonrandom distribution of the sounds of (a) language begins to figure in an important way in theoretical phonological analysis. The human factor, however, is generally limited to that of "the principle of least effort" in relation to a fundamental need to achieve symmetry or harmony.

Le Roy (1967: 71–72) concisely summarizes the fundamental principles of Martinet's theory as follows: "We must make it clear that by 'economy' Martinet means the principle of 'least effort' (or of 'least expenditure') as well as that of internal organization thanks to which a balance is struck between the fundamental antinomic tendencies he observes between 'man's need to communicate and express himself' and 'his tendency to reduce to a minimum his mental and physical activity.' Martinet sees too in the inertia and asymmetry of the speech organs a decisive reason why equilibrium never results in complete symmetry; that is why he substitutes for the 'teleological' notion of harmony envisaged by the early phonologists that of a tendency towards stabilizing the system by integrating the phonemes: indeed, isolated phonemes, not integrated in correlations or bundles, seem somewhat unstable and tend either to disappear or to find a correlative partner."

Lepschy (1970: 104) further elaborates on this basic point of the importance of finding systematic explanations for sound change and discusses the differences between Martinet's approach and that of the Prague school phonologists:

Phonology for Martinet must interpret *phonetic* facts; these are the basic data, and not just one of several realizations of an abstract system. But phonology must concentrate on a particular aspect of phonetic facts: i.e., the linguistic *functions* of sound differences [the communication factor] (and) the way in which they are used [the human factor] in the linguistic system.

In Martinet's phonological work an important part is devoted to the study of diachronic problems. He tries here to go beyond the purely descriptive phase in which phonologizations and dephonologizations are recorded, and attempts to provide *explanations* of the changes according to general principles. A basic criterion of interpretation is offered by two contrasting elements: efficiency in communication (using as many units as possible, as different from each other as possible) and tendency to minimum effort (using as few units as possible, as similar to each other as possible). There is a tendency to reconcile these two opposing requirements. This tendency (which is not interpreted in the "teleological" terms familiar to the School of Prague) can be conceived as a striving for *economy,* i.e., towards attaining an improved functional load. Why then do all languages not reach an identical, economically optimum, phonological system? Optimum economy can never be reached because there are physiological disturbing factors such as inertia and assymmetry of the speech organs.

The introduction of the human factor into phonological analysis (even in the limited guise of Martinet's economy) has several far-reaching theoretical and methodological consequences for the structuralist paradigm: a respect for and reliance on "real" (as opposed to contrived or totally introspective) language data; the potential importance of frequency counts involving statistics or quantitative methods of linguistic validation; and the need for "external" (extralinguistic) support as a necessary control for linguistic explanations. These theoretical and methodological implications resulting from the inclusion of the human factor have been discussed in Le Roy's evaluation of Martinet's role in modern linguistic theory:

> We are therefore brought back to the primordial question that every linguist comes up against in attempting to make a classification, whatever the plan of his research, namely that of choosing and evaluating criteria: which facts are relevant, how can their importance be assessed, how can one avoid arbitrariness? As Martinet has said, "it must be repeated yet again that it is not up to language to conform to the edicts of linguistics, it is up to linguists to adapt their methods if they do not do full justice to the language being studied." (Le Roy 1967: 74, citing Martinet 1955: 125–26)

> However, there has been a salutory reaction on the part of some linguists who are very sympathetic to the structuralist trend but are anxious not to be carried away by sterile and gratuitous intellectualism. We have already shown how Martinet thanks to his realistic approach to diachronic phonology, has very felicitously bridged the gap between traditional comparative grammar and the new conceptions, and it is well worth quoting his statement that "it is high time that linguists became aware of the independence of their discipline and got rid of the inferiority complex that impels them to relate every step that they take to some great philosophical principle; in this way they only succeed in blurring the contours of reality instead of sharpening them." . . . In Martinet's *Éléments de linguistique générale,* he insists, and rightly, on the need to establish a liaison between pure speculation and the exploitation of the data so as to strike a balance—"more realism and less formalism"—between theory and practice. (Le Roy 1967: 82–83, citing Martinet 1955: 18)

Martinet realizes that *explanation* may not be language internal and that other external factors must be appealed to as well. He views these external factors necessary for explanation as being "historical" in nature rather than appealing directly to the human factor as a primary source for explanation or control. This may be explained by the fact that Martinet only began to incorporate the human factor into his analysis (mostly limited to the "minimax" principle of least effort employed to maintain maximum contrastive oppositions).

As we shall see in chapter 2, William Diver broadens the appeal to the human factor—in the form of the ability to learn and produce two fundamental classes of consonants (stable and mobile) in certain linguistic environments)—validated by statistical skewings and compared to other extralinguistic aspects of human behavior in order to better explain the nonrandom phonotactic distribution of sounds within a language.[11] However, before I introduce the theory of phonology as human behavior, I will first explain the synergetic interaction of the communication and human factors in language on which the theory is based.

Defining Language Synergetically

In the beginning of this chapter, I defined language semiotically as a system of systems that is composed of various subsystems (revolving around the notion of the linguistic sign) that are organized internally and systematically related to each other and that is used by human beings to communicate. This particular definition of language and the theoretical and methodological implications with regard to *langue* and *parole* that I have previously discussed provide the semiotic or sign-oriented linguist with a holistic or isomorphic view of language, one based on the following two fundamental factors: the communication factor and the human factor. Both these factors can be further related to the larger holistic concept of *synergesis,* which may be defined as the cooperative action of discrete agencies with the result that the total effect is greater than the sum of the discrete effects taken independently.

Put more simply with regard to the semiotic or sign-oriented view of language, the linguistic whole (language) is greater than the sum of its individual parts (i.e., the various units that may be related to signals and meanings and their use: phonemes, syllables, morphemes, stems, roots, words, word classes, meanings, phrases, clauses, sentences, utterances, contexts, texts, etc.). Furthermore, concerning the communication and human factors, successful linguistic communication can be achieved only through the combined effort of an encoder and a decoder cooperating together. Thus, synergesis is a fundamental concept underlying language and the behavior of language use(rs), one that may be appealed to in order to explain disparate linguistic phenomena in a systematic, holistic, and isomorphic way.[12]

Concerning phonetics versus phonology—the signifier half of the linguistic sign—the communication factor includes the following basic principles:

1. There is an invariant sound unit on the abstract phonological level of *langue*—the *phoneme*—composed of distinctive articulatory and acoustic features from which communicative oppositions (usually determined by minimal pairs: e.g., *pit* vs. *bit*) are derived.[13]

2. The phonemes of a language—each signifying "mere otherness"—are in a tight paradigmatic relation, one based on their communicative oppositions.

3. The syntagmatic distribution of the phonemes of a language is part of a relatively open system allowing for as many communicative oppositions as possible in as many phonetic environments as possible in a language.

4. Therefore, it has generally been believed that the distribution of the invariant phonemes in a language is random and unpredictable.

5. There are variant realizations of the abstract phoneme produced on the concrete phonetic level (*allophones*); each allophone appears in a single, specific pho-

netic environment, and together (complementary distribution) they represent all the concrete realizations of the abstract phoneme in the language.

6. In addition to the primary distinctive features associated with the phoneme represented, allophones also contain secondary features associated with the specific phonetic environments within which they appear that are nondistinctive and do not create communicative oppositions.

7. The allophones of a phoneme are in a tight paradigmatic relation, one based on the closed syntagmatic system and composed of the specific phonetic environments in which the allophones appear.

8. Therefore, it is generally believed that the distribution of the variant allophones of an invariant phoneme is nonrandom and predictable.

Concerning phonetics versus phonology, the human factor includes the following basic principles, principles that can be further related to the various laws of synergesis:

1. *Human intelligence.* Human beings can draw far-reaching abstract conclusions from minimally salient concrete cues through the cognitive process of inference: we infer (i.e., perceive and are aware of) the abstract phoneme despite the fact that we heard the concrete allophone that was actually uttered.

2. *Human efficiency.* Human beings invest minimal effort for maximal results in the semiotic communication process: by inferring abstract phonemes rather than concrete allophones, we have to invest just enough to perceive only those articulatory and acoustic features necessary for communication, rather than all the primary and secondary features associated with each individual allophone.

3. *Memory limitations.* Human beings have large but limited memories that can be directly related to human intelligence and human efficiency.

These same synergetic principles linking the communication and the human factors for phonetics and phonology connect all the so-called independent and autonomous levels of language as well. Phonemes are determined by minimal pairs that rely on semantic lexical distinctions. Minimal morphological forms may appear as single phonemes (e.g., plural nominal, or third-person-singular verb, or genetive /s/ in English) that rely on semantic grammatical distinctions.

Zipf (1949) established the fundamental synergetic principle of least effort (or economy) in all domains of language, the principle that leads language users to unifications or diversifications of the elements of language units in order to alleviate their physical and mental effort. Some of the more obvious examples of Zipf's law concerning the lexicon include the relation between the frequency and length of words and the number of possible messages (dictionary or contextual meanings) that they convey.

According to Zipf, the frequent use of a word results in a reduction in its size, on the one hand, and an increase in the number of messages that it may convey, on the other. Thus, from the point of view of the encoder, linguistic economy is best realized by a highly compressed lexicon composed of exclusively short words conveying a multiplicity of messages, or what Zipf calls *the force of unification.* From the point of view of the decoder, on the other hand, linguistic economy is best realized by a lexicon composed of words maximally distinct in form and restricted to one exclusive message, or what Zipf calls *the force of diversification.*

Therefore, it is possible to claim that the semiotic act of communication can be seen as a "mini-max" struggle: the desire to create maximum communication with minimal effort. However, this mini-max struggle is reflected by two converse communication processes engaged in by encoders and decoders who stand in opposed and mirror-image-like positions. Minimal effort on the part of the encoder will place a heavier burden on the decoder's inferential abilities. The opposite is also true. Minimal effort on the part of the decoder may result in a breakdown in communication that most often can be remedied by an increased effort on the part of the encoder: that is, by forcing him to choose his signs in a way that may be inferred with less effort on the part of the decoder. In short, this mini-max struggle of linguistic communication is controlled by the first synergetic principle (adapted from Tobin 1990c: 59):

Synergetic Principle 1. The more cooperation there is between the encoder and the decoder, the greater the chance there is for successful communication.

This synergetic relation between the encoder and the decoder is presented schematically in figure 1.3.

Concerning phonetics versus phonology, the synergetic relation between the encoder and the decoder is found in the encoder's production of a large number of allophones that are perceived as a more limited number of phonemes by the decoder, as is illustrated by the phoneme /p/ and its four allophones [p^h], [p'], [p‘], and [p^-] for American English (list adapted from Bronstein 1960: 80):

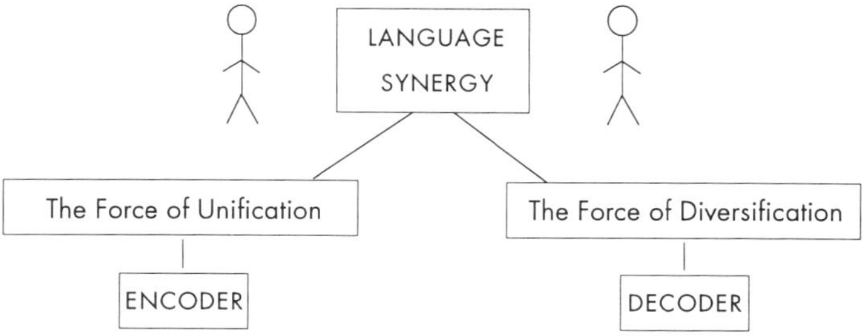

Figure 1.3 The synergetic relation between the encoder and the decoder.

1. [p^h], a fully aspirated /p/ before a stressed vowel, as in *pen;*
2. [p'], a slightly aspirated /p/ before an unstressed vowel, as in *pajamas,* or sometimes finally, as in *hip;*
3. [p‘], the unaspirated /p/, commonly after /s/, as in *spend;* and
4. [p^{-}], an unreleased /p/, as in *hip boot,* and sometimes finally, as in *map.*

If we examine the complementary distribution of these allophones from the point of view of language synergy, we observe that this distribution is both predictable and nonrandom. Each particular allophone appears precisely in that specific phonetic environment in which it is produced most naturally by the encoder. Not unsurprisingly, the amount of energy invested by the encoder in a specific phonetic environment directly matches the effort that has to be expended by the decoder in order to create successful communication.

1. [p^h]: The allophone with full aspiration appears in the environment of a stressed vowel, which—for English, believed to be a stress-timed language in which the vowel in a stressed syllable is longer than the vowels in nonstressed syllables—requires the most effort by the encoder.[14]

Therefore, the allophone requiring the greatest amount of effort on the part of the encoder appears precisely in that environment in which he or she is already investing most of his or her energy. Furthermore, it is not a coincidence that this same phonetic environment also provides the most salient acoustic and communicative information, thus making it worthy of the expenditure of maximum effort by the decoder as well.

2. [p']: The allophone produced with slight aspiration, requiring less effort on the part of the encoder, most naturally appears before an unstressed vowel or sometimes word finally.

Therefore, the allophone requiring less effort for aspiration on the part of the encoder appears precisely in that environment in which he or she is already investing less energy. Not surprisingly, again there is a direct match between the amount of effort expended by the encoder and the decoder and the communicative role of the phonetic environment: the smaller the communicative force of the environment, the less the amount of energy invested by the encoder and the decoder.

3. [p‘]: The unaspirated allophone requiring the least effort for aspiration appears in the environment of a consonant cluster following a sibilant, a phonetic environment that requires a greater general effort and a larger expenditure of air on the part of the encoder.

Therefore, the allophone requiring the least effort for aspiration on the part of the encoder appears precisely in that environment in which he or she is already investing most of his or her energy and releasing the largest amount of air. Once again, there is a direct match between the amount of effort expended by the encoder and the decoder and the communicative role of the phonetic environment: in those environments requiring maximum effort—such as a consonant cluster—there is a trade-off or compromise between the effort invested to produce the minimal number of primary and that invested to produce the minimal number of secondary cues necessary for efficient communication.

4. [p˺]: The allophone in which there is no release whatsoever—the allophone requiring the least effort altogether—appears in those environments where a release of air is least necessary for communication by both the encoder and the decoder: that is, syllable- or word-final position.

In short, the synergetic relation between phonemes and their allophones may be seen as the primary example of the search for maximum communication with minimal effort on which all of human language is based.

Summary and Conclusions

In this chapter, I have tried to show how the distinction between phonetics and phonology has developed in this century from Saussure to the Prague and functionalist schools that preceded William Diver's theory of phonology as human behavior. In particular, I have concentrated on the gradual interaction between the communication and the human factors and their incorporation in phonological theory.

To review, Saussure basically provided us with the notion of *system,* the abstract level of *langue* versus the concrete level of *parole,* synchrony versus diachrony, and a distinction between what he called phonetics (historical change) and phonology (the articulatory and acoustic features of sounds). The Prague school relegated phonetics to the study of sounds on the concrete level (*parole*) and phonology to the abstract sound system of *langue.* This was done by introducing the teleological, functional communication orientation to linguistics. This resulted in the development of modern phonemic analysis and, subsequently, the development of distinctive feature theory. Martinet continued this functionalist approach and began to recognize the crucial role that the human factor played in diachronic phonological explanation through his therapeutic approach to sound change from the point of view of *economy.*

As we shall see in the next chapter, Diver has extended this formerly limited view of the human factor to that of a means of explaining the nonrandom, combinatory phonotactic distribution of phonemes in a language. The theory of phonology as human behavior has created different views of, or new kinds of, distinctive features. These new distinctive features can now be directly related to human physiology and our ability to learn, which involves human perception, cognition, and behavior. Diver has also introduced the notion of quantitative statistical observation and analysis of favored and disfavored phonotactic skewings, which can be supported by similar skewings of observed human behavior in extralinguistic contexts.

In chapter 2, I will introduce the theory of phonology as human behavior as first presented in Diver (1979) for English and further extended to Italian and Latin by Davis (1984/1987). I will then apply the theory to the triconsonantal (CCC) root system of Hebrew (Tobin 1990a, 1990c) and to initial consonant clusters in Hebrew and Yiddish monosyllables (Miron 1990; Bernholtz-Priner 1993); to a major problem in Hebrew diachronic phonology; to a poetic text; to teaching phonetics as human behavior; to language acquisition; and, finally, to the fields of speech pathology and audiology.

2 Phonology as Human Behavior

With regard to the empirical facts that constitute our everyday language: some "facts" which seemed to be obvious may turn out, on closer inspection, to be far from self-evident. They raise complicated questions of interpretation, analysis, and understanding. It depends largely on one's theoretical interpretation which of the many facts appear as important, and which of the data will be selected and observed out of the "buzzing confusion" of daily experience. A change of viewpoint may bring about a re-evaluation of what is known and shed new light about phenomena which never attracted attention. —T. Thass-Thinemann (1973: 23)

Other sciences work with objects that are given in advance and that can be considered from different viewpoints; but not linguistics. . . . Far from it being the object that antedates the viewpoint, it would seem that it is the viewpoint that creates the object; besides, nothing tells us in advance that one way of considering the fact in question takes precedence over the others or is in any way superior to them.—Ferdinand de Saussure ([1916] 1966: 8)

The Columbia School

William Diver is the founder of the Columbia school of linguistics, also referred to as form-content analysis, which espouses a Saussurian-based sign-oriented linguistic theory developed over the last thirty years at Columbia University.[1] This theory is based on the rather obvious but often overlooked premise that language is a device of human communication. Its basic theoretical and methodological orientation is that the structure and the very nature of language are a direct result of its communicative function and ecologically reflect the nature of human beings. The two basic premises of the theory are that language is an instance of human behavior and a device for communication.

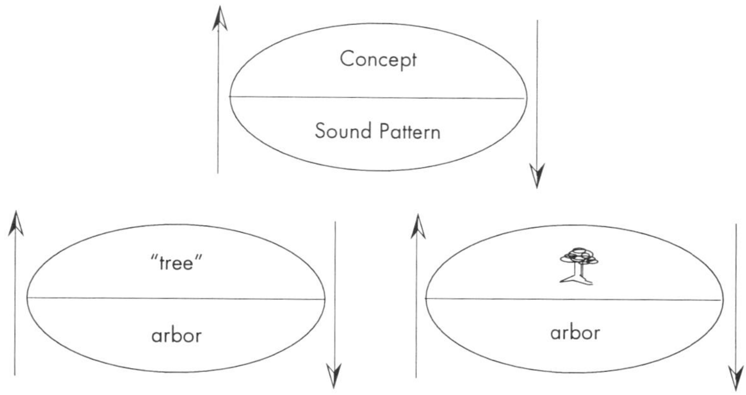

Figure 2.1 The linguistic sign (from Saussure 1916 [1983]).

For the Columbia school, the sign-oriented definition of language as a system of systems used by human beings to communicate implies that signals and invariant meanings are the primary theoretical units of analysis. Therefore, in language, as in other communication systems, the sign is composed of a distinct signal to which a single unitary meaning is invariably paired. Neither the signals nor the invariant meanings are known in advance of the analysis. On the contrary, the first task confronting the linguist is the postulation of each signal and its invariant meaning (see fig. 2.1).

The postulation of the linguistic sign must be viewed as a unified process, as the simultaneous postulation of both signifier and signified. This requires the analyst to approach specific linguistic problems and data—usually distinct morphological or lexical forms—isolate them, postulate an invariant meaning for each form, and then determine inductively how the invariant meaning directly or indirectly motivates the occurrence of its invariably paired signal every time and within every context in which it appears.

The precise nature of the signals—be they individual speech sounds, independent or segmentable linguistic forms, abstract signals such as word-order position or zero (0), prosodic cues, written words or entire sentences, or texts—and their postulated invariant meanings must be determined by observing human needs in interaction with communicative needs through inductive generalizations about language data. Through inference, context, and knowledge of the word, human behavior and intelligence must be taken into account to explain how the sequence of signs—each composed of a signal and an abstract and often imprecise invariant meaning—can fit together to communicate relatively precise messages in different linguistic and situational contexts.[2]

Phonetics and Phonology in the Columbia School

As may be inferred from the above, most of the work done within the framework of the Columbia school has been in the realm of the lexicon and the grammar. The phonetic-phonological areas of language, however, have not been totally neglected, and the basic orientations of this theory, namely, the communication and the human factors, have also been applied to the sound system of language.

The question of the nature of the relation between phonetics and phonology discussed in the previous chapter has been viewed by Diver (1979: 161–63) in the following way:

> Do we, in linguistics, need both a phonetics and a phonology? And if we do, what is the relation? The question of the extent to which phonetics is relevant to phonology has long been debated, and the extreme position, that phonetics is entirely irrelevant, has been taken by such otherwise diametrically opposed scholars as Trubetzkoy (1949) and Bloomfield (1933). But the opposite view may also be taken: If phonetic research provides us with an accurate acoustic and physiological description of speech sounds, what do we need phonology for?
>
> As between the two positions, there is no doubt that phonetics has the stronger prima facie case. It is all very well to say that physics is not a science of meter reading, but it is equally true that without its meter readings the science of physics would not exist; it would not be physics, but metaphysics. As for phonetics and phonology, it is phonetics that has the meter readings, and the great weakness in the case of phonology is the curious uncertainty of its relation to the meter readings of phonetics. No linguist, to be sure, would agree that we can dispense with phonology, and phoneticians implicitly agree, in that it is the awareness of phonological problems that generally motivates the exact course of phonetic research.
>
> But what motivates phonology? . . .
>
> This brings us to the great paradox of phonemic analysis. There has never been any great difficulty, either for modern phonemicists or ancient alphabet makers, in establishing the existence and identity of phonemes. The area of disagreement in phonemic analysis is small, and the task of reducing languages to writing does not

produce widely disparate results. And yet it is by no means clear exactly what it is that is being done when a phonemic analysis is carried out. Most phonemicists have been avowedly descriptive linguists; their task, they say, is to state the facts. But is that what they are doing? Are phonemes facts, in the sense of observations that can be recorded without recourse to abstraction or explanation? Surely not. That hope was forever exploded with the development of the spectrograph, when it became clear that there was no one-to-one relation between the discrete phonemes and acoustic reality. Is it the phonetic facts they are describing? Obviously not. The trouble with the spectrogram is just that; it presents us with phonetic facts, it describes them for us, and does nothing more. Indeed, much of the point of modern phonemics has been to escape, in the words of Martin Joos (1975: 115), the gooey continuity of the phenomena—that is the phonetics. The meter readings of the phonetician have never been of direct interest to the phonemicist, either in the laboratory or in the field. Even the narrowest of phonetic transcriptions, so-called, is implicitly phonemic; this is indeed as it should be, a first approximation of a phonemic description.

The paradox, then, is that the phonemicist can neither get along with phonetics, nor get along without it. And a corollary paradox is that the descriptive linguist is not a descriptive linguist—the reason being that the units, or categories, that he is presumably describing are in fact not directly observable.

The descriptive linguist, among linguists, is the one who has most determinedly refused to entertain a priori assumptions about language in the conduct of his analysis and has most rigorously persisted in a methodology that begins with raw data; if even he is, in fact, depending on something other than observation. It would appear to be a good idea to take a careful look at the identity of what are regarded as the fundamental units of language and linguistic analysis.

It is precisely this, the determination of what constitute the raw data of sound units, what the norm is, and how the sound units are measured and determined, that Diver views as only a part of the problem of phonology versus phonetics.

The Identification of Unobservable Units

Once one takes as one's fundamental hypothesis that phonological and phonetic analysis may be viewed as an attempt to describe and understand the units of language and linguistic analysis, then one's theoretical orientations come into play. The particular problem, as pointed out by Diver, however, is that the units of sound are inherently unobservable. When dealing with unobservable units, description cannot precede explanation: unobservable units cannot be described until they are understood.

Unobservable units may first be understood through the communication factor:

Let us now return to the problem of the phoneme as a unit. The phoneme being unobservable, as we see on the spectrogram, we cannot reasonably expect to describe it without doing anything else, such as to understand it, to explain it, to come to some comprehension of its characteristics. . . .

The ancient alphabet maker [as well as the modern phonemicist], apparently, was aware that there was a skewing in the distribution of the speech sounds, an irregularity in the phonetics, and that this skewing correlated with certain characteristics of messages that were communicated thereby. He [like native speakers of any language; see chap. 1, n. 9] was apparently able to establish that certain gross phonetic characteristics of the sounds were used distinctly in that particular language, and that others were not. This ability is clearly attested to by the changes alphabets undergo as they move from one language to another in the ancient [or modern] world. There is no suggestion that the alphabet maker, or the alphabet user, was a skilled phonetician or was interested in nice phonetic details, but we can tell from his alphabetic behavior that the early writer of Latin, for example, could hear the difference between [k] and [g], even though the distinction was not made in the alphabet he had borrowed, and he could ignore the differences among [ci], [ka], and [qu], even though these alphabet distinctions were available to him.

The ability of a user of a language to establish the existence of unobservable units in this way is very suggestive, particularly to what it is that he is correlating with the phonemic skewing. The ideal terrain for the phonemicist is the minimal pair: two "words" or "morphemes" that are minimally distinct in sound and are also different in meaning. We are thus confronted by, and dependent on, a signal-meaning pair, the same kind of thing in principle, that we see in forms of communication outside of language, as in the familiar case of the language of bees; that is, we are confronted by an ingredient in an act of communication. It has been a considerably moot point for a long time now as to whether communication is a controlling factor in the structure of language. Many have argued that it is not [see chap. 1, n. 6]. But this unobservable unit, the phoneme, comes to light only when approached by way of distinctiveness—that is, communication—and it regularly comes to light when it is approached in this way. This has by now happened so often that it is difficult to escape the inference that it is not just coincidence, and that, at least so far as phonology is concerned, communication lies at the heart of linguistic structure, and that what motivates phonemics is the need to establish a relationship between communication and phonetics. (Diver 1979: 165, 167)

Despite the fact that we can attribute part of the explanation of the concept of the phoneme to the communication factor, we are still left with the manner in which the phoneme can be optimally characterized: "In the case of the phoneme we are assured only of the fact of its existence: in a particular language, there is a particular number of distinct units. From phonemic analysis alone, we do not know the characteristics of those units, nor even what it means to be a significant characteristic; we only know they are distinct from each other" (Diver 1979: 167).[3] Furthermore, two fundamental questions—how to characterize the unobservable sound unit, the phoneme, and whether the traditional articulatory and acoustic characterizations are indeed the optimal way to describe phonemes—lie at the heart of the theory of phonology as human behavior: "It is not surprising that there should be a great uncertainty as to the relation of the phoneme to its phonetic base. (For example, should the phoneme be identified in terms of articulatory or acoustic features [or both?]? Should *l* be called a liquid or a lateral? Should *p* be called fortis or voiceless? Should we, with the ancients, continue to call *s* a sibilant because it sounds like the hissing of a snake?) Nor is it surprising that for the pure phonemicist there should be a temptation to assert that there is no relationship at all between the phoneme and its phonetic base: as far as distinctiveness alone is concerned, it may be enough to be an abstract unit" (Diver 1979: 167).

Thus, we can see that Diver is critical both of the descriptivist phonemicists (who recognized the phoneme as a unit of phonological analysis) and of the generative phonologists (who rejected the phoneme as a unit of phonological analysis) concerning the theoretical and methodological implications of their conclusions regarding the relation between phonetics and phonology.

The Statement of the Problem

The fundamental difference between the theory of phonology as human behavior and other phonological theories is how they define the primary problem of phonological research. For Diver (1979: 167–69), the statement of the problem of phonological research lies in discovering both the optimal characterization of the abstract sound unit, the phoneme, and an explanation for the nonrandom skewing of the sound units within language:

> In moving into the next stage of the problem—that of establishing the characteristics in addition to the identity of the distinctive units—it is reasonable to . . . observe a skewing or irregularity, establish an appropriate orientation to act as an external constraint, and devise hypothetical characteristics that . . . will provide us with an understanding of the skewed observations against the background of the orientation. Specifically, then, what is the skewing that poses the problem? What is the orientation? And what are the characteristics that provide a solution to the problem?
>
> First, the skewing. We saw earlier that the skewing in the phonetics posed a problem that, against the background of the communication factor, has led to the hypothesizing of phonemes, the phonemes thus being the solution to the problem posed by the phonetic skewing. But the phonemes themselves, once hypothesized, are found to have a skewing of their own; namely, that asymmetry in distribution and combination that we study under the name of phonotactics. Let me rephrase the phonotactic problem. . . . Given a stock of distinctive units and a large corpus of phonemic transcription, it might be expected that, other things being equal, the phonemes would be distributed symmetrically within the larger linguistic units that they serve to differentiate: the morphemes, words, phrases, of the language. We know, of course, that they are not distributed symmetrically, and it is the motivation for the particular skewing we find that constitutes the phonological problem. (Diver 1979: 167–68)

The communication factor alone, however, does not provide the orientation to explain the nonrandom phonetic skewing of the sound units of language: "As to orientation, we have seen that communication as an orientation is crucial for providing us with a basis for establishing the list of distinctive units, but that the phonemic procedure does not do more than that. To go beyond this point, it has been found necessary . . . to introduce additional orientations. The additional orientations are three in number; they behave in the same way as a single one but with the added complication that they interact with and to some extent contradict each other, adding considerably to the complexity of the problem" (Diver 1979: 168–69). The four orientations underlying the theory of phonology as human behavior are

1. the communicative,
2. the physiological (the physiology of the vocal tract),

3. the acoustic (the medium that is used for transmission), and
4. the human (adapted from Diver 1979: 168–69).

Thus, we now have a summary of the orientations behind Diver's (1975: 13) earlier definition of phonology:

> Non-random distribution of the signal serves for us as the problem to be solved in grammatical analysis, and solutions to the problem are offered in the form of hypotheses about meaning. But within the signal there is another non-random distribution, that of the "phonemes" in the varying arrangements that Bloomfield referred to as making up the "phonetic structure" of the language, and to which later the term "phonotactics" was widely applied. This non-random distribution, too, calls for an attempt at understanding. Why is it that in English, as in many other languages, such combinations as *sr* and *tl* occur either not at all or with very low frequency in initial position in the signals of the language? Here again, hypotheses are called for, since the phonetic continuum—articulatory and acoustic alike—does not do us the favor of dividing itself up into observable categories. And here again we find the human factor and the act of communication—as well as the articulatory and acoustic realities—playing a role in our speech for an understanding of the non-random distributions.
>
> Phonology, then, is for us an attempt to understand the non-random distribution within the signal, and grammar is the attempt to understand the non-random distribution of the signals themselves.

The Fundamental Analytic Position

The fundamental analytic position of the theory of phonology as human behavior may be summarized by the following principles:

(i) Users of a language behave as though they have learned certain distinctive units, the phonemes, which they deploy for communicative purposes.

(ii) We cannot observe directly what it is that they behave as though they have learned.

(iii) We can however observe the phonotactic skewing, a skewing that has been built up over the centuries and millenia in the very mouths of the speakers.

(iv) We can infer that these long-range skewings represent favorings and disfavorings on the part of users of the language. (It is to be observed that the skewings are not idiosyncratic to particular languages; their general characteristics recur from language to language.)

(v) We can then examine the favorings and disfavorings against the background of the orientation—which means with independent knowledge of what kinds of favorings and disfavorings humans are prone to in areas other than the use of language.

(vi) We can infer that a disfavoring, for example, represents a difficulty in a learning process, and by a close examination of what it is that constitutes a difficulty in the way of a particular learning process, we can infer what it is that is being learned.

(vii) What it is that is being learned we may identify as a characteristic of the distinctive units. (Diver 1979: 170)

The Analysis

The fundamental problem posed by Diver for the theory of phonology as human behavior is a search for an explanation of the observable phonotactic skewings of the unobservable distinctive sound units of language (which can be verified both synchronically and diachronically as they have developed over centuries by users of the language). If we take one of the classic examples of phonotactic skewings—the relative infrequency of *tl* and *sr* in word-initial position, both in English (where it does not occur) and in such other languages as modern Hebrew (where it has a relatively low frequency of occurrence)—we may assume that these long-range, nonrandom recurrent skewings represent favorings and disfavorings of certain collocations of distinctive sound units.[4]

We are also aware of the fact that human beings exhibit similar favorings and disfavorings in other areas of their behavior (such as performing common daily tasks or sports), which, like language, are learned. Thus, as can be seen in the analytic principles underlying the theory of phonology as human behavior listed above, we may infer that a disfavoring may represent a difficulty in the learning process, and, by examining what constitutes a difficulty in a particular learning process, we can infer what is being learned. What is being learned may then be identified as a characteristic of the distinctive units. Thus, an explanation of the particular skewings of initial consonant clusters in English and other languages may provide us with distinctive features of sounds in a way that will allow them to be compared to other areas of human behavior (to be discussed further in this chapter and chaps. 3 and 6 below), therefore allowing us to view phonology as an instance of human behavior.

Table 2.1 Frequency Distributions for Occurrence of *l* and *r* in Initial Clusters in English

	p	b	t	d	k	g	f	s	ʃ	θ	Totals	Cross-Totals
l	38	42	0	0	54	24					158	
r	42	62	54	40	61	51					310	
l							55	54			109	190
r							32	0			32	419
l									0	0		
r									17	19		

Consonant Clusters in English

The actual skewing of word-initial consonant clusters whose second member is either *r* or *l* in monosyllabic words in English as presented in Diver (1979: 170) clearly indicates nonrandom favorings of what are traditionally called stops or occlusives to cluster initially with *r* (the absence of *tl* and *dl* being the extreme case) and nonrandom favoring of nonstops that are traditionally called fricatives and sibilants or spirants to cluster initially with *l* (the absence of *sr* being the extreme case).[5] The statistical favorings can be seen in table 2.1 (which reproduces Diver 1979: 170, table 6.1).

Stable versus Mobile

If we examine the various classifications and categorizations of the particular sound units found in table 2.1 (according to the various distinctive features postulated by Saussure and the Prague school onward: stop, occlusive, obstruent, consonant, fricative, spirant, sibilant, liquid, lateral, resonant, etc.), we can see that none of these features serves to illuminate or explain the nonrandom skewings of these distinctive sound units. In light of his orientation, Diver, on the other hand, proposes two alternative distinctive features—*stable* versus *mobile*—that he claims can explain the favorings and disfavorings of the observed phenomena (Diver 1979: 171–72):

Stable indicates that the articulatory organ employed in the production of the sound is relatively stationary during excitation of the resonant cavity. Thus, the lip and apex, respectively, are stationary during the production of *fff, sss,* and *lll.*

Mobile indicates the opposite: the articulator is necessary in motion during sound production. For the stops there is an explosion of the pent-up air, and the lip, apex, and dorsum, respectively, are violently displaced. A trilled *r* is vigorously vibrated, and we shall see in a moment that it is a trilled *r,* characteristic of an earlier stage of the language, that we are here concerned with.

Returning now to the skewings, in terms of stable versus mobile, we can make the single statement that combinations of sames are favored and combinations of differents are disfavored. That is, the rows containing zero and the lower numbers are mobile plus stable and stable plus mobile; those with the higher numbers are mobile plus mobile and stable plus stable:

	Stable (l)	Mobile (r)
Mobile (p, t, k) (b, d, g)	–	+
Stable (f, s)	+	–

Bearing in mind the preference of likes, that is, the higher frequencies of "mobile + mobile" or "stable + stable" collocational combinations, let us look at the instances of ʃ and θ:

	l	r	
ʃ	0	17	*ʃl– < OE skl– ʃr, OE skr – (shrine, scrin)
θ	0	19	θr – <tr– (three = tres) *θl (tl–θ disfavored)

In the case of *ʃ,* we see that a sound change within the recorded history of the language has produced a realignment of the stable-mobile relations. As *sk* > *ʃ,* a stable rather than a mobile becomes juxtaposed to the following *l* or *r,* and the modern frequencies, 0 *ʃl* < *skl* and 17 *ʃr* < *skr* still reflect the older distribution and the preference for sames: stops favor *r* and disfavor *l.* At the same time it is an interesting point that the recouping of clusters since the sound change also favors the formula: already in English we have, coming in from various sources, vocabulary items beginning with the favored combinations *skr-,* as in *scribble,* but not with the disfavored combination *skl-.*

The case of *θr* and *θl* represents in part a variant on the same theme, although there are additional complications. *θr-*, which occurs, has as its major etymological source a favored combination by way of Grimm's law, *tr-*, as we see in comparison of *three* with Latin *tres*. We may assume that the presently disfavored *θr-*, has lost a considerable amount of ground in the interim—compare its 19 with the 54 of the presently favored *tr*—but it is still hanging on. In contrast, the presently disfavored *θl-* comes by way of Grimm's law from *tl-*, obviously disfavored, and it would have to do a great deal of recouping to overcome this initial disadvantage. That has been prevented, however, by the general disfavoring of *θ* itself, which has a low frequency status in the language as a whole (for reasons not being discussed here, but compare its total instances of 99 with the 315 of *f*) and in some dialects has been eliminated outright by phonological change.

Returning now to the formula, we see that the zeros associated with *f* and *θ*, which seem to be turning up in the wrong column, are reflections of additional factors playing a role in these particular instances, and we can with some security restate the position that in respect to stable and mobile, sames are favored and differents are disfavored. (Diver 1979: 172–73)

Likes Are Favored, and Differents Are Disfavored

Diver (1979: 173) then shows how the interrelation between the physiological and the human factor orientations may now be appealed to to explain the nonrandom phonotactic distribution of the data:

We require, then, an external source for an understanding of the particular nature of the skewing, and once we have addressed ourselves directly to the problem, the source is not difficult to find. In this instance we are concerned with an interaction between the physiological orientation and the human factor orientation. A certain musculature, the physiological factor, is being controlled—that is where the human factor comes in—to produce a sequence of articulatory gestures that will in turn produce sounds. We would naturally suppose, in terms of the human factor, that combinations of gestures that are easier to learn to control will be preferred over combinations that are more difficult to learn to control. In the present case, the skewings seem to support this supposition. With *tl-*, for example, we have a violent motion, the explosion that must immediately be quelled and brought under control so that a gesture of a very different kind can be made. With *tr-*, on the other hand, the violence of the motion can continue unchecked; it is merely transmuted—"steered" perhaps is the term—in another gesture equally violent, and the control problem is greatly lessened. Where we begin with a stable gesture, *s* or *f*, we have the same problem of control in reverse.

Active Articulators versus Place of Articulation and the Adroitness of the Apex

This explanation of the general skewing—relying on the physiological and human factor orientations—which is based on the relative degree of ease or difficulty of the control of musculature, can even be applied further to explain the subskewings within the larger skewings, thus providing us with a single linguistic generalization that will account for all the data in the simplest way possible: "Further, that it is the problem of control of the musculature that is involved is supported by the subskewings within the skewings. The strongest disfavorings, the zeros, occur where it is exactly the same musculature that has to be brought under control, the apex in both elements of *tl, dl,* and *sr.* Where there is only a change in kind of motion, such as violent to nonviolent, but with different musculatures, the skewing is milder as in the labial plus apical combinations, *pr* and *br,* or dorsal plus apical combinations in *kr* and *gr.* Here the switch to a somewhat different musculature relieves the problem of control, although the change in degree of violence of motion is still playing a role" (Diver 1979: 173).

Diver then presents a parallel kind of control to his phonological hypothesis, the fact that in other areas of human behavior involving muscular control, abrupt, jerky transitions from one movement to another are usually considered to be awkward and uncoordinated. Thus, in sports such as golf and tennis, such movements (e.g., a hitch in the swing in baseball) result in a lack of control over the ball and are discouraged. It may very well be that, in speech, speakers have learned to avoid such uncoordinated different movements in favor of the same preferred skewings that we indeed find in language: "It is by now apparent that explicit introduction of the human factor leads to a consideration of the problem in the terms of precision of control over gestures, gestures that in turn produce sounds. For our understanding of skewings we therefore naturally begin to look at well-known variables—outside language—that have an effect on precision of control. For example, a person is called right-handed because his right hand is more adroit than his left; confronted by any task requiring precision of control, wielding a tennis racquet or a pencil, the right-handed person uses his right hand. Similarly, as among lip, apex of the tongue, and dorsum [the active articulators], it is apparent that the apex is the most adroit of the three. It is not surprising then that, as has often been remarked, the apical sounds are generally more frequent than the others" (Diver 1979: 174).[6]

By concentrating on precision or degree of control as a result of his focusing on the human factor orientation, Diver paves the way for distinguishing between active articulators and passive receptors—articulators requiring control as opposed to those that do not—and thus further distinguishes between phonetic and phonological features and their role in linguistic analysis: "Note that attributing to these sounds a characteristic of dental or alveolar [the traditional classification of place of articulation based on passive receptors] rather than apical [the active articulator] does not provide us with an understanding of a greater degree of exploitation based on adroitness; the teeth and alvoelae cannot be said to be adroit. The problem with phonetics, of course, is that it gives us a great deal more information about speech sounds than is required by a phonology (hence the controversy about how phonemes are to be labeled), and it is just the task of the phonology to demonstrate that, of all those phonetic characteristics that are undeniably there, only certain ones are of significance for the understanding of the skewing. As seen in the present example, given the importance of precision of control it is evident that the part of the physiology that is subject to control—the articulator rather than the place of articulation—will in general be the provider of the significant characteristic" (Diver 1979: 174).

Number of Articulators versus Voiced-Voiceless

Diver also provides us with a further explanation of the subskewings of the data on the basis of the traditional opposition of voiced and voiceless obstruents (which may be seen to overlap the other two traditional categories of place and manner of articulation). Once again, this new explanation exploits the same linguistic generalization based on the human factor orientation that can be attributed to another extralinguistic example of human behavior serving as a parallel control: "Another example of physical control outside language is to be seen in the childhood trick of trying to pat your stomach and rub your head at the same time; that is, trying to perform two different actions at once. This difficulty, too, is reflected in the skewings. In the case of what is called a voiceless stop—*t,* for example—a single articulator both shapes and excites the resonant cavity; for *d* on the other hand, an additional articulator—the glottis—is invoked to provide additional excitation, thus changing the character of the acoustic product and adding another distinctive unit to the inventory. But coordination of the glottis with the apex, doing two things at once, requires more control, and the voiced stops suffer in frequency accordingly, another well-known observation" (Diver 1979: 174–75).[7]

Diver then points out the connection between the simultaneous excitations of the oral tract and the glottis for voicing and relates it to the important phonetic issue of voice-onset time (VOT):

> This matter of "voicing" in terms of the control of two simultaneous movements is closely associated with the phonetic research that has been done on voice-onset time, variation in onset time being obviously related to simultaneity. When we compare different languages, we see that the extent to which "voicing" consists of doing two things at once is a matter of degree, varying from language to language, rather than an absolute. A schematic version of this may be seen in the following where —— represents the gesture of one articulator, closure and release, and ..... represents the other, vibration of the glottis:
>
> | | | | |
> |---|---|---|---|
> | *Romance* | *b* | *p* | |
> | | —— ..... | —— ..... | —— ..... |
> | *English* | | *b* | *p* |
>
> In each language category the sound that is written with the letter *p* and that shows greater frequency in frequency counts has a later voice onset, which in turn means that the gesture produced by the glottis is to a lesser extent simultaneous with the gestures of the other articulator. Conversely, the *b* in each category has an earlier voice onset; that means "doing two things at once" to a greater degree, and *b* is accordingly disfavored. The middle number of the trio above is therefore either favored or disfavored depending on the option available in the particular language. (Diver 1979: 175)[8]

Diver then discusses the theoretical and methodological implications of this new approach to the simultaneous control of different sets of articulators and contrasts it to the traditional notions of voiced-voiceless and fortis-lenis: "If now we turn to the controversy of whether voice-voiceless or fortis-lenis is the more appropriate characterization of such pairs of sounds—

both, again, being phonetically accurate statements—we see from the above that it is the phonetic factor of voice onset that is also a factor in phonology. By contributing directly to the variable of one articulator vs. two in the makeup of the phonological gesture, it motivates skewings. The fortis-lenis difference, on the other hand, appears to be a consequence of phonological factors rather than a motivator. With only one articulator both shaping and exciting the cavity, as with *p,* crispness of articulation is desirable for optimum excitation; but when a second articulator, the glottis, is assisting with the excitation we can relax, literally, and (here comes the human factor) a lenis articulation results. Lenis, in other words, is merely a failure to do something, when we can get away with it, that would be required under other circumstances" (Diver 1979: 175–76).

Diver then discusses the direct implications of the control of one and two sets of articulators with regard to the problem at hand:

> We may use the figures in Table 6.1 [see table 2.1 above] for a first look at the actual skewings involved as we move from one articulator per gesture (both shaping and exciting) to two articulators per gesture. Comparison of the favored and disfavored combinations, the sames and the differents, in terms of voiced vs. voiceless, reveals that the voiced member of the pair drops much further in frequency than does the voiceless:
>
> | | r | l | |
> |---|---|---|---|
> | p | 42 | 38 | –4 |
> | b | 62 | 42 | –20 |
> | t | 54 | 0 | |
> | d | 40 | 0 | |
> | k | 51 | 54 | –7 |
> | g | 51 | 24 | –27 |
>
> For *p* there is a drop of 4, from 42 to 38, in going from the favored to the disfavored combination; for *b* there is a drop of 20, from 62 to 42, *t* and *d,* of course, are not usable, since both drop as far as they can, to 0, *k* drops 7, from 61 to 54, but *g,* combining two articulators, drops 27, from 51 to 24. (Diver 1979: 176)

The Disfavoring of the Same Musculature and the Human Factor

At this stage, all the subskewings in the data have been presented and explained by the theoretical and methodological consequences of the human factor orientation. Diver (1979: 176) can now compare and contrast the differences in the skewings and subskewings and determine the relative contribution of the various disfavorings and the elements of the human factor orientation that motivated these skewings:

These figures indicate not only the effect of the combination of two articulators in one gesture as a disfavoring, they also show that we must take into account how many disfavorings are present in a given instance: here, two disfavorings have greater consequence than one. A third disfavoring (already mentioned) is to be seen in the drop of *tl* and *dl* to zero, one that arises when the same musculature is involved in the transition from mobile to stable. Direct comparison of the three disfavorings shows how the drop in frequency accelerates as the difficulties pile up:

		Average Amount of Drop	Percentage of Average Drop
One disfavoring (mobile + stable)	*pl kl*	5.5	10.7
Two (+ two articulators)	*bl gl*	23.5	41.6
Two or three, one strong (+ same musculature)	*tl dl*	47.0	100.0

The application of the human factor thus allows us to explain all the skewings in general; to rank them in order to further explain the subskewings according to the same theoretical and methodological principles; and to extend the analysis beyond initial consonant clusters to the level of the word and the process of word formation, which will be used to introduce the communication orientation and the interplay between the human factor and the communication orientations.

The Disfavoring of the Same Musculature and the Communication Factor

Diver then explains the connection between the number and the ranking of difficulties based on the human factor and introduces the role of the communication factor as the data are extended to words and the process of word formation in the following way (Diver 1979: 176–78):

In the case of *dl* all three disfavorings are at work, but it is to be noted that *tl* drops to zero with only two disfavorings, not being voiced. This, of course, suggests that the third disfavoring is stronger than the second, since *bl* and *gl,* also with two, do not drop nearly as far. In fact, reuse of the same articulator—i.e., the same musculature—seems itself to be disfavored, even in instances where the reuse is delayed sufficiently so that the considerations of abrupt transition cannot be involved. Examples follow, and it will be seen that here, too, the amount of disfavoring is correlated with the degree of additional disfavoring and the consequent piling up of difficulties.

The first two examples, containing a relatively strong additional disfavoring, show an articulator being reused in word-final [position] after appearing in an initial cluster (as will be seen in a moment, it is the cluster that constitutes the extra disfavoring).

ClVC	189	*slip*	CNVC	60	*snip*
CCVl	40	*spill*	CCVN	98	*spin*
ClVl	1	*flail*	CNVN	0	*smin*

First with *l* there are 189 of the type *slip,* with *l* in the initial cluster, and 40 words of the type *spill,* with *l* in final position, in the presence of an initial cluster. But there is only one word, *flail,* with *l* in both the initial cluster and final position.

So also with nasals—i.e., with reuse of the musculature that opens and closes the nasal passage. There are 60 words of the type *snip,* with *any* nasal in the initial cluster, and 98 of the type *spin,* with any nasal in final position, but no words of the type *smin,* with any nasal in the initial cluster and any nasal in final position.[9]

We may now reduce the extra disfavoring by moving from the examples of the type CCVC to examples in CVC. (For the purpose of the present chapter we shall merely infer the disfavoring of CC- in comparison with C- from the well-known difference in frequency without going into the question of motivation; the actual numbers of CC- are a much smaller percentage of their mathematical potential than is the case with C-).[10]

We are now down to the single disfavoring of reuse of the same articulator at the beginning and end of the word, and we may expect that, as proves to be the case, the drop in frequency will be less marked.

For this example, the labial, apical and dorsal articulators will be examined as they appear in *p t k* and *b d g,* the type *pit.*

1. Observed initial: labial 86 + apical 72 + dorsal 71 = 229
2. Observed final: labial 59 + apical 108 + dorsal 62 = 229

Of the 229 words both beginning and ending with any of the six sounds indicated, 86 began with labials (*p b*), 72 with apicals (*t d*), and 71 with dorsals (*k g*). Of the same 229 words, 59 end with labials, 108 with apicals, and 62 with dorsals. If on this basis we calculate a symmetrical distribution in the combination of initials and finals, assuming that there is no influence from one end of the word to the other, we get the figures that Diver reports for the co-occurrence of initial and final stops:

L+A	L+D	A+L	A+D	D+L	D+A	:	L+L	A+A	D+D	Total
41	23	19	20	18	33		22	34	19	299

The calculated values are of course obtained by taking, for example, the proportion of initial labials (86/229) and multiplying that by the proportion of final apicals (108/229), giving the proportion of labial plus apical that could be expected to occur if all initials and finals combined freely with each other:

$$86/229\ (.376) \times 108/229\ (.427) = .177$$
$$.177 \times 229 = 41$$

The left part [of the display of calculated values shown above] shows combinations of different articulators at the beginning and end of the word, of the types *bat* (L+A), *pick* (L+D), *tap* (A+L), *dock* (A+D), *cab* (D+L), and *get* (D+A); on the right are combinations of the same articulators, of the types *pep* (L+L), *debt* (A+A), and *cog* (D+D). (Diver 1979: 177–78)

Diver then reports a comparison of the calculated co-occurrences with the actual numbers:

	L+A	L+D	A+L	A+D	D+L	D+A	:	L+L	A+A	D+D	Total
Calc.	41	23	19	20	18	33		22	34	19	= 299
Obs.	43	26	21	23	21	37		17	28	13	= 229
Diff.	+2	+3	+2	+3	+3	+4		−5	−6	−6	

The actual figures for the 229 words show slight departures from the calculation based on symmetry. With different articulators—the left part [of the display of calculated values shown above]—43 rather than 41 for an increase of 2; 26 for an increase of 3; and continuing with an increase in each category of 2, 3, 3, and 4. But with same articulators the direction of departure reverses, and we have drops of 5, 6, and 6. That is all those with different articulators increase a little, and all those with the same articulators drop. Now if our hypothesis were in fact entirely ungrounded, we would expect that in each category there would be a 50-50 chance of departing from the calculated amount either in the direction predicted by the hypothesis or in the opposite direction, just as in a single toss of a coin we have a 50-50 chance for

> heads and for tails. But with every individual category departing in the same direction—that is, in the direction predicted by the hypothesis—we have the equivalent of throwing heads nine times in a row. It would appear that even in the absence of other disfavorings there is a significant avoidance of reuse of the same musculature from one end of the word to the other. (Diver 1979: 178)[11]

This skewing, which indicates avoidance of repeatedly doing the same thing, like the other skewings that have been discussed, can also be extended to other areas of human behavior: for example, the use of "the educated left jab" of a skilled boxer (i.e., alternating with skill and precision the use of both hands in order to win a match) and the familiar interaction of attention span, boredom, and monotony (i.e., the common penchant for either doing more than one thing at a time, or taking breaks from a single task, or, possibly, seeking alternative ways of doing the same thing). All the skewings in general, and the subskewings in particular, indeed show that various traits of the human factor that are applicable to human behavior outside language are also present in our language behavior as well—most obviously in phonology when viewed as human behavior.[12]

Visible Phonemes Are Preferred in Initial Position; Apical Phonemes Are Preferred in Final Position

It is also interesting to note another aspect of the human factor, this time on the word level. If we look at the statistics of initial and final consonants in CVC sequences, we see that there are even further subskewings that represent the interaction between the communication and the human factor orientations: in word-initial position, the difference in frequency among articulators is not very great (86, 72, 71), with a slight preference for labials; in word-final position, however, there is a clear-cut preference for the apicals (108) as opposed to the labials and dorsals (59, 62, respectively).

It is common knowledge that labials—sounds that can be seen as well as heard—are best suited for lipreading because they appeal to both our senses of vision and hearing (Garfunkel-Aloufy 1992; Zeitchik 1992). The adroitness of the apex as an articulator has already been established. Therefore, there are two questions that need to be asked as a result of the above skewing: Why should there be an almost random distribution of active articulators with a slight skewing for labials in word-initial position? Why should there be a strong skewing for apicals in word-final position?[13]

Diver (1979: 179) answers these questions by directly appealing to the communication orientation: "To understand this we must come back to the communication orientation. As we proceed through an individual communication, the accumulation of the information makes it progressively easier to anticipate what will come next; in fact, we all know people who, as hearers, come in in sympathetic chorus on the final words of sentences. In words, too, in any particular context, the early part of the word is likely to give us as much information as we really need to identify the word. Even with a minimal pair differentiated in final position—say *cat* and *cap*—both words of the pair are not likely to make equally good sense in the particular message: "I have a dog and a c——." The beginnings of words, then, contain a much greater burden of distinctiveness than do the ends."

Here lies the answer to the first question. In word-initial or utterance-initial position, there is the greatest burden on communication—both for the encoder and, especially, for the decoder. Therefore, the system of phonology—the phonemic inventory with all its distinctive articulatory and acoustic features—must be exploited to the fullest. Phonemes that can be seen as well as heard will make face-to-face communication easier and more efficient. Therefore, it is not surprising that there is a slight preference for visible phonemes in initial position.[14]

Diver (1979: 179–80) then goes on to answer the second question by appealing to the communication orientation of the theory once more: "It is entirely understandable that if different gestures present different degrees of difficulty, the more difficult gestures will be disfavored where the motivation for maintaining distinctiveness is lessened, as in final position. In the present case, the greater ease of control inherent in the more adroit articulator accounts for its considerably higher frequency in a position of low communicative load."

Here lies the answer to the second question. In word-final or utterance-final position, there is the least burden on communication—both for the encoder and for the decoder. Therefore, the system of phonology—the phonemic inventory with all its distinctive articulatory and acoustic features—does not have to be exploited to the fullest. Indeed, in the mini-max struggle for maximum communication with minimal effort, it is here where the encoder does not have to exercise too much effort at all. Therefore, it is not surprising that there is a significant skewing for apicals in final position.[15]

The different communicative role of initial and final positions can also be tested and verified with another variable previously discussed: voicing, or the number of articulators or sets of articulators to be activated simultaneously. Diver states the following on this matter:

> So also in final position for another variable we have already examined: one articulator vs. a combination of two articulators; that is voiceless vs. voiced.
>
> | | *One Articulator* (*p t k*) | *Two Articulators* (*b d g*) |
> |---|---|---|
> | Initial | 417 | 412 |
> | Final | 616 | 357 |
>
> In initial position (high communicative load) there is practical equality between the voiceless stops, 417, and the voiced, 412. But as the need for distinctiveness drops in final position the more difficult task of coordinating two articulators asserts itself, as it were, and leads to a drop in frequency, 616 to 357. Here again we can note an extreme case, the classic examples of German and Russian, where the voiced stops go down to zero frequency in final position. (Diver 1979: 180)

Diver then summarizes the role that communication has in determining the structure of language—one of the basic tenets of the Columbia school, along with viewing language as an instance of human behavior—mentioned at the beginning of this chapter: "Earlier, apropos of the methodology of phonemics, reference was made to the question of whether communication is a significant ingredient in determining the structure of language. Here, as there, the answer seems to be a clear affirmative. Not only is communication an essential motivator for the existence of distinctive units in language; it is also a controlling factor in the phonotactic structure of those same units" (Diver 1979: 180).

Thus, once again, we return to the basic motto underlying the theory of language and phonology as human behavior: language in general—and phonology in particular—can be seen as a mini-max struggle, the desire to create maximum communication with minimal effort.

Summary and Conclusions

I will conclude with the major principles of the theory of phonology as human behavior as presented in Diver (1979: 180–81):

> 1. We begin with the phonetic observations, articulatory and acoustic, within which there are no observable units.

2. By means of the communication orientation we can establish the *number* of distinctive units in a particular language. This is the standard procedure of the phonemicist.

3. Consideration of the acoustic and physiological characteristics associated with these units suggests a variety of possible characterizations; that is, a nonunique terminology for describing the units.

4. In choosing among these possibilities, it is apparent that the characteristics of the units must be of such a kind that the human user of the language can learn them.

5. This means that either

a) the human learner has an innate capacity for learning these particular characteristics that is entirely independent of his usual ways of learning, or that

b) the human factor, in the ordinary acceptance of the term, is relevant to this learning process, too.

6. The innateness hypothesis is essentially untestable, it is of use only as a residual hypothesis after all others have failed.

7. Proceeding with the human factor hypothesis, because it can be tested, we do not know in advance, deductively, in exactly what way the human factor will interact with the communication and other factors.

8. Therefore, we must have some inductive source of information by means of which to assess the degree of penetration of the human factor.

9. That inductive source is the phonotactic skewing, the result of the accumulated learning of many generations.

10. The skewing, viewed in ways that are consistent with the human factor, against the background of communication, acoustics, and physiology, informs us of the kinds of characteristics with which we are confronted.

The conclusions that can be drawn from the theory and that will underlie the rest of the analyses found in this volume are basically the following.

1. Phonology is not random but motivated; the frequencies of the phonological units and the ways they combine are determined both by their phonetic makeup and by the speaker's exploitation of—or coping with—that phonetic makeup in the act of communication.

2. Gestures enhancing communicative distinctiveness are favored, and articulatorily more difficult gestures are disfavored.

3. There is a conflict between the communication and the human factors in the search for maximum communication with minimal effort in the diachronic development of a language and in its current synchronic state.

4. This conflict is even more keenly felt in language acquisition, where func-

tional errors and processes may be observed, and even more so in the clinic, where functional and organic errors and processes show an even more extreme conflict between the communication and the human factors.

5. The theory of phonology as human behavior can explain the connection and interaction between the phylogeny, ontogeny, and pathology of the development of sound systems in human language in a principled way.

In the following chapters, I will show how the theory of phonology as human behavior has been applied to other languages, diachronic problems, a text, teaching phonetics as human behavior, language acquisition, and the speech and hearing clinic. It should be clear that the human factor being discussed here seriously questions the innateness hypothesis underlying rationalist theories of linguistics in favor of a more empiricist point of view. The issue of rationalist versus empiricist linguistic and phonological theories is a hard one to resolve and has been much debated.

According to Sampson (1980: 158, 160–61):

> Here again the answer lies largely in the contrast between rationalist and empiricist methodology. Empiricism tells us to regard our opinions as fallible, and continually to seek counter-evidence to them; rationalism tells us that we are born with true knowledge already in us. . . .
>
> In general, empiricism encourages one always to think "I may be wrong, and the other man may well be right"; rationalism encourages one to think "I know the truth, so the only point in talking to the other man is in order to show him the light". When scholars of these contrasting frames of mind encounter one another, it is clear which man is likely to win the debate.
>
> Another consequence of the constrast between rationalist and empiricist intellectual styles is a tendency for Chomskyan linguists to abandon the principle that science is cumulative. An empiricist takes for granted that, although his predecessors in any given field may have been wrong in many ways, he is able to progress as far as he can only because of the work they have already done. We advance in knowledge by criticising and replacing elements of the framework of ideas we inherit from previous generations. . . .
>
> The rationalist does not see matters that way; he thinks of the individual as "inheriting" true knowledge in a genetic sense, the main problem being to draw out into the open knowledge which is already there inside one—the thought of previous generations is redundant insofar as it is correct, and merely misleading where it is wrong.

Be that as it may, no single theory has a patent on truth—and I shall continue here to explore the possibilities opened by the theory of phonology as human behavior to explain the combinatory phonology of different languages, language acquisition, and elements of both functional and organic speech errors and processes in the clinic.

Postscript

> The patterns assumed by consonant phonemes are usually rather more complicated and considerably less symmetrical than are those of vowels.
> —Robert A. Hall Jr. (1964: 93)

At the time that the manuscript for this book was being completed, research was being done on the initial consonant clusters of the type examined in this chapter for English and in the subsequent chapters for Italian, Hebrew, and Yiddish for the following languages: Indo-European: German (Middle High/Modern), Yiddish, Dutch, Afrikaans, Swedish, Norwegian, Danish, (Germanic); Latin (Vulgar/Classical), French, Spanish, Portuguese, Catalan, Romansch, Sardinian, Romanian, (Romance); Russian, Ukrainian, Polish, Czech, Slovak, Serbo-Croatian, Bulgarian, (Slavic); Greek (Classical/Modern), (Hellenic); Lithuanian, (Baltic); Bukharian (Judaeo-Persian)(Indo-Iranian); Semitic: Hebrew, Arabic (Classical/Moroccan), Aramaic; Finno-Ugric: Finnish, Estonian, Hungarian; Caucasian: Georgian (Grusinski); Esperanto and Klingon by my undergraduate and graduate students at the Ben-Gurion University of the Negev and Haifa University. These initial findings support the basic principles discussed for English and the other languages with different statistical skewings across languages and have been reported in Tobin (1995). In addition, the theory has also been applied to the Rio de Janeiro dialect of Brazilian Portuguese (Rosenthal 1995) and to two Palestinian Arabic dialects (Himis 1995).

II

Phonology as Human Behavior across Languages

Phonotactics is the term used to refer to the way in which phonemes combine together in a particular language. It is possible to imagine two different languages with the same inventory of phonemes but whose phonemes combine together in quite different ways, and it is therefore not sufficient merely to list the phonemes. If in languages any phoneme could follow any other phoneme with equal probability there would be no place for phonotactics, but in fact there are powerful constraints operating in all languages, and each language has different rules governing the sequences of phonemes which may or may not occur.
—J. D. O'Connor (1973: 229)

In any given language, not all phonemes occur in all positions with respect to the syllable on which they are uttered or with respect to each other. The statement of these limitations is part of the analyst's task in describing the phonological pattern of the language.—Robert A. Hall Jr. (1964: 103)

The consonant patterns of most languages, when taken as a whole, simply do not lend themselves to formulation in overtly neat patterns. As Edward Sapir said, no language forms a water-tight system, and we should be suspicious if too pretty a picture results from the phonemic analysis of a phonetically asymmetrical situation.
—Robert A. Hall Jr. (1964: 97)

3 The Italian and Latin Connections

The general question that confronts us is, how far will such well-known traits of human behavior penetrate into the structure of language? Our only answer lies in the skewed distributions, and the skewings we have been looking at suggest that, in the case of phonology at least, they penetrate very deeply indeed. —William Diver (1979: 179)

Description cannot precede understanding. —William Diver (1979: 182)

Combinatory Phonology

In the first application of the theory of phonology as human behavior to the larger combinatory phonological (phonotactic) system of a language—Italian—Davis (1984/1987: 1–4) eloquently presents the theoretical and methodological tenets underlying his analysis. He first introduces and justifies the phoneme as the unit of analysis in his combinatory phonology: "If the phoneme is the minimal distinctive unit of speech, then the phonemic inventory of a language is the point of departure for a study of the sound system of the language, its phonology. If phonemes are the building blocks, then phonology is a sort of linguistic architecture, with phonemes for stones of various cut, languages for cathedrals, and the principles of phonetics, communication, and human biology providing the external control that engineering, symbolism, and esthetics bring to the study of building. But while stones do not exist, presumably, for the sake of building, ashlars, quoins, and cornice stones do. And while sound waves per se have language as the tiniest of their domains, phonemes have communication as their raison d'être. Unlike cathedrals, languages are not consciously constructed, and unlike stones, phonemes are not directly observable" (Davis 1984/1987: 1). He then returns to the fundamental question of the relation between phonetics and phonology and the role of phonology in traditional and in combinatory phonological theories: "Traditional phonology, therefore, has usually treated phonemic transcriptions as arbitrary codes and has expended most of its resources in the mere identification of phonemes. Recent work in combinatory phonology initiated by William Diver, however, has demonstrated that phonology is more accountable to phonetics than has generally been recognized, and that, just as with other aspects of human culture, language bears the imprint of the mind of the species" (Davis 1984/1987: 1).

Davis comes to grips with the crucial question of the unobservability of phonemic units and the consequence that this has on structural studies, both theoretically and methodologically: "Phonemes have two loyalties, one to phonology, and one to phonetics. The skewings of sound waves within the continuous and aperiodic stream of speech do suggest some sort of underlying discreteness, but it is only the communicative distinctiveness of phonemes that permits their identification. A phoneme is a hypothesis, something not directly—that is, phonetically—observable, yet real nevertheless: the formula behind the phenomenon" (Davis 1984/1987: 2). He then deals with the issue of the phonemic inventory of a language, its role and importance to phonemics and traditional phonology, and its questionable place in creating a theory of language: "A phoneme is a model for a phone. A phonemic inventory, it follows, might be understood as a body of related hypotheses, a theory about a language. Structuralist linguistics shows both the fruitfulness of this phonemic level of analysis (in successful transcription) and its inadequacy: the identification of a phonemic inventory, in itself, reveals nothing about the operation of a language—no more than the stonemason's inventory gives us the plan of St. John the Divine" (Davis 1984/1987: 2). The inadequacy of traditional and structuralist phonemic analyses and the very little that has been done with phonemic inventories of languages are then blamed on the general disregard for the communication and human factor orientations inherent in the definition of language and of the theory of phonology as human behavior: "Implicit in the very existence of the phonemic inventory, however, though little has been made of this, is the function of language as a tool of human communication. The differential employment of phonemes to that end, moreover, can easily be shown, in any natural language, to be non-random" (Davis 1984/1987: 2).

The need to establish—in addition to a phonemic analysis and inventory—a new theory dealing with nonrandom phonotactic distribution—a combinatory phonology—was sensed by many of the great linguists early in this century. Davis first quotes Saussure's position (found in the opening epigraphs to this volume) and then proceeds to show how others felt the need for a combinatory phonology to deal with the dynamics of sound units, even though they did not do it themselves:

The early linguists suspected that something more than simple permutation was involved.

Sapir (1921: 53–54):
The phonetic habits of a given language are not exhaustively defined by stating that it makes use of such and such particular sounds out of the all but endless gamut that we have briefly surveyed. There remains the important question of the dynamics of those phonetic elements. Two languages may, theoretically, be built up of precisely the same series of consonants and vowels and yet produce utterly different acoustic effects. . . . (Sapir mentions the dynamic effects of length, stress, pitch and syllabification.) Most important of all, perhaps, are the very different possibilities of combining the phonetic elements. Each language has its peculiarities. . . . These dynamic factors in their totality, are as important for the proper understanding of the phonetic genius of a language as the sound system itself, often far more so.

And Bloomfield (1933: 129–30, 137–37):
Tables like these [standard phonemic tables], even when they exclude non-distinctive features, are nevertheless irrelevant to the structure of the language, because they group the phonemes according to the linguist's notion of their physiological character, and not according to the parts which the several phonemes play in the working of the language. . . .

Once we have defined the phonemes as the smallest units which make a difference in meaning, we can usually define each individual phoneme according to the part it plays in the structural pattern of the speech forms. . . .

The phonemes so defined are the units of signaling; the meaningful forms of a language can be described as arrangements of primary and secondary phonemes [i.e., including stress and pitch]. If we take a large body of speech, we can count out the relative frequencies of phonemes and of combinations of phonemes. This task has been neglected by linguists. . . .

. . . A serious study of this matter is much to be desired. (Davis 1984/1987: 3–4)

Davis then claims that combinatory phonology first and foremost lends an explanatory dimension to linguistic theory, which, of course, also implies that combinatory phonology provides a broader and more coherent theory of phonology:

Given such a build-up, it is indeed remarkable that linguists have so ignored that area of study to which all their work on phonemicization naturally leads. The result of this failure has been the limitation of linguistics to description. Rather than saying that "linguistics is not prescriptive, but descriptive," we should say that "linguistics is both descriptive and explanatory." [1] . . . For explanation is in fact possible. Diver's work on the distribution of phonemes has shown that their behavior is a function of their completely human nature: their articulation by human vocal organs, their audition by human ears, and their conception and perception by human minds. Our knowledge of articulatory and acoustic phonetics, and of human behavior, becomes at this level of analysis no longer peripheral but central to phonology. But these independent bodies of knowledge not only make explanatory phonology possible; they make it responsible. The result is a more coherent phonology in terms of its own principles and a less isolated phonology with regard to science in general. The tool of communication turns out to be an extension of its user.

The Study

Davis (1984/1987) represents the first application of the theory of phonology as human behavior to the entire phonemic system of a language. Davis defines his research in the following way: "In this study, the phonemes of Modern Standard Italian are identified and categorized by traditional means and with reference to earlier analyses. Then the simplest entries in the lexicon—essentially, monosyllabic stems—are collected, transcribed, and analyzed for phonemic skewings. The highly non-random distribution of the phonemes is immediately apparent as a fact of the language that must be addressed. The attempt to establish a motivation for the distribution results, *a posteriori,* in appeals to the phonetic composition and acoustic transmission of the phonemes and what Diver has dubbed 'the human factor,' the peculiar strengths and weaknesses of human intelligence from what language is, from what communication might be" (Davis 1984/1987: 4–5). He then describes, defines, and explains why he chose the methodology used in Diver (1979) to collect lexical data from a recently published standard Italian dictionary (*Dizionario Garzanti* 1977) rather than spoken data (the advantages of which were mentioned in chap. 2, n. 5 above):

> The data for this study are lexical, not discursive or textual. Frequencies given refer to the distributions of the phonemes on the basis of the lexical items, not its frequency of use in conversation and literature. Each unique lexical item is counted

> once, regardless of its popularity or obscurity. In that respect, the study is an analysis of the Italian lexicon, not of Italian speech.
>
> The discursive-textual approach has been rejected as unsuitable for the problem at hand. Speakers and writers choose lexical items, not phonemes. In the course of their communication, they must constantly select words that are appropriate to the context, and this appropriateness will depend primarily on the meaning of the words, not on their sound. Of course in some literature, such as poetry, the sound of words does matter, but in mainstream communication it must be almost irrelevant. And even though it is likely that in ordinary conversation, speakers avoid words that they find difficult to pronounce, they must, to get their message across, ultimately choose words that convey certain concepts.[2] . . . Historical change may alleviate difficulties that speakers in general have with certain articulations, but at any given synchronic state of a language, speakers have to select from among givens. (Davis 1984/1987: 6)

Davis then specifies the particular advantages of his methodology with regard to the goals of his study: "A lexical approach to the distribution of phonemes, on the other hand, permits an evaluation of the forces that operate phonologically within the word, largely independent of semantic content. If phonemes are not distributed there at random, then what determines the patterns? This study provides evidence that the evolution of lexical items, at least, proceeds according to the principles of communication by humans through means of articulatory production and acoustic perception" (Davis 1984/1987: 6). Furthermore, in addition to the diachronic implications of choosing a lexical approach, Davis also points out the anthropological implications of his methodological choice:

> The lexicon is indeed a product of cultural evolution. Sapir (1921: 4) grouped languages with religion, custom, and art when he wrote that speech "varies as all creative effort varies—not as consciously, perhaps, but none the less as truly." Words are seldom created outright, but even coinage is usually derivative (Bolinger and Sears 1981: 4). The lexicon takes shape gradually and continuously through the very act of speech.
>
> For this reason, lexical frequencies and discursive-textual frequencies are probably highly correlated in any given language. Two detractors from correlation come to mind. In onomatopoeia, the sound of a word somehow suggests its meaning. Even among the few words of true onomatopoetic origin, however, the relation is only imperfect. It is said that in German bells go "bim-bam," while in English they go "ding-dong," regardless of the provenance of the bells. Another discrepancy

Table 3.1 Phonemic Inventory of Italian (Hypothesized)

	Labial	Dental	Palatal	Velar	Labialized-Velar
Nasal	m	n	ɲ		
Stop	p b	t d		k g	kʷ gʷ
Affricate		t͜s d͜z	t͜ʃ d͜ʒ		
Fricative	f v	s z	ʃ		
Lateral		l	ʎ		
Trill		r			
Semiconsonant			y		

	Front			Back
Close	i			u
	e			o
		ɛ	ɔ	
Open		a		

between the two kinds of counts arises when certain phonemes in a language are associated with particular morphological types. For example, the English fricative /ð/ is ubiquitous in speech, primarily because of the extreme demand for the word *the;* yet relatively few words contain /ð/. In Italian, a similar situation obtains with the sound *qu,* which is associated with demonstratives, relatives and the like.

In short, phonology, like grammar, is hardly concerned with frequency of use. The future-perfect tense is just as secure in the grammars of English and Italian as the present. Conversely /ð/ and /q/ are no more secure in their respective phonologies by virtue of their semantic advantage.[3] (Davis 1984/1987: 6–7)

Davis (1984/1987: 19) presents the phonemic inventory for his analysis as a system proposed as adequate to describe distinctively (phonemically) any utterance in standard Italian.[4] (I reproduce his table 2 here as table 3.1, with slightly altered transcription.) He further points out that, "as of yet, nothing has been said of the distribution of these units, and Table 2 [see table 3.1] gives no clue as to what form that distribution might take" (Davis 1984/1987: 18). Davis then defines the object of his study as follows, once again noting the interconnection between phonetics and phonology crucial to the theory of phonology as human behavior: "The second phase of this investigation (the phonological phase) states the distribution and proposes explanatory motivations which, if correct, disprove the supposed arbitrariness of the code and thereby suggest a natural integration of phonetics into phonology" (Davis 1984/1987: 18–19).

The Analysis

Determining the Analytic Approach

Davis (1984/1987: 33) defines the first step in the analysis as determining the appropriate comparisons to be made among the thirty-one phonemes of Italian. In discussing these issues, he clarifies the different functions that the seven vowels—now labeled as phonemes of aperture—and twenty-four consonants—now labeled as phonemes of constriction—play in the phonotactics of Italian monosyllabic stems (see chap. 2, n. 10 above).

This redefining of consonants and vowels according to their relative degrees of constriction and aperture allows for the establishment of a single hierarchy for all phonemes based on a fixed set of parameters of stricture and airflow—what underlies the traditional category of manner of articulation—without having unclear, ambiguous, or dubious terms such as *semivowels, liquids, approximants,* etc., discussed in the previous chapters.

Davis states the following concerning aperture and constriction:

> The role of a phoneme in providing aperture or constriction relates, albeit imperfectly, to the phoneme's degree of stricture, in the phonetic sense. The seven phonemes of aperture all have degrees of stricture low enough to permit non-turbulent airflow through the oral cavity. Among the phonemes of constriction, on the other hand, five, /s, z, f, v, ʃ/, have degrees of stricture that produce turbulent airflow—"fricatives," in phonetic terminology. Eight, /p, t, k, b, d, g, kʷ, gʷ/, have complete stricture, with stoppage of airflow—"stops." Four, /t͡s, ʧ, d͡z, ʤ/, have two degrees of stricture each, first complete stricture, then a transition to turbulent airflow—"affricates." The "trill" /r/ has variable stricture, "intermediate between the tight, maintained closure of stop, and the narrow, maintained open channel of fricative," in Catford's [1977: 128] words. For /r/, excitation of the oral cavity is accomplished not so much by means of aerodynamic friction as by the physical, periodic flapping of the apex of the tongue against the alveolar ridge. Six phonemes of constriction,

Table 3.2 Phonetic Characterization by Stricture and Airflow

Stricture	Phonemes	Airflow
0°	p t k b d g kʷ gʷ	0°: stopped
0°	m n ɲ	2°: nonturbulent
0°–1°	t͜s d͜z t͜ʃ d͜ʒ	0°–1°: stopped, then turbulent
[a]	r	periodic[a]
1°	f s ʃ v z	1°: turbulent
2°	l ʎ y i u	2°: nonturbulent, potentially turbulent
3°	e o	3°: nonturbulent
4°	ɛ ɔ	4°: nonturbulent
5°	a	5°: nonturbulent

[a]Stricture and airflow for /r/ might be said to vary around half.

like the phonemes of aperture, have non-turbulent airflow: /l, y, m, n, ɲ, ʎ/. In phonetic terminology [Catford 1977: 117–22], these along with /i, u/ are "approximants," phonemes that, due to their degree of stricture, are either non-turbulent (when voiced) or turbulent (when devoiced). If phonemes of aperture and constriction fall into the same category in terms of stricture, then that phonetic variable alone cannot differentiate phonologically between them. And, in general, phonetic terminology may not coincide with phonological classes. Although /i/ and /y/ have identical stricture, they pattern differently. The crucial difference for them is duration. . . . /y/ is necessarily fleeting, transitional to or from maximal aperture; /i/ is prolongable, in fact sometimes phonetically long at the point of maximal aperture. The importance of maximal aperture, maximal constriction, and transitional states is emphasized by the fact that lengthening in Italian occurs precisely at the extremes of aperture and constriction: [fatto, faato] "deed, done"; [bɛllo] 'beautiful; but not *[kalldo]. (Davis 1984/1987: 32–33)

He then presents his table 3 (reproduced here as table 3.2, with slightly altered transcription), which shows how the thirty-one phonemes of Italian are characterized phonetically by six hierarchically distinct degrees of stricture as well as six types of airflow.

The twenty-four phonemes of constriction that can occur in some position in the stem before maximal aperture are presented. On the basis of the distribution of initial consonant groups (which Davis [1984/1987: 37] presents in a table that is not reproduced here), the phonemes of constriction can now be reclassified into three classes and five subgroups based on the descending order of their frequency of distribution in initial consonant groups:

By distribution, the phonemes fall rather neatly into five groups: (Class I) the Siamese twins /s, z/, which alone can occur before a second group (Class IIa), /p, k, f, t, b, g, d/, which, in turn, alone occur before third (Class III), /r, y, l/, except for 11 instances of /y/ elsewhere (these are the diphthong /yɛ/) and for 3 instances of /zl/. Five phonemes (Class IIb) /kʷ, v, m, n, gʷ/, occur after Class I but not before Class III. The last group (Class IIc) [/ʧ, ʤ, ʃ, t͜s, d͜z, ɲ, ʎ/] does not occur in combination. Classes IIa, IIb, and IIc (Class II) have in common the invariable role of providing maximal constriction at the front end of the stem. Members of Classes I and III may or may not provide maximal constriction. When they do not, Class I occurs before II (e.g., /sp/), and Class III occurs after Class II (e.g., /pr/). This patterning is not unmotivated; rather, the classes created in response to the distribution correlate rather well with the phonetic facts of stricture and airflow. Class I includes the most turbulent of the Italian phonemes /s/ [see Catford 1977: 37–38, 153–58]. Class II includes all phonemes with complete or first degree stricture and aperiodic airflow, minus /s, z/ and plus the unique instance of ʎ/. The phonemes of Class III have second degree stricture (y, l/), minus /ʎ/, or percussive excitation of the oral cavity (/r/); that is, nonnasal phonemes characterized as lacking aerodynamic stoppage or turbulence. Furthermore, the phonemes of Class III, always occurring immediately before a voiced phoneme of aperture, are themselves voiced. The phonemes of Class I (/s, z/), are voiced or not depending on the voicing of the following phoneme of constriction and voiceless when immediately preceding a phoneme of aperture (contrast German). (Davis 1984/1987: 36–38)

Just as the phonotactic distribution of initial consonant clusters in English reflected diachronic aspects of language (as we saw in the preceding chapter), the same holds true for the patterning of the distribution of initial consonant groups in Italian vis-à-vis Latin: "The patterning [of initial consonant groups] also shows the effects of diachronic language change. /v/ does not fall with /f/, but /v/ was [w] in Classical Latin [where the data are available]. . . . Nor do /ɲ, n; ʎ, l; ʃ, s/, respectively fall together, but the first of each pair is a diachronically new phoneme, absent from Latin, as were /t͜s, d͜z, ʧ, ʤ/. In all these cases, a recent phonetic change has not yet been followed by a corresponding distributional adjustment; the current distri-

Table 3.3 Frequencies of Phonemes of Constriction by Class

Class I		Class II						Class III	
s	426	p	318	v	130	ʃ	49	r	500
z	32	t	314	g	128	k^w	33	l	209
		k	305	d	103	g^w	25	y	119
		f	229	n	81	t͜s	22		
		b	193	ʧ	74	d͜z	16		
		m	17/1	ʤ	55	ɲ	7		
						ʎ	1		

bution still reflects an earlier phonetic state of affairs" (Davis 1984/1987: 38–39)

The justification of Davis's new subclassifications based on the frequency of the distribution in initial consonant groups further reduces and simplifies (theoretical linguistic economy?) the traditional categories of consonants and reflects their roles in Italian phonology:

> We are now in a position to further reduce the number of comparisons to be made among phonemes. Classes I, II, and III play different roles in the phonology of Italian, just as phonemes of constriction and aperture play different roles. Class I [/s, z/] stands out acoustically and may serve as a sort of phonetic prefix before the initial maximal constriction, which is usually Class II [/p, k, f, t, b, g, d/; /k^w, v, m, n, g^w/; /ʧ, ʤ, ʃ, t͜s, d͜z, ɲ, ʎ/]. Class III [/r, y, l/] shares with the phonemes of aperture non-turbulent oral airflow and may provide transition between constriction and aperture. To proceed by analyzing the distribution of the C_1's as such, then the C_2's, and then the C_3's would seem ill-advised (in fact, this was attempted, with unsatisfactory results). An /s/ as C_1 is not at all the same thing as a /p/ as C_1; nor is an /r/ as C_1 the same thing as an /s/ or a /p/. Notice, too, . . . that the distribution of Class II in combination with I and III (i.e., in clusters) resembles its distribution when it stands alone at the beginning of the stem. We shall see how the differences, in fact, result from the effects of clustering. But the similarities suggest that each phoneme, in whatever ordinal position, should be treated as a member of a class. Rather than by absolute ordinal position (C_1, C_2, C_3), then, we shall offer an analysis motivated by functional class (I, II, III). So all the occurrences of each phoneme can be combined as in Table 5 [reproduced as table 3.3 here], and we may procede to make comparisons within classes. (Davis 1984/1987: 39–40)

Simple Pairwise Comparisons

The number of different sets of articulators that have to be controlled to create maximum communication and sound distinctions and the preference for those sounds that require less effort and control—when there is a choice between these oppositions—present the most striking and consistent contrast. Davis considers the theoretical and methodological implications of this principle, discussed in the previous chapter (Davis 1984/1987: 40–41):

> The most striking and consistent contrast—and one which has been noticed before about language in general (Bloomfield 1933: 137)—is that between voiceless and voiced members of minimally contrasting pairs of phonemes:
>
> | | | | | | | | |
> |---|---|---|---|---|---|---|---|
> | p 318 | t 314 | k 305 | f 229 | s 426 | t͡ʃ 74 | t͡s 22 | kʷ 44 |
> | b 193 | d 103 | g 128 | v 130 | z 32 | d͡ʒ 55 | d͡z 16 | gʷ 25 |
>
> In no case is a voiced phoneme more frequent in initial position than its voiceless counterpart. One might conclude confidently: "Voiceless phonemes are more frequent in initial position than their voiced counterparts"; but that statement merely describes the distribution. We require to know how voicing makes such a difference. Evidence is near at hand. Consider the three member opposition below:
>
> | | |
> |---|---|
> | p 318 | t 314 |
> | b 193 | d 103 |
> | m 171 | n 81 |
>
> The nasals are least frequent. A hypothesis emerges: In each case, the addition of one additional articulator (voicing and then nasality) corresponds to a decrease in frequency. Put differently, the addition of one articulating organ (the larynx and then the velum) corresponds to a decrease in frequency. The two gradients voiceless-to-voiced and voiced-to-nasal are seen to be one. Now if this observation were not consistent with some independently known and relevant principle, it would still amount to little more than description, but in fact the coordination of different activities is known to be a problem in human behavior in general. Diver uses the analogy of simultaneously patting the head and rubbing the tummy, or vice-versa. One also thinks of the accomplished pianist who sets out to learn to play the organ and spends several frustrating weeks trying to coordinate hands and feet. Of course, the difficulty involved in activating the larynx is much less severe, and people pronounce b's and even m's with no appreciable difficulty; yet in the long life of language, the disfavoring produced by the extra articulator has its effect on frequency. That very slight difficulty is encountered over and over in every speaker's linguistic lifetime,

with the result that the common repository of words used by speakers—the lexicon—when viewed at one point in time records the cumulative effect. We conclude that in general (calling this Factor A for "Articulators"):

A. Additional articulators are disfavored.

The disfavoring of additional articulators must be viewed in the perspective of the communication and human factors together. As I have previously stated (see chap. 2, nn. 7–9):

1. The voiced-voiceless distinction in consonants is often relevant only for the obstruents—stops, fricatives, affricates—which require the highest degree of muscular control and are therefore at the top of the hierarchy of constriction. The other major consonant class—the resonants (semivowels, liquids, approximants, etc.)—at the bottom of the hierarchy of constriction are all usually voiced as are vowels.

2. This, of course, leads to the question, If voiced sounds are harder to make, then why are there more voiced sounds than unvoiced ones in all human languages?[5]

3. The answer lies in the acoustic and communication orientations: vowels and resonants have acoustic formants that provide more auditory and perceptual information—they provide resonance and have acoustic formants that provide the primary auditory and communicative information most necessary for speech perception. In other words, they are easier to hear in general and over distances in particular.

4. The production of nasals involves three sets of articulators: nasals are all voiced (+1), oral stops (+2), produced with the uvula (+3), which lowers to allow most of the air to enter the nasal passage but leaves enough air in the oral passage to determine which set of active oral articulators is being used: bilabial *m,* apical *n,* or dorsal ŋ.

5. Despite the fact that nasals are complex sounds articulatorily, they are also, first and foremost, natural sounds and are very rarely problematic in language acquisition and in the clinic. As we know, the vocal and nasal tracts were originally designed for eating and breathing, respectively.

6. Nasals are closest to vowels as far as the primary auditory and perceptual acoustic information that they provide is concerned. That is, nasals have a unique pattern of formants like vowels but give strong acoustic cues (sometimes even stronger than vowels) in speech production and reception (Raphael et al. 1974, 1975; Dorman et al. 1974).

The disfavoring of additional articulators goes beyond voicing and nasality as well, which leads to a second principle that coarticulation by near articulators is disfavored. According to Davis (1984/1987: 42):

This effect is not limited to the larynx and velum but applies as well to two oral articulators, specifically the lips and dorsum of the tongue:

k	305	g	128
k^w	33	g^w	25

The sharp fall-offs here suggest an additional advantage for /k^w, g^w/. Two oral articulators, it appears, are especially disfavored, due to the greater coordination required than for the more distant larynx—an explanation supported by the (non-minimal) comparisons /b : k^w (193 : 33) and /g : k^w/ (128 : 33) where both phonemes have two articulators, but only /k^w/ has two oral articulators.[6]

. . . Since the difference here is not additive, it will be necessary to propose a separate factor, say Q. [in honor of the phoneme /k^w/, which he transcribed as /q/; see n. 4 this chapter]:

Q. Co-articulation by near articulators is disfavored.

Davis (1984/1987: 42) then extends the first two principles—the disfavoring of additional articulators (A) and the disfavoring of coarticulation by near articulators (Q)—even further and introduces a third: Visible articulators are favored (V). Following Diver's lead, he then relates all these phonological principles to general principles of human behavior, both theoretically and methodologically:

It has been demonstrated that an observed skewing in the data can be plausibly explained with references to the phonetics of the units in question and in terms of a general principle of human behavior. This simplest of comparisons shows at the very outset of the analysis the interplay of phonetics and the "human factor"—a relationship that permeates phonology, forcing us to acknowledge these two external bodies of knowledge as requisite for the solving of the phonological problem. They account for the observations, and the observations are not accounted for without them. They serve as external controls on hypotheses: we cannot hypothesize any principle at odds with what human beings can do with their mouths and their minds. They make phonology responsible, and not speculative. We call them "orientations" of phonology.

The same data from a different perspective:

p	318	b	193	m	171
t	314	g	128	n	81
k	305	d	103	ɲ	7

In simple oppositions, labials are more frequent than their non-labial counterparts. In each of the above gradients, the number of articulators remains constant, but the place of articulation—actually, the articulator itself—changes. Why should the lips be favored as articulators in initial position? Speakers who are mildly irritated at not being understood [or speakers who want to emphasize their point] have been known to instruct the inattentive [or skeptical] listener: "Watch [or read] my lips!" and the hard-of-hearing regularly resort to lip-reading. In addition to the primarily acoustic transmission of speech, the visibility of labial articulations can be an aid in comprehension. True, speakers cannot always see each other, especially now with the telephone, but the ordinary conversational situation has always allowed for visual reinforcement of an acoustic impression. (It might also be noted that human beings are exceptionally visual creatures who sometimes resort to manual and facial gestures to help get a message across, and who have developed a secondary, purely visual, method of communication in writing.) We can now propose Factor V, for "Visibility"):

V. Visible articulations are favored.[7]

As we have seen in the previous chapter, the theoretical and methodological implications of the favoring of visible articulations naturally leads us into the interplay of the human and the communication factors and their cooperative or synergetic role in linguistic analysis (as was discussed in chap. 1):

The introduction of factor V raises two important and related issues: cooperation and communication. Speech has long been recognized as a cooperative effort between speaker and hearer, the former providing clues to the latter in order to communicate a message, and the latter blocking out distractions in order to concentrate and understand. We know that cooperation involves compromise: that speakers give only as much assistance as they think necessary, being torn between the need for communication and the desire to take the easy way out (the Human Factor again). Some linguists [particularly of the generative kind], for example, Lightfoot (1982: 31–32), have argued that communication is not particularly important in language, that language is used for other purposes as well (most of which are themselves actually communicative). Common sense and evidence alike refute this position. Could anyone seriously propose that poetry and the arousal of emotions (to use two of Lightfoot's purported counterexamples) play any large role in determining the form of language? And does not the very existence of distinctive units on the one hand (phonemes, morphemes) and meaning on the other imply communication? Lightfoot's analogy between language and the heart is absurd and shows a poor understanding of evolution: It is true that a heart does not develop "because it would be useful to pump blood," but we know that individuals born with hearts that do not pump blood do not survive to contribute to the genetic pool. Similarly, language that fails to communicate must be replaced with something more effective ("What did you say?"). Communication is, in fact, so essential to language—and to the analysis of language—that we regard it as the primary orientation of linguistics. Factor V demonstrates the importance of communication in phonology by positing a favoring for Visibility in initial position of the word, just where most of the distinctiveness of the word is at stake: Initially, the hearer knows nothing; once he knows that the word begins with /p/, he is well on his way to comprehension, having eliminated a couple of dozen other possibilities.[8]

The two factors of A and V alone account for 17 of the possible 171 comparisons within Class II.[9] . . . By the algebraic property of transivity (if $x > y$ and $y > z$, then $x > z$, Factors A and V account for an additional 6 comparisons . . . For example, /p/ > /b/ by Factor A, and /b/ > /d/ by Factor V; therefore /p/ > /d/ by transitivity through /b/. (Davis 1984/1987: 44–46)

Davis then points out that the following three phonological principles represent different theoretical orientations: the disfavoring of additional articulators (A); the disfavoring of coarticulation by near articulators (Q); and the favoring of visible articulators (V). The first two principles represent the effect of the human factor orientation. The third principle represents the effect of the communication orientation. In the previous chapters, I have expressed the view that language is a constant struggle for maximum communication with minimal effort.

The following two questions then arise both theoretically and methodologically: How do these two factors or orientations interact with each other? and, How do we determine what is a demonstrably valid factor? Davis then provides us with the following answers based on pairwise comparisons of factors A and V for the phonemic inventory of Italian (found in his table 6, which is not reproduced here). After he discusses the clear-cut cases of favorings for factors A and V previously discussed, he then turns to those examples where the factors appear to be confounded owing to the frequencies when studying what he calls a minimal comparison of a shared distinctive feature. With regard to the question of how the two factors interact with each other:

Here, no prediction in terms of frequency can be made on the basis of factors A, Q, and V, since there is no way of knowing *a priori,* which factor is most important. (In fact, Q does not appear at all in the table, since the only direct comparisons are confounded. Q will be important, however, later.) In those cases, we can only make empirical observations. For example, in the pair /k : b/, Factor A [the human orientation] wins out over Factor V, but in /m : g/, Visibility [the communication orientation] comes out on top. It is likely that other factors are involved in the distribution of many of these pairs, but whatever they turn out to be, the conflict between A and V will remain. This is not to say that such pairs cannot be used for discovering valid factors (We have already seen how /k : k^w, g : g^w/ contribute to the determination of factor A; they do not contribute to the determination of Factor V because the comparison is not minimal, being confounded by involvement of different articulators); no, it is only that, because of a real conflict between demonstrably valid factors, no hypothesis can be advanced with regard to such pairs.

With regard to how one determines what is a demonstrably valid factor:

> A "demonstrably valid factor" is a phonologically relevant principle (i.e., an explanatory statement) with extra-phonological support. Thus Factor A accounts for all minimal comparisons involving Number of Articulators; it is supported by principles of human behavior with regard to coordinating activities. Factor V accounts for all minimal comparisons involving Visibility; it is supported by sensual reinforcement of impressions. A "minimal comparison" involves a set (two or more) of phonemes differing only along one feature. Heretofore, we have operated with an intuitive definition of "feature"; it might be well now to make that more explicit. (Davis 1984/1987: 47)

The idea of making the concept of feature more explicit brings us back, of course, to the differences between phonetics and phonology, which, in turn, respectively imply the different abstract and concrete levels of unobservable and observable phenomena discussed in the previous chapters. I return now to the different quantitative and qualitative attributes of phonetic and phonological features discussed by Diver. Davis distinguishes between phonetic and phonological features and their role in the creation of an explanatory phonology in the following way (Davis 1984/1987: 48):

> The science of phonetics provides detailed descriptions of a great many articulations. The detail, in fact, exceeds the demands of phonemics, and the phonemic inventory of any language can have various characterizations. Phonetics describes phones, which are observable. Phonology deals with phonemes, which are unob-

servable, but characterizable only through their mutual distinctiveness. "Observable units," says Diver (1979: 165), "cannot be described before they are understood. Description cannot precede explanation." As an [extralinguistic] example of an unobservable unit, he uses the planet Neptune, which was discovered only because of its disturbing effect on the orbit of the planet Uranus. Neptune was known before it was seen. Similarly, the electrical charges of subatomic particles were identified through their behavior without the atom ever being seen. So the phonemes of a language can be characterized only as their distribution in the language is understood. Table 2 [reproduced as table 3.1 above] gave the hypothesized phonemes of Italian as traditionally characterized by Place of Articulation and Manner of Articulation. Factors A and V have shown that the identification of the articulating organs of a phoneme is essential to an explanatory phonology. "Articulatory organ" is a feature. It seems desirable, then, to characterize phonemes on the basis of the articulating organs, not Place of Articulation; in other words, in terms of the active articulator, not the passive receptor [see chap. 2, n. 6]. We have also seen, in the division of the consonants into functional classes, the importance of Stricture and of Airflow. With these features, we can recategorize the phonemic inventory as in Table 7 [reproduced here as table 3.4] (refer to Table 3) [reproduced here as table 3.2 above].

By replacing the traditional place of articulation with the concept of active articulator and the traditional manner of articulation with the concept of relative degree of stricture and airflow, we can approach explanatory phonology in the same way as was previously done by replacing the traditional labels of voicing and nasality with the concept of number of sets of articulators. Davis reiterated the theoretical and methodological implications of these changes in the following way (Davis 1984/1987: 48):

The tongue has been divided into three regions on the basis of the distinctiveness of the phonemes articulated by the apex, the anterodorsum, and the posterodorsum. For Italian, no fewer divisions are adequate, and no more are necessary. The triplet /ʎ, y, i/ have elsewhere been discussed distributionally, but not phonetically. We have seen that /y/ is phonologically transitional and phonetically momentary, while /ʎ, i/ are phonologically maximal (in terms of relative constriction and aperture) and phonetically prolongable. As for distinguishing /ʎ/ and /i/, phonologically /ʎ/ provides constriction, and /i/ provides aperture; phonetically, airflow for /ʎ/ occurs around the sides of the tongue, while for /i/ it occurs through a small central channel. The acoustic difference is a change in formant structure. Happily, the one stem in the corpus with initial /ʎ/ also contains /i/: in *gli* /ʎi/ "the, him," the airflow varies along the transverse dimension from lateral for /ʎ/ to central for /i/ with an

Table 3.4 Phonemes Characterized by Articulators, Aperture, and Airflow

Coarticulators		Oral Articulator(s)														
		Lip			Apex			A-Dorsum			P-Dorsum			Lips + P-Dorsum		
Stricture	Airflow	0	L	V	0	L	V	0	L	V	0	L	V	0	L	V
0	0	p	b		t	d					k	g		kʷ	gʷ	
0	2			m			n						ɲ			
0–1	0–1				t͜s	d͜z		ʧ	ʤ							
1/2	1/2					r										
1	1	f	v		s	z		ʃ								
2	2					l			ʎyi						u	
3	3								e						o	
4	3								ɛ						ɔ	
5	3								(a)			(a)				

Note: "A-Dorsum" refers to the anterodorsum, "P-Dorsum" to the posterodorsum. The division is trivial for /a/. For the phonetic terminology, see Catford (1977: 144). "0" is null, "L" is larynx, and "V" is velum. "1/2" is to be understood as "periodic between 0 and 1."

accompanying rise in the second acoustic formant, so that /i/ "sounds higher" than /ʎ/.[10] . . . Why should lateral airflow be associated with constriction and central airflow with aperture? All the other phonemes of aperture, like /i/, have central airflow. The only comparable phoneme of constriction, /l/, has lateral airflow, non-turbulent around the apex. Most likely, /ʎ/ operates on the model of /l/; in fact, they are historically related.[11]

Davis then explores how the new concepts related to phonology as human behavior can allow for the postulation of even further explanatory or demonstrably valid phonological principles. The first of these is related to stricture and airflow and the favoring of explosive phonemes in initial position (Davis 1984/1987: 50–52):

The analysis has gotten a lot of mileage out of three factors. It might be tempting to stop here, since the introduction of more factors is likely to create more contradictions and, paradoxically, block more comparisons. But quite a few cells in Table 6 [not reproduced here] remain completely empty—unaccounted for. Motivated "No

Predictions" are better—more explanatory—than unmotivated "No Predictions," so let us continue with more comparisons.

The following comparison involves a change in stricture.

p	324	b	193
f	229	v	130

The two phonemes with complete constriction (0°) are more frequent in initial position than their turbulent (1°) counterparts. [The] place of articulation is not constant here, but the change from the upper lip /p, b/ to the upper teeth /f, v/ appears to respond to the change in Aperture, not the other way around. All four phonemes are Visible, with the lower lip as articulator. These being the only such pairs in Class II, supporting evidence from pairs across classes might be brought to bear. When the instances of /s, z/ occurring before a Class II phoneme are subtracted from their totals, two additional comparisons emerge:

t	315	d	103
s	155	z	0

Again, the 0° phonemes are more frequent. This difference between /t/ and /s/ is due almost entirely to the /tr-/ clusters, but that is no explanation. We turn later to the question of *why* there are 60 /tr-/ clusters and no /sr-/ clusters [the answer to which we have learned in the previous chapter regarding mobile + mobile and stable + stable preferences in initial consonant clusters]. Two other interclass pairs, however, offer what appears to be counterevidence.

l	137	r	132
d	103	d	103

Here, those instances of /l, r/ occurring after a Class II phoneme have been subtracted, and the 2° phonemes are more frequent than the 0° /d/. But this third set may not belong with the other two. [l, r] are, by virtue of their degree of stricture, particularly suited to laryngeal co-articulation. Some languages do have voiceless [l̥ r̥], which are turbulent, but the turbulence is acoustically weak enough for these phones to be disfavored in language in general. By contrast, voiced [l, r] have a resonance that gives them acoustical favoring. On the other hand, [d] is relatively unsuited to voicing, since laryngeal articulation requires a forward flow of air through the glottis, a flow which is arrested in the oral activity by the complete constriction on the part of the apex in the articulation of [d]. [b, g] are similarly disfavored. [p, t, k] involve no conflict of laryngeal articulation and airflow [cf. the allophones of /p/ in chap. 1 and chap. 2, n. 8]; nor do phonemes of degree one (f, v, s, z, ʃ). In a more detailed study, perhaps with other languages with other patternings, this favoring of voiced degree two over voiced degree zero might need to be made explicit; here it is offered only in support of the following hypothesis concerning the above comparisons of /p, f; b, v/, factor E, for "Explosion":

E. Explosive phonemes are favored in initial position.[12]

By transitivity, Factor E accounts for one more comparison:

p f > v

We can see from the data presented above how the various factors representing different orientations interact. /p/ being greater than /f/ supports the favoring of initial explosive phonemes (E), while /f/ being greater than /v/ illustrates the disfavoring of additional articulators (A). The fact that all three of these phonemes are visible neutralizes the visibility factor (V), although it may be hypothesized that bilabial /p/ may be even more visible than labiodental /f/ and /v/.

Comparing Italian and Latin

Davis points out the importance of language-specific and comparative and contrastive cross-linguistic phonological analyses as well, in order to put a broader perspective on the phonological factors being postulated: "There is some danger of over-analyzing the data and of regarding the phonological factors as some sort of inviolable laws. Different languages have different rankings of phonemic frequencies, and until thorough analysis has been done of several unrelated languages the degree to which the factors proposed in this study are restricted to Italian, rather than applicable generally, cannot be known. Data from other languages will also be helpful in determining which factor predominates when two or more conflict for a phoneme" (Davis 1984/1987: 54).

As we shall see in the next chapter, such an analysis has been made for Hebrew. Davis, himself, has also made an analysis for Latin, which he uses to compare and contrast initial Latin phonemes of constriction: "The Italian language itself shows significant diachronic change in the relative frequencies of phonemes in initial position. Table 8 [not reproduced here] gives the distribution for Classical Latin [from *Cassell's Latin Dictionary*], from

Table 3.5 Frequencies of Initial Latin Phonemes of Constriction, by Class

Class I		Class II								Class III	
s	2/1	p	231	m	114	d	50			r	212
		t	179	w	100	b	48			l	199
		k	170	n	81	k^w	45			h	90
		f	161	g	59	y	25				

Note: For the sake of simplicity, the clusters /sw, ps, ks, gn, rh/ have been omitted.

a count performed under guidelines as comparable as possible to those of Italian. At the risk of simplistic analysis, Table 8 has been arranged similarly to Table 4 [also not reproduced here], with again three classes of phonemes of constriction. . . . /h/ has disappeared since Classical times, and /w/ has become /v/, wholesale. Other well-known major changes are /k/ > ʧ and /g/ > ʤ, both in restricted environments. Table 9 [reproduced here as table 3.5] gives the distribution by class" (Davis 1984/1987: 54–56).

Davis then compares and contrasts the frequencies of the shared initial phonemes between the two languages (Davis 1984/1987: 56):

The Class II phonemes held in common by the two languages, in order of decreasing frequency in Latin, rank as follows:

	p	t	k	f	m	w>v	n	g	d	b	k^w
Latin:	1	2	3	4	5	6	7	8	9	10	11
Italian:	1	2	3	4	6	7	10	8	9	5	11

He explains the slight differences in frequencies in the following way (Davis 1984/1987: 56–57): "In the evolution of Latin to Italian (not to forget foreign invasions and the *questione della lingua*) /b/ has overtaken /m, w > v, n, g, d/ and /n/ has fallen behind /g, d/. In Latin, neither Factor A nor Factor V was operating fully (although Factor E holds for /p : f/). /m/ is more frequent than /b/. As is widely known (e.g. Buck 1933: 121), historical reconstruction has shown that Indo-European **b* was extremely rare in initial position, and it is the only reconstructed IE source of Latin initial /b/. The ratio of b/p for Latin is only .21, while for Italian it is .61. The ratios for the other 0° phonemes are more comparable: Latin d/t = .28, Italian d/t = .33; Latin g/k = .35, Italian g/k = .42. Rather than Italian /b/ being abnormally high,

Table 3.6 Proportions of Stems from Sources Other than Classical Latin, from a Random Sample

Class II Italian Phoneme	No. of Stems from Classical Latin	No. of Stems from Other Sources[a]	Proportion from Other Sources[a]
b	21	34	.6
g	18	19	.5
m	40	27	.4
d	16	7	.3
v	39	7	.2
n	19	3	.1

[a]The other sources were French (twenty); late, medieval, and vulgar Latin and other Italian (eighteen); Greek (thirteen); English (ten); other Germanic (fifteen); Spanish (six); Provençal (five); and others (eighteen).

it appears that Latin /b/ was abnormally low due to its IE heritage. Indeed, Italian seems to have borrowed an unusually large number of b-stems, mainly from French and Germanic languages. A random number of stems in the corpus yielded the following statistics on borrowing."[13] These statistics are presented in Davis (1984/1987: 57) as table 10, reproduced here as table 3.6. These statistics are then described and explained in the following way with regard to the theoretical and methodological implications of the frequencies with the postulated phonological principles:

In the sample, /b/ is proportionally the most borrowed of the six, testing significantly higher than /d, v, n/ (but not /g, m/). /n/ is the least borrowed, testing significantly lower than /g/ (but not /d/).[14] . . . /n/ appears actually to have [lost] ground (Latin n/m = .71, Italian n/m = .47) while /g, d/ gained slightly (again, Latin g/k = .35, Italian g/k = .42; Latin d/t = .28, Italian d/t = .33). The high ratio for /n/ in Latin may be due to its proliferation among stems with "negative" semantic content. By contrast, Latin was underutilizing /b/ in initial position. Borrowing in the past two millenia has been selective in correcting that imbalance. It is futile, but logical, to ask why Indo-European should have been so deficient in initial /b/ in the first place, in violation of phonological principles. The point is that the Factors are violable, and individual languages at points in their histories will deviate from them, mainly because of pressures on the phonemic system from whatever direction and also because of the development of semantic associations with certain phonemes. (Davis 1984/1987: 57–58)

The problem of historical fluctuations and their effect on phonological data is not totally lost, however, and actually leads to an additional factor called T, for *Transition:*

Comparisons among the diachronically recent phonemes, and between them and the longer-established ones, run an especially high risk of falling victim to just such historical fluctuations as Latin /b, n/. Nevertheless, one factor that has been noted in other languages (Diver, personal communication) and that involves new Italian phonemes finds support here, too. This is Factor T, for "Transition":

T. Transitions from one distinct constriction to another within a single phoneme are disfavored.

Four phonemes in Italian have this characteristic of Transition (from 0° to 1°: /t͜s, d͜z, ʧ, ʤ/. The two articulators with the anterodorsum /ʧ, ʤ/ do not lend themselves to comparison, there being no anterodorsal 0° phonemes in the inventory.[15] . . . The two apicals of Transition /ts, dz/, however, oppose the 0° apicals:

t	314	d	103
t͜s	22	d͜z	16

The difficulty of performing two distinct tasks, even consecutively, with one organ in one gesture is responsible for Factor T—a little like trying to open a bottle of champagne gradually. (Davis 1984/1987: 58–59)

Indirect Comparisons

After having exhausted most of the pairwise comparisons of related phonemes, Davis takes it on himself to perform indirect comparisons on unrelated phonemes crossing over traditional phonological classes:

The time has come to make some indirect comparisons, that is, comparisons between phonemes that are too different for simple, one-dimensional gradients. For this, phonemes will be characterized in terms of the five factors established thus far, then examined for agreement and disagreement of favorings, and then subjected to association between mutual favorings and disfavorings and relative frequency.

Table 3.7 Class II Phonemes Evaluated for Factors A, Q, V, E, and T

	Articulators (Disfavored)	Q-Coarticulation (Disfavored)	Visibility (Favored)	Explosion (Favored)	Transition (Disfavored)
p	+	+	+	+	+
t	+	+	−	+	+
k	+	+	−	+	+
f	+	+	+	−	+
b	0	+	+	+	+
m	−	+	+	−	+
v	0	+	+	−	+
g	0	+	−	+	+
d	0	+	−	+	+
n	−	+	−	−	+
ʧ	+	+	−	+	−
ʤ	0	+	−	+	−
ʃ	+	+	−	−	+
k^w	0	−	+	+	+
g^w	−	−	+	+	+
t͡s	+	+	−	+	−
d͡z	0	+	−	+	−
ɲ	−	+	−	−	+
ʎ	0	+	−	−	+

Table 11 [not reproduced here], an update of table 6 [also not reproduced here], shows which comparisons have yet to be made (mostly among the new phonemes). Table 12 [reproduced here as table 3.7] evaluates the phonemes in terms of the five factors. (Evaluation is by favoring only—the inverse of disfavoring, in the cases of A, Q, and T—so that signs mean the same thing throughout the table.) And Table 13 [not reproduced here] adds to Table 11 indications of mutual favoring (+), mutual disfavoring (−), and disagreement (0). For example, in the comparison /t : g/, /t/ is favored for Factor A, and the other factors are equal between the two, so the cell receives (+); the observed ranking for this pair is as predicted. In the comparison of /n: ʃ/, /n/ is disfavored by Factor A, and the other factors are equal, so (−) is assigned; the observed ranking is not as predicted. In the comparison /f: ʧ/, /f/ is favored by V and T, but /ʧ/ is favored by E, and (o) is assigned; no prediction is possible. Such indirect comparisons account for 45 correct predictions (+), and show that 65 pairs cannot be compared (o). Indirect comparisons are required for only 7 of the 45 "top ten" pairs, and these are all positive. (Davis 1984/1987: 59)

In table 3.7 we have all the Class II phonemes evaluated for Factors A (number of articulators), Q (coarticulation), V (visibility), E (explosion), and T (transition). Establishing all the values for each phoneme does not solve all the problems, however, which leads us to observing how the phonemes of constriction cluster together as a means of solving the remaining problems. Davis introduces the problem in the following way: "Two kinds of residual problems remain. No predictions have been made—and no blockages motivated—for five pairs: /k : t, g : d, n : ɲ, ʧ : t͜s, ʤ : d͜z/; these all involve simply a change in articulator. Incorrect predictions have been made for four pairs: / n : ʃ, n : ʎ, ʤ : t͜s, ɲ : ʎ; these are complex comparisons. To solve these nine residual problems, it will be necessary to look for the first time at clustering of phonemes of constriction" (Davis 1984/1987: 60–62).

Consonant Clusters

Davis first presents the descriptive facts concerning which consonants from which classes cluster together (Davis 1984/1987: 62–64):

Clusters between Classes II and III as seen in Table 4 [not reproduced here] occur almost exclusively with seven members of Class II, viz. /p, k, f, t, b, g, d/ (we shall return to the few exceptions /sy, zl, my, ly, vy/). The only old, established phonemes that do not cluster are /s, m, n, v, k^w/; nor do /r, y, l/ cluster among themselves. /m, n, k^w/ and, formerly /v/ in the form of /w/, all involve three articulators. Clustering among these four phonemes seems to be ruled out by a combination of Factor A (Number of Articulators) and an avoidance of coordination of complex tasks, thanks to the Human Factor. /r, y, l/, however, require only two articulators each, and /s/ only one. These four phonemes have in common continuous airflow, and, as was remarked earlier, stems in Italian prefer to begin with complete constriction (Factor E). Being thus disfavored, these phonemes are less likely to occur in combination with other incompletely constricted phonemes during a transition from relative constriction to relative aperture. Such a combination would require the maintaining of an intermediate degree of stricture. (This is not to say that such combinations do not occur at all; see Diver [previous chapter] for the data on English

Table 3.8 Distribution of Clusters of Classes I and II

	r	y	l	Total
t	96	2	0	98
p	50	24	20	94
k	54	27	12	93
f	51	16	17	84
b	51	6	10	67
g	52	5	10	67
d	13	1	0	14
Total	367	81	69	517

sl-clusters.) Among the phonemes that do cluster, however, one seems to refute the hypothesis that incomplete constriction is disfavored in clustering in initial position: /f/ has no trouble clustering whatsoever. /f/ in initial position descends from various Indo-European "stops," mainly **bh* and **dh* (Buck 1933: 121, 126), and it probably retains the old distribution. We shall soon see another reason why /s, r, y, l/ should not cluster among themselves, while /f/ might cluster with them.

The three cases of /zl/ in Table 4 [not reproduced here] are new stems borrowed since the time of Classical Latin (*slip* "brief", *slitt* - "sled", and *slav* - "Slav"). All the exceptions with /y/ have the diphthong /yɛ/; in fact, a total of 38 of the 113 instances of /y/ as C_2 or C_3 are due to /yɛ/. Attributing the distribution of /y/ in these cases to the distribution of the diphthong leaves a distribution of II–III clusters (again adding in the s- and z- clusters) as given in Table 14 [reproduced here as table 3.8].

The results and the theoretical and methodological implications of the figures in table 3.8 are described and explained by Davis as follows after he observes each column separately:

Except for the rise of /t/ from second rank to first, the ranking of the totals for clusters is the same as for overall totals as given in Table 5 [table 3.3 above here], suggesting that Factors A, V, and E are operating also in this more restricted environment (Factors Q and T are not applicable, except that those phonemes disfavored by them /kʷ, gʷ, t͜s, ʧ, d͜z, ʤ/, do not cluster with Class III). These factors alone, however, cannot account for the supremacy of /t/ in clusters or for the distribu-

Table 3.9 Distribution of Clusters of Classes II and III, by Class III Phoneme

r		y		l		y, l	
t	96	k	27	p	20	p	44
k	54	p	24	f	17	k	39
g	52	f	16	k	12	f	33
f	51	b	6	b	10	b	16
b	51	g	5	g	10	g	15
p	50	t	2	t	0	t	2
d	13	d	1	d	0	d	1

tion within Table 14 [table 3.8 here]. It will be necessary to look at each column separately, as in Table 15 [table 3.9 here].

For clusters with /r/, the frequencies hang closely around the median 51 except for the two extremes, /t/ with almost twice as many as /d/ with only a quarter as many. It appears that /r/ occurs freely with this subclass (IIa) of phonemes unless the apex is the articulator (/t, d/). And it is precisely the apex which articulates /r/. The combined frequencies for /y, l/, column "y, l," show a completely different picture. (If, as Austerlitz [1983: 21–22] says, there is a [w] "born of" [b] and a [w] "born of" [u], then Italian has a [y] born of [l] and a [y] born of [i]—though perhaps not in Austerlitz'[s] original phonetic sense.) /y/ in this environment is a development from /l/. Words with l-clusters tend to be literary or archaic, that is Latinate. There exist even a few doublets (such as the common *chiamare* "to call," with /ky-/, and the obsolete and literary *clamare* "to cry out," with /kl-/). In the column "y, l," the two apicals sit at the bottom of the ranking, and otherwise, Factors A, V, and E operate. The first task, then, is to explain the difference between column "r" and column "y, l." If it were not for the eccentric behavior of /t/, one might pursue the idea that combinations involving the same articulator are disfavored. That, as it turns out, is quite near the mark, but the problem of the behavior of /t/ is best approached through the side door.

The side door, as it were, turns out to be Diver's (1979) analysis of initial consonant clusters in English and the new features stable and mobile presented in the previous chapter (Davis 1984/1987: 66–67):

Diver has shown (p. 171), for English (which, however, no longer has a trill), that phonemes of complete constriction prefer /r/, while phonemes of incomplete constriction prefer /l/. His analysis depends on the preference of /p, b, t, d, k, g/ for /r/ versus the preference of /f, s/ for /l/. He concludes that the decisive factor is the coordination of like gestures:

A phonetically accurate characteristic of these sounds that is not included in the usual repertoire of phonetic features is that they differ among themselves in being either *stable* or *mobile*. *Stable* indicates that the articulatory organ employed in the production of the sound is relatively stationary during excitation of the resonant cavity. Thus, the lip and apex, respectively, are stationary during the production of *fff, sss,* and *lll*. *Mobile* indicates the opposite: the articulator is necessary in motion during sound production. For the stops there is an explosion of the pent-up air, and the lip, apex, and dorsum, respectively, are violently displaced. A trilled *r* is vigorously vibrated. . . .

. . . We are concerned with an interaction between the physiological orientation and the human factor orientation. A certain musculature, the physiological factor, is being controlled—that is where the human factor comes in—to produce a sequence of articulatory gestures that will in turn produce sounds. We would naturally suppose, in terms of the human factor, that combinations of gestures that are easier to learn to control will be preferred over combinations that are more difficult to learn to control. In the present case, the skewings seem to support this supposition. With *tl-*, for example, we have a violent motion, the explosion that must immediately be quelled and brought under control so that a gesture of a very different kind can be made. With *tr-*, on the other hand, the violence of the motion can continue unchecked; it is merely transmuted—"steered" perhaps is the term—in another gesture equally violent, and the control problem is greatly lessened. Where we begin with a stable gesture, *s* or *f*, we have the same problem of control in reverse. Further, that it is a problem of control of the musculature that is involved is supported by the subskewings within the skewings. The strongest disfavorings, the zeros, occur where it is exactly the same musculature that has to be brought under control, the apex in both elements of *tl, dl,* and *sr*. Where there is only a change in kind of motion, such as violent to non-violent, but with different musculatures, the skewing is milder, as in the labial plus apical combinations, *pr* and *br,* or dorsal plus apical *kr* and *gr*. Here the switch to a somewhat different musculature relieves the problem of control, although the change in degree of violence or motion is still playing a role. (Pp. 171, 173).

Table 3.10 Stable and Mobile Coordination

	Observed			Expected		Skewing	
	r	y, l	Total	r	y, l	r	y, l
0°	316	117	433	307.4	125.6	+	–
f	51	33	84	59.6	24.4	–	+
Total	367	150	517				

Note: $\chi^2 = 5.10$, $\chi^2 = 2.71$.

Likes Are Favored; Differents are Disfavored

Davis then compares and contrasts Diver's findings indicating the principle that likes are favored and differents disfavored for English with the Italian data to show that the same principle is working in each language (Davis 1984/1987: 67):

> Italian has no /sl/ clusters, but the skewing is strong enough with /f/ alone, as shown in Table 16 [reproduced here as table 3.10]. Under "Observed," the "o°" row contains the sums of the frequencies of the o° phonemes in Table 15 [3.9 above here] clustering with /r/ (= 316) and /y/ or /l/ (= 117); the sums for /f/ are in a separate row. "Expected" frequencies for each cell are calculated by multiplying the marginal totals for that cell and dividing by the grand total (= 517). χ^2 (chi-squared) is the sum over the four cells of $(\text{Obs} - \text{Exp})^2/\text{Exp}$. Here, χ^2 is a descriptive measure of association that quantifies the observed skewing. As an object of comparison let us use the measure of the most extreme hypothetical distribution that could reasonably be expected by chance, a χ^2 of 2.71, as given in any standard statistics text. The observed χ^2, 5.10, is greater than expected,[16] and we can conclude with Diver that:
>
> M. Mobile-plus-stable and stable-plus-mobile clusters are more disfavored than clusters of like mobility or stability

Active Articulators and Consonant Clusters

These new features of stable and mobile—a simplification of the traditional manner of articulation—clearly go hand in hand with the reclassification of phonemes by active articulator, a more efficient category than the passive receptor. Davis (1984/1987: 67–68) links their connection while quoting Diver (1979: 174): "This skewing also supports the earlier decision to recategorize the phonemic inventory in terms of articulators: 'As seen in the present example, given the importance of precision of control it is evident that the part of the physiology that is subject to control—the articulator rather than the place of articulation—will in general be the provider of the significant characteristic.' "

This general statement concerning the important role of the active articulator rather than the passive receptor is then applied to the Italian data and compared and contrasted with Diver's English data: "Now returning to Table 15 [table 3.9 above here]; we see that the ranking of /t, d/ at the bottom of the 'y, l' column is due to the Mobility of Class II and the Stability of /l/, and to the re-use of the apex as articulator. The 'r' column reveals something more. Not only are /t/ and /d/ more frequent there than with 'y, l,' but /t/ is ranked first, and /d/ last. Diver noted that the violence of /t/ is 'steered' into the violence of /r/. Italian supports an even stronger statement: that the violence of /t/ and the violence of /r/ actually join forces for the common good. In other words, /t/ acts as a kind of springboard for the trilled /r/: the explosion of /t/ propels the trill of /r/. This initial explosion is somewhat wasted with /p/ and /k/, since they are physically too far away from /r/ to give it any spring. With /d/, by contrast, the weakened energy of explosion, relative to /t/, is insufficient to propel the trill, and the voiced apical becomes not a springboard but a stumbling-block [cf. chap. 2, n. 8]" (Davis 1984/1987: 68–69).

The interface of stable-mobile and active articulators is also exploited successfully to explain other nonrandom distributions in consonant clusters: "The distributions of the 'y' and 'l' columns of Table 15 [table 3.9 above here] are similar but interestingly different. Under 'l,' /k/ is ranked third, after /p, f/; under 'y,' it moves into first place. /k/ and /l/ are formed with adjacent articulators, the dorsum and the apex, whereas /pl, fl/ involve the more independent lips and apex. Of these three clusters, /kl/ has the least compatible members in terms of coordination of gestures. With /y/ as an alternative to /l/, /k/ has historically tended to reject the l-cluster and has adjusted its own articulation forward along the tongue, so that the cluster /ky/ can be articulated in what is almost a single gesture: phonetically, a palatized /k'/. This option is unavailable to /p, f/, which have retained to a greater extent the old l-clusters. /g/, with its lower explosive energy, relative to /k/, is less inclined to avoid the stable /l/, and it too has kept l-clusters" (Davis 1984/1987: 69).

Apical Adroitness and Consonant Clusters

An additional observation linked to the principle of active articulators can also be used to explain the nonrandom distribution of consonant clusters more fully:

> One more observation on clustering, the membership of /s/ in Class I, of /r, l/ in Class III, and the facility with which /t/ and also /st/ combine with /r/ suggest that apicals in general may have claim to some phonological principle relating to clustering, somewhat as labials have visibility. Diver (1979: 174) has recognized the "adroitness" of the apex, as opposed, say, to the lips and the dorsum, as a factor to be reckoned with. This property appears (personal communication) to play a greater role in the distribution of stem-final rather than stem-initial position, where [for the latter] the communicative load is greater and speakers make fuller use of the phonemic inventory, including those phonemes articulated by less talented organs. From the analysis of Italian, it is clear that Adroitness, more than the other factors presented here, interacts in complex ways with several phonological considerations. Recall the first-rank /tr-/ and the last-rank /dr-/, a difference so great between these two apicals that, in the overall distribution (Table 5) [table 3.3 above here], /t/ ranks above /k/ but /g/ ranks above /d/. (Davis 1984/1987: 69–70)

The Complexity of Interacting Factors

Davis then ties up the loose ends of phonemes of constriction and the complexity of the interaction of the principles of clustering before he turns to phonemes of aperture.

> The complex principles of clustering cannot, without great difficulty, be incorporated into the record-keeping of pairwise comparisons (last version, Table 13) [not reproduced here]. Suffice it to state here that the important comparisons /t : k, g : d/, which previously could not even be made indirectly, are accounted for by clustering. /t/ combines so readily with /s-/ and /-r/ that it surpasses the respectable combination of /k/ with all of /s, r, y, l/ and overcomes its own handicap with regard to /y, l/. Notice (Table 4, column "o") [not reproduced here] that where there is no clustering the two comparisons reverse:
>
> | | | | |
> |---|---|---|---|
> | k | 154 | d | 85 |
> | t | 148 | g | 57 |
>
> The quadruplet gives a good picture of the complexity of interacting factors. /k/ is advantaged (+) over /t/ (o) for Explosion, having a smaller super-laryngeal volume

behind the constriction, that is, between the larynx and the dorsum-to-velum contact, and hence a greater potential energy. Where clustering is not of concern, /k/ is more frequent than /t/. By contrast, /g/ is disadvantaged (−) for Explosion with respect to /d/ (o) for just the same reason: /g/ has a smaller super-laryngeal volume than /d/, but because of that volume, the dorsum-to-velum constriction of /g/ conflicts all the more with the airflow generated by laryngeal vibration—the air has nowhere to go. If the Adroitness of /t, d/ is operating in this no-cluster environment (and presumably it is, the musculature of the apex being constant), then it is masked by the effects of super-laryngeal volume on another factor, Explosion.

The three other empty cells in Table 14 [table 3.8 above here] cannot be filled with reference to clustering. /t͜s, d͜z, t͜ʃ, d͜ʒ, n, ɲ/ do not cluster in initial position. Of these, /n/ is the oldest, and /t͜ʃ, d͜ʒ/, too, are rather well established. /t͜s, d͜z, ɲ/, on the other hand, are, one might say, historically disadvantaged in initial position (though more regular in medial position). They are newcomers into the race for representation in the lexicon, and no major diachronic change has pushed them in this environment like the famous palatalization of Latin /k, g/ that gave birth to /t͜ʃ, d͜ʒ/.

The four incorrectly predicted (−) cells have similar problems. /ʃ, ʎ/, too, are diachronically special, the former all bound up in morphophonology and the latter occurring in initial position only in the free morpheme *gli* "the, him" (and in its combining form *glie-* "him, her"). If it has taken stalwart /b/ thousands of years to regain its rightful place, we should not expect quick lexical action in the case of the more exotic /t͜s/ and company. (Davis 1984/1987: 70–72)

If nothing else, Davis's work on phonemes of constriction reveals how the theoretical and methodological model introduced in chapter 1 allows for the postulation of a limited number of abstract theoretical hypotheses and principles that will account for the nonrandom distribution of as large and broad a corpus of concrete data as possible.

Phonemes of Aperture

Davis says the following about phonemes of aperture: "Aperture brings respite from constriction. The phoneme of aperture is a relative maximum in the stem, the point of slope zero, to take an analogy from analytic geometry, in a curve that is concave downward from initial to final (or medial constriction)" (Davis 1984/1987: 72). Put in more basic terms, phonemes of aperture allow for maximum airflow and compose the nucleus of syllables in human speech. This central role in communication also implies that the collocation of phonemes of aperture is freer with respect to neighboring phonemes than that of phonemes of constriction.

Just as with phonemes of constriction, the theory of phonology as human behavior replaces many of the traditional categories previously applied to phonetics and phonology:

1. "Front" and "back" vowels indicate the relative position of the anterodorsum and posterodorsum—the active articulators—of phonemes of aperture.
2. "Open" and "close" and very often "high," "mid," and "low" refer to different degrees of aperture resulting from the position and movement of the lips—the other active articulators for phonemes of aperture—as well as the anterodorsum and posterodorsum.
3. Both in their form and in their relative frequency, diphthongs may be compared with other complex units such as affricates and support factor T: transition of stricture within phoneme, extending it to the realm of aperture in addition to constriction.

Davis further compared the frequencies of phonemes of aperture and did not find the same clear-cut tendencies to favor the factors of number of articulators or visibility that worked so well with phonemes of constriction. This might be attributed to the fact that the phonemes of aperture form an articulatory and acoustic continuum or cline and the distinctions between them are less acute than those of phonemes of constriction. Acoustically speaking, the changes in the formant frequencies of phonemes of aperture appear in their transitions to and from other phonemes. Therefore, it is not surprising that the principles obtained from Davis's data reflect these collocational phenomena.

It should also be noted that Davis's Italian data show a highly significant favoring of the neutral, low central /a/ vowel over what are traditionally referred to as the individual front and back vowels. Not unsurprisingly, there is also a preference for front vowels over back vowels in his data. These results are consistent with the theory of phonology as human behavior and have been attested to in more general terms elsewhere (e.g., Levitt 1984: 136).

Summary and Conclusions

In this chapter, the theory of phonology as human behavior, introduced by Diver (1979), was extended and applied to Italian and, to a more limited extent, to Latin. The importance of combinatory phonology and the key role of the phoneme in phonology were defended. The crucial role of lexical versus discourse data was justified. The importance of replacing traditional phonetic and phonological categories and classifications and replacing them with new—more human behavioral-, cognitive-, and communication-oriented—ones was validated.

The following principles concerning phonemes of constrictions were postulated and validated:

1. additional articulators are disfavored;
2. coarticulation by near articulators is disfavored;
3. visible articulations are favored;
4. explosive phonemes are favored in initial position;
5. transitions from one distinct constriction to another within a single phoneme are disfavored; and
6. mobile-plus-stable and stable-plus-mobile clusters are more disfavored than clusters of like mobility and stability.

Two additional principles regarding phonemes of aperture and the interaction and transitions between the two kinds of phonemes were obtained by Davis:

7. among constrictions, maximal constriction is favored, and, among apertures, maximal aperture is favored; and
8. sequences of phonemes with the same articulator are disfavored unless their juxtaposition is, by virtue of some other factor, mutually beneficial.[17]

In his conclusion, Davis states the following concerning the implications of applying the theory of phonology as human behavior to a single language as well as to other languages: "The results of the phonological analysis in this study are of two kinds: technically phonological and generally linguistic. The 'soft' phonemic data of the Italian lexicon—soft by virtue of resulting from an earlier, phonemic, analysis—support a small number of simple principles (factors) that explain the observed distribution of units by reference to pertinent but independent bodies of knowledge.

These technical hypotheses arising from real skewings in one language tell us something about that language, about how it works. Thus anyone especially interested in the Italian language might find something of use here. But the shape that these hypotheses have taken—with reference to such universals as the configuration of the human vocal tract, the transmission of sound, communication as a biological phenomenon, and the species-specific and species-general character of intelligent human behavior—the shape of these hypotheses promises no small applicability to other languages and to language in general" (Davis 1984/1987: 89). In the spirit of the above, in the following chapter analyses of the nonrandom distribution of the phonemes of constriction forming the triconsonantal (CCC) root system, the lexical base of the Hebrew language, as well as initial consonant clusters in monosyllables in Hebrew and Yiddish will be presented.[18]

4 The Hebrew and Yiddish Connections

Theory dictates which observations, of the infinite observations that *could* be made, *should* be made. Without theory there would be no indication of what to observe and how to interpret it once observed.
—J. J. Ohala and J. J. Jaeger (1986b: 3)

There is some danger of over-analyzing the data and of regarding the phonological factors as some sort of inviolable laws. Different languages have different rankings of phonemic frequencies, and until thorough analysis has been done of several unrelated languages the degree to which the factors proposed in this study are restricted to Italian, rather than applicable generally, cannot be known. Data from other languages will also be helpful in determining which factor predominates when two or more conflict for a phoneme. —Joseph Clair Davis Jr. (1984/1987: 54)

It is interesting to observe that in the Semitic languages, in the consonantal structure of the root, there is a widespread avoidance of the same item occurring both at the beginning and at the end of the root, another instance of an extreme case where elsewhere we see only a trend.
—William Diver (1979: 178)

Theoretical and Methodological Background

In this chapter, I will present quantitative analyses of the phonotactic distribution of the Hebrew triconsonantal (CCC) root system (adapted from Tobin 1990a, 1990b) and of initial consonant clusters in monosyllabic words in Hebrew (adapted from Miron 1990) and Yiddish (adapted from Bernholtz-Priner 1993). These analyses were inspired by the epigraphs to this chapter, taken from Diver's and Davis's analyses of English and Italian discussed in the previous chapters. This study may also be compared and contrasted to other quantitative approaches to sign-oriented linguistics and phonology (e.g., Herdan 1966; Shannon and Weaver 1949), phonometrics (Zwirner and Zwirner 1970), phonometric-based phonotactics (Bluhme 1964), and language synergetics (Altmann 1978; Altmann and Lehfeldt 1980) as well as other phonological theories such as those discussed in Tobin (1988a, 1988b, 1988c, 1988d).

The Triconsonantal (CCC) Root System

The Data

I will present here a partial analysis of the combinatory phonology of the triconsonantal (CCC) root system of a generalized (panchronic) view of Hebrew, leaving a more complete analysis of different periods and dialects of Hebrew for future research. My analysis entails the application of general phonological principles that were previously postulated and examined for all the monosyllabic words and stems found in English and Italian dictionaries, respectively, to the more abstract prelexical notion of the triconsonantal (CCC) root system of Hebrew. In other words, the data presented here represent abstract linguistic signs prior to the lexicalization process of word formation.

This difference in the unit of analysis has certain theoretical and methodological implications. Much of the research on English and Italian focused on word/stem-initial and word/stem-final consonants. Therefore, these consonants were being examined at the beginnings and ends of clearly defined and relatively well-segmented independent or bound units. This is not the case with the Hebrew triconsonantal (CCC) root system. Hebrew roots do not appear *as* words or stems but rather *in* words or stems.

Unlike words and stems, however, these roots are not clearly defined, well-segmented, continuous independent or bound units. The first and third consonants of a triconsonantal (CCC) root do not necessarily appear in word/stem-initial and word/stem-final positions. Not all triconsonantal (CCC) roots are transparent, nor are they always easily segmented within words. Thus, the successful application of phonological principles previously applied to the more concrete unit of monosyllabic words and stems to this more abstract, prelexicalized level of discontinuous triconsonantal (CCC) roots should provide a strong confirmation of their theoretical and methodological validity.

My database consists of all the (2,773) triconsonantal (CCC) roots appearing in a recent edition of a Condensed Hebrew Dictionary (Even Shoshan 1988), a standard dictionary used in Israel today. This particular dictionary was chosen because it lists the roots and indicates the historical period (biblical, talmudic, mishnaic, medieval, modern, or contemporary) of entries and also includes the entire range of spoken and written registers.

The use of a dictionary as a database forces one to rely on a standard Hebrew orthography, which, like most alphabets (or syllabaries), represents a fairly accurate phonemic analysis of the sounds (or consonants) of the language spoken when the writing system was developed. Such a standardized orthography may best represent a general or panchronic view of the sound system of a language.

The choice of all the triconsonantal (CCC) roots found in the lexicon is motivated by the principle of "the least possible evil." It provides a reasonable representation of the various diachronic and synchronic stages of both spoken and written Hebrew and represents as broad a database as possible to yield significant statistical generalizations about Hebrew.[1]

Active Articulators, Stricture, and Airflow

Research in phonology as human behavior has found the traditional and neotraditional consonantal categories (e.g., place of articulation, manner of articulation, voicing) previously used in studies of the patterning of root phonemes in Semitic and Hebrew root systems from both structural and generative approaches (e.g., Greenberg 1950; Herdan 1962; Morgenbrod and Serifi 1981; Weissman-Gordon 1978) to be wanting for the following reasons.

1. Place of articulation often merely labels a passive receptor (e.g., dental, alveolar, palatal or posteroalveolar, velar, etc.) rather than an active articulator (e.g., lips, apex, anterodorsum, posterodorsum, etc.).

2. Manner of articulation often includes specific place information, together with labels indicating different degrees of stricture and airflow (e.g., oral vs. nasal stops, central vs. lateral [alveolar] fricatives and/or approximants), and also includes place-oriented and/or articulator-oriented phonation processes (e.g., labialization, dentalization, palatalization, velarization, nasalization, glottalization, etc.).

3. These and other manner categories (e.g., consonants vs. vowels, semivowels, liquids, glides, approximants, and/or obstruents vs. resonants, etc.) often depend on

Table 4.1 The Hebrew Consonant System: Active Articulators

Lips	/p, b, m/
Apex	/t-T, d, n, t͜s, r, s, z, l/
Anterodorsum	/ʃ, j/
Posterodorsum	/k, g/
(Lips/velum +) posterodorsum	/w, q/
Pharynx	/ħ, ʕ/
Glottis	/ʔ, h/

the concept of voicing and are all directly or indirectly related to different degrees of stricture and airflow.

4. Voicing also spans the opposition of place and manner and is related to both specific articulators (the larynx, glottis, vocal folds) and different degrees of the control of airflow (fortis vs. lenis).

Therefore, these imprecise traditional categories have been replaced by such alternative concepts as active articulators versus passive receptors, scales of relative degrees of stricture and airflow, and the number of sets of articulators being utilized, which support the communication and human factors inherent to this approach.[2]

The Analysis

The Hebrew Consonant System: The Active Articulators

I first examined the Hebrew consonant system according to the concept of active articulators. The six active articulators that can be postulated for Hebrew are the lips, the tongue (divided into three parts: apex, anterodorsum, posterodorsum), the pharynx, and the glottis. The distribution of the Hebrew consonants with regard to active articulators is found in table 4.1.

The first basic tenet of phonology as human behavior is that speakers of a language are learning how to control the musculature of different articulators in order systematically to produce distinctive sounds composed of relative degrees and patterns of stricture and airflow and thereby to communicate.

The Disfavoring of Additional Articulators

The second basic tenet of phonology as human behavior is that there should also be a direct connection between the relative difficulty involved in learning how to control the musculature of the various articulators needed to produce distinctive sounds and the nonrandom distribution of those sounds within the language. If, for example, we examine what are traditionally called the voiceless-voiced-nasal triads of the Hebrew labials /p-b-m/ and apicals /t-d-n/ according to the number of active articulators that speakers must learn to control, we find that they form the following tridimensional hierarchy:

1. voiceless (0) = active (oral) articulators only;
2. laryngeal (+1) (L) = active (oral) articulator(s) + vocal folds; and
3. nasal or velar (+2) (V) = active (oral) articulator(s) + vocal folds + uvula.

An examination of the twenty-two phonemes of constriction in Hebrew with the number of sets of active articulators that speakers must learn to control reveals the following distribution: 0 (/p, t-T, t͜s, s, ʃ, k, q, ħ, ʔ, h/) = 11; +1 (L) (/b, d, r, l, z, j, g, w, ʕ/) = 9; and +2 (V) (/m, n/) = 2.

The largest number of phonemes of constriction in Hebrew (11) entails the fewest active articulators needed to be controlled (0); closely followed (9) by those phonemes of constriction where only one additional set of active articulators needs to be controlled (+1); followed by a sharp drop (2) for those phonemes of constriction where a second additional set of active articulators needs to be controlled (+2). There is a direct connection between the Hebrew consonant system and this tridimensional hierarchy clearly indicating a consistent disfavoring of those phonemes of constriction for which speakers have to learn to control additional sets of active articulators. Therefore, the Hebrew triconsonantal (CCC) root system reflects the well-known synergetic principle of linguistic economy: the need for communicative efficiency (a maximum number of distinctive communicative oppositions) maintained with a minimum of effort.[3]

The Disfavoring of Additional Articulators in Adjacent Phonetic Environments

This disfavoring of additional articulators not only may be observed within the phonemic system but also may have wider implications for the combinatory phonology or phonotactics of a language. It has been shown, for example, that there is a general and significant disfavoring of the use of additional articulators in adjacent phonetic environments. The specific adjacent phonetic environments examined include consonants composing word-initial consonant clusters in English monosyllables; word-initial consonant clusters and word-final consonants and consonant clusters in English monosyllables; and word/stem-initial and word/stem-final consonants in English and Italian monosyllables.

An examination of the first and third consonants of the Hebrew triconsonantal (CCC) root system according to the tridimensional hierarchy of the number of active articulators reveals the following distribution:

	0		L (+1)		V (+2)	
	N	%	*N*	%	*N*	%
I	1,537	55.4	917	33.1	319	11.5
III	1,284	46.3	1,084	39.1	405	14.6

1. Approximately half of all the initial and final root consonants involve only one set of active articulators (0).
2. Approximately one-third to 40 percent of all the initial and final root consonants involve one additional set of active articulators (+1).
3. Approximately 10–15 percent of all the initial and final root consonants involve the use of a further additional set of active articulators (+2).

This disfavoring of additional articulators in the Hebrew C-I and C-III positions both reflects the distribution of the Hebrew consonants within the phonemic system and supports the previous research done for English and Italian.

The Hebrew Consonant System: Stricture and Airflow

Before I could further examine the skewed phonotactic distribution of the Hebrew consonants within the triconsonantal (CCC) root system, I had to look at the other important features of consonants: scales of relative degrees of stricture and airflow. Three degrees of airflow and five degrees of stricture have been postulated for both the phonemes of constriction (consonants) and the phonemes of aperture (vowels) of Italian. However, since we are dealing here exclusively with phonemes of constriction, I will need to present only two degrees of each.

The Hebrew phonemes of constriction can be classified in the following way, on the basis of a hierarchical scale (0–2) of stricture and airflow:

1. complete stricture (0) and complete obstruction of the airflow (0): /p, t-T, k, ʔ, q, b, d, g/;
2. complete stricture (0) and partial (nonturbulent) obstruction of the airflow (2): /m, n/;
3. incomplete stricture (1) and (turbulent) airflow (1): /(f-v), s, ʃ, (x) h, ħ, z, ʕ/;
4. transitory (complete-incomplete) stricture (0-1) and (obstruction-turbulent) airflow (0-1): /t͜s/;
5. incomplete stricture (2) and (nonturbulent) airflow (2): /l, j, w/; and
6. an intermediate degree of stricture (1/2) and (turbulent) airflow (1/2): /r/.

There is an integral connection between the active articulators and the relative scale of stricture and airflow. Both sets of features must be taken into account when studying the combinatory phonology of the Hebrew triconsonantal (CCC) root system.

The Disfavoring of Additional Articulators in Adjacent Phonetic Environments for Different Articulators

I first observed the general disfavoring of additional sets of active articulators for what traditionally has been referred to as voiceless-voiced-nasal oppositions. I then examined whether a similar disfavoring can also be found for what is usually referred to as voiced versus voiceless obstruents. A comparison of those phonemes of constriction sharing the same active articulators and the same degrees of stricture and airflow, but differing (0, +1) within the tridimensional hierarchy, is found in table 4.2.

These data indicate a further across-the-board disfavoring of additional articulators (0, +1) (voicing) in the phonetic environment of C-I and C-III

Table 4.2 The Disfavoring of Additional Articulators in Adjacent Phonetic Environments

	First Position: C-I									
	Lip		Apex				P-Dorsum		Pharynx	
			T	77			q	139		
(0)	p	166	t	144	s	144	k	110	ħ	175
Total				221				249		
(+1)	b	127	d	103	z	77	g	121	ʕ	159
Difference		(−39)		(−118)		(−67)		(−128)		(−16)
	Third Position: C-III									
			T	99			q	148		
(0)	p	141	t	73	s	105	k	81	ħ	126
Total				172				229		

positions for phonemes of constriction sharing the same active articulators and the same degree of stricture (0-0 mobile stops) (1-1 stable fricatives), for the following active articulators:

lips	/p-b/	(I-39), (III-4)
apex	/t+T-d/	(I-118), (III-103)
	/s-z/	(I-67), (III-44)
p-dorsum	/k+q-g/	(I-128), (III-162)
pharynx	/ħ-ʕ/	(I-16), (III-7)

This further disfavoring of additional articulators within adjacent phonetic environments supports the previous research done for English and Italian. It must be mentioned, however, that these data are particularly vulnerable to the methodological problems previously discussed.[4]

Table 4.3 The Favoring of Phonemes with Complete Constriction in Root-Initial and Root-Final Positions

Stricture		Number of Roots	%
First Position: C-I			
0	/p, t-T, k, q, b, d, g, ʔ, m, n/	1,477	53.3
0–1	/t͜s/	95	3.4
1/2	/r/	146	5.3
1	/s, z, ʃ, ħ, ʕ, h/	871	31.4
2	/l, j, w/	184	6.6
		2,773	100
Third Position: C-III			
0	/p, t-T, k, q, b, d, g, ʔ, m, n/	1,358	49
0–1	/t͜s/	91	3.3
1/2	/r/	320	11.5
1	/s, z, ʃ, ħ, ʕ, h/	768	27.7
2	/l, j, w/	236	8.5
		2,773	100

The Favoring of Phonemes with Complete Stricture in Root-Initial and Root-Final Positions

An examination of the distribution of root-initial and root-final phonemes of constriction with regard to degree of stricture (0-2) reveals a clear favoring of phonemes with complete stricture (0) both in C-I and C-III positions, as seen in table 4.3. The data in table 4.3 indicate the following:

1. Approximately half of all the root-initial and root-final phonemes of constriction are those with complete stricture (0).

2. Approximately 30 percent of all the root-initial and root-final phonemes of constriction are those with incomplete stricture of the first degree (1).

3. Approximately 15–20 percent of all the root-initial and root-final phonemes of constriction are those with varying degrees of stricture (0-1, 1/2, 2).

It must be noted again, however, that these data are open to the methodological problems previously mentioned.

The Favoring of Stricture over Active Articulators in Root-Initial and Root-Final Positions

This favoring of complete stricture may be shown to be even stronger than that of the number of active articulators, particularly if we take the following theoretical and methodological issues into account: the problem of the historical occlusive-spirant allophonic alternations, [p-f, b-v, k-x], etc. (see chap. 3, nn. 1, 4, and chap. 5, n. 12) and the fact that we are dealing here with roots, not words.

The crux of the problem is, of course, that we cannot always predict which degree of stricture these C-I and C-III phonemes will have when they occur in words. There is, however, one class of Hebrew consonants with consistent complete stricture regardless of phonetic environment: the nasal consonants. The nasal consonants also involve the control of two sets of additional articulators and are therefore generally disfavored—despite their naturalness (discussed in chap. 2, n. 9). Indeed, I have already demonstrated this general disfavoring in the phonemic system and in the phonotactic distribution of all phonemes of constriction in C-I and C-III positions.

To test the relative strengths of the number of active articulators and complete stricture, I examined the distribution of the voiceless-voiced-nasal labial and apical triads (/p-b-m/, /t-d-n/) in C-I and C-III positions and found:

	C-I		C-III	
	Lip	Apex	Lip	Apex
0	p-166	t+T-221	p-141	t+T-172
(L) +1	b-127	d-103	b-137	d-144
(V) +2	m-152	n-167	m-177	n-228

1. The nasal consonants (+2) with consistent complete stricture are favored over the voiced consonants (+1) with variable stricture in both root-initial and root-final positions.

2. The nasal consonants (+2) are the most favored in the voiceless (0), voiced (+1), nasal (+2) triad in root-final position (where there may be a general tendency for root-final consonants to appear in their spirantized form with incomplete stricture).

C-I	C-III
most favored 0 -387 (p, t+T)	V (+2)-405 (m, n)
less favored V (+2) -319 (m, n)	0-313 (p, t+T)
least favored L (+1) -230 (b, d)	L (+1)-281 (b, d)

This preference for complete stricture is also found in the consistent favoring of apical stops (t + T-d) over apical fricatives (s-z) in C-I and C-III positions:

	C-I	C-III
0 Stricture	t-1 - 221	t-1 - 172
	d - 103	d - 144
	—	—
	324	316
1 Stricture	s - 144	s - 105
	z - 77	z - 61
	—	—
	221	166

This stronger preference for complete stricture in C-I and C-III positions is worthy of further study in relation to the diachronic development of the synergetic connection between the human and the communication factors.

The Disfavoring of the Same Articulators in Adjacent Phonetic Environments

Previous research also has shown that there is a significant avoidance of phonemes of constriction made by the same active articulators in word/stem-initial and word/stem-final positions for English and Italian

Table 4.4 The Disfavoring of the Same Articulators in Adjacent Phonetic Environments

Articulator	Phoneme	C-I	C-II	C-III
Lip	p	166	3	17
	b	127	2	9
	m	152	5	7
Apex	t	144	25	78
	T	77	43	35
	d	103	23	36
	n	167	52	72
	r	146	41	55
	l	82	11	39
	t͡s	95	34	26
	s	144	57	54
	z	77	25	31
A-Dorsum	ʃ	265	7	5
	j	92	7	6
P-Dorsum	k	110	1	2
	g	121	0	3
Lip + P-Dorsum	q	139	11	2
	w	10	0	1
Pharynx	ħ	175	0	1
	ʕ	159	1	4
Glottis	ʔ	171	5	14
	h	51	0	10
		2,773	353	507
% of C = C-I		100	12	18

monosyllables. An examination of the Hebrew triconsonantal (CCC) root system reveals a similar avoidance of the use of the same active articulators in all root positions. The distribution of consonants according to active articulators in the triconsonantal (CCC) root system indicating a disfavoring of the same articulators in adjacent phonetic environments is found in table 4.4.

The disfavoring of the same articulators in adjacent phonetic environments in the Hebrew triconsonantal (CCC) root system may be summarized in the following way: First, the use of the same active articulators is consistently disfavored in both C-1 + C-II and C-I + C-III positions, with a stronger disfavoring for the more adjacent C-I + C-II position. The number of phonemes of constriction made by the same articulators in the triconsonantal (CCC) root C-I + C-II positions is 353 (12 percent), as opposed to 507 (18 percent) C-I + C-III of 2,773 C-1 phonemes of constriction.[5] Second, I already have shown a consistent disfavoring in the use of additional sets of articulators for phonemes of constriction in the triconsonantal (CCC) root system according to the tridimensional hierarchy of voiceless (0), voicing (+1), nasals (+2) in general. This disfavoring also exists in those phonemes of constriction made by the same set of articulators within the triconsonantal (CCC) root system:

		C-I		C-II		C-III	
		N	%	*N*	%	*N*	%
(0)	(voiceless)	1,537	55.4	186	53	244	48
(+1)	(voiced)	917	33.1	110	31	184	36
(+2)	(nasal)	319	11.5	57	16	79	16
		2,773	100	353	100	507	100

These consistent favorings and disfavorings throughout the triconsonantal (CCC) root system may be attributed to the great difficulty of learning to control the same set of articulators in close proximity. The more difficult it is to control the musculature within limited and restricted space and time, the less frequent the use of the same set of active articulators, the more proximate the environment, the greater the disfavoring. These data support the previous research done for English and Italian.

The Disfavoring of the Same Phoneme in Adjacent Phonetic Environments

Previous research has shown that this disfavoring of the use of the same set of active articulators in adjacent phonetic environments is even greater in its most extreme case: the specific avoidance of the same phoneme in adjacent phonetic environments. An examination of the Hebrew triconsonantal (CCC) root system for the repetition of the same phoneme in adjacent phonetic environments is found in table 4.5. The distribution revealed by table 4.5 can be summarized as follows:

1. This general disfavoring of the same sets of active articulators is even greater in its most extreme case: the specific avoidance of the same phoneme in all triconsonantal (CCC) positions.

2. The nine repeated phonemes in both C-I and C-II positions appear eleven times (0.4 percent of C-I 2,773, 3 percent of C-II 353). The eighteen repeated phonemes in C-I = C-III positions appear fifty-seven times (2 percent of C-I 2,773, 11 percent of C-III 507). This disfavoring is not as strong in C-II and C-III positions, where there are 147 examples of nineteen repeated phonemes (5 percent of C-I 2,773, 29 percent of C-III 507).

3. The disfavoring of additional sets of active articulators in the tridimensional hierarchy holds for the same phonemes in C-I = C-III positions and for almost all the voiced-voiceless oppositions as well.[6]

4. Of the fifty-seven instances of repeated phonemes in C-I and C-III positions, thirty-seven (65 percent) are (0) voiceless, eleven (19 percent) are (+1) voiced, and nine (16 percent) are (+2) nasals.

5. This disfavoring of additional sets of active articulators does not hold for the same phonemes in C-II medial positions in general but basically holds for the voiced-voiceless oppositions.

6. Of the eleven instances of repeated phonemes in C-I and C-II positions, four (36.4 percent) are both (0) voiceless and (+1) voiced, and three (27.2 percent) are nasals; the voiced-voiceless opposition holds only for the /k-g/ pair.

7. Of the 147 repeated phonemes in C-II and C-III positions, there are sixty-two (42.2 percent) (0) voiceless, sixty-three (42.9 percent) (+1) voiced, and twenty-two (14.9 percent) nasals; the voiced-voiceless opposition is almost complete.[7]

	C-I = C-III		C-I = C-II		C-II = C-III	
	N	%	*N*	%	*N*	%
(0)	37	65	4	36.4	62	42.2
(+1)	11	19	4	36.4	63	42.9
(+2)	9	16	3	27.2	22	14.9
	57	100	11	100	147	100

Table 4.5 The Disfavoring of the Same Phoneme in Adjacent Phonetic Environments

Articulator	Phoneme	C-I = C-II	C-I = C-III	C-II = C-III
Lip	p	1	3	9
	b	1	1	14
	m	2	3	10
Apex	t	0	8	10
	T	0	2	5
	d	1	0	12
	n	1	6	12
	r	0	2	11
	l	1	1	14
	t͜s	0	2	5
	s	0	4	7
	z	0	2	6
A-Dorsum	ʃ	2	5	7
	j	0	0	0
P-Dorsum	k	1	2	1
	g	0	1	4
Lip + P-Dorsum	q	0	1	5
	w	0	0	0
Pharynx	ħ	0	0	6
	ʕ	1	4	2
Glottis	ʔ	0	1	0
	h	0	9	7
		11	57	147
% of C-I = C-II / C-III,				
C-II = C-III: C-I (2,773),		0.4	2	5
C-II (353), C-III (507)		3	11	29

Table 4.6 The Favoring of the Apex in the Phonemic Inventory of Hebrew

Articulator	Number of Consonants	%
Lip	3	14
Apex	9	41
A-Dorsum	2	9
P-Dorsum	4	18
Pharynx	2	9
Glottis	2	9
	22	100

The same reason accounts for the observed disfavoring of the repetition of the same phoneme (most consistently in C-I and C-III positions). If it is difficult to control the same active articulators in adjacent environments, it is even more difficult to do so in the extreme case of repeating the very same phoneme. These data also support the previous research done for English and Italian.

The Favoring of Apical Consonants

A skewing of the number of phonemes of constriction produced by each of the different active articulators may also be observed. Indeed, both the previously cited research and a cursory glance at the International Phonetic Alphabet and other phonetic charts show a strong favoring for those phonemes of constriction produced by the apex. An examination of the consonant system of Hebrew reveals that the apex controls 40 percent or more than twice to four times as many phonemes of constriction as any other active articulator, as seen in table 4.6.

An examination of the relation among the active articulators, the number of phonemes per articulator, and the number and percentage of triconsonantal (CCC) roots per articulator in C-I position is found in table 4.7. The data for C-I position indicate that phonemes of constriction produced by the apex are favored and account for over 37 percent of the roots, followed by the lips (16 percent), the posterodorsum (14 percent), the anterodorsum (13 percent), the pharynx (12 percent), and the glottis (8 percent).

An examination of the relation among the active articulators, the number of phonemes per articulator, and the number and percentage of triconsonantal (CCC) roots made by the same articulator in C-II position is found in table 4.8. The data for C-II position indicate that phonemes of constriction produced by the apex are even more clearly favored and account for 88 percent of the roots, followed by the anterodorsum (4 percent), the lips and the posterodorsum (3 percent), the glottis (1.4 percent), and the pharynx (0.3 percent).

An examination of the relation among the active articulators, the number

Table 4.7 The Favoring of the Apex in C-I Position

Articulator	Phonemes	Roots	%
Lip	3	445	16.1
Apex	9	1,035	37.3
A-Dorsum	3	357	12.9
P-Dorsum	2	231	8.3
(L + V) + P-Dorsum	2	149	5.4
Pharynx	2	334	12
Glottis	2	222	8
	22	2,773	100

Table 4.8 The Favoring of the Apex in C-II Position

Articulator	Phonemes	Roots	%
Lip	3	10	3
Apex	9	311	88
A-Dorsum	3	14	4
P-Dorsum	2	1	0.3
(L + V) + P-Dorsum	2	11	3
Pharynx	2	1	0.3
Glottis	2	5	1.4
	22	353	100

Table 4.9 The Favoring of the Apex in C-III Position

Articulator	Phonemes	Roots	%
Lip	3	33	6.5
Apex	9	426	84
A-Dorsum	3	11	2.2
P-Dorsum	2	5	1
(L + V) + P-Dorsum	2	3	0.6
Pharynx	2	5	1
Glottis	2	24	4.7
	22	507	100

of phonemes per articulator, and the number and percentage of triconsonantal (CCC) roots made by the same articulator in C-III position is found in table 4.9. The data for C-III position indicate that phonemes of constriction produced by the apex are also more clearly favored and account for 84 percent of the roots, followed by the lips (6.5 percent), the glottis (4.7 percent), the anterodorsum (2.2 percent), the posterodorsum (1.6 percent), and the pharynx (1 percent).

These data indicate that the apex—the most adroit and easily controlled of the active articulators—is the most highly favored articulator. In other words, that articulator that is the easiest one to learn to control is the one that is the most exploited by speakers of the language.

The Favoring of Labial Consonants in Root-Initial Positions

An examination of the distribution of the repeated phonemes in the triconsonantal (CCC) root system reveals, not unsurprisingly, a similar favoring of apical phonemes of constriction. There was, however, a slight favoring of the labial phonemes of constriction in initial/medial C-I = C-II position, which is found in table 4.10.

This preference for labials in the first two root positions is similar to the favoring of visible phonemes found for word/stem-initial position for both English and Italian monosyllables. Labials, unlike children, should be seen *and* heard. Therefore, a tendency for the favoring of visible phonemes in initial positions—precisely where the largest number of clues are neces-

Table 4.10 The Favoring of Visible Phonemes in C-I = C-II Position

	I = II		I = III		II = III	
	Roots	%	Roots	%	Roots	%
Lip	4	36.4	7	12.3	33	22.4
Apex	3	27.2	27	47.4	82	55.8
A-Dorsum	2	18.2	5	8.8	7	4.8
P-Dorsum	1	9.1	4	7	10	6.8
Pharynx	1	9.1	4	7	8	5.4
Glottis	0		10	17.5	7	4.8
	11	100	57	100	147	100

sary for effective communication—should not be too surprising when we take the synergetic connection between the communication and the human factors into account. Indeed, a comparison of the labial stops with their simple apical and posterodorsal counterparts reveals a similar favoring for more clearly visible sounds in C-I position: lip: p-166, b-127; apex: t-144, d-103; and p-dorsum: k-110, g-121. This visibility factor in root-initial and root-medial position is, of course, susceptible to various diachronic and methodological considerations as well.[8]

Consonant Clusters in Hebrew

The Data

Miron (1990) collected initial consonant clusters found in monosyllabic words in Hebrew of the $C_1C_2VC_3$ type.[9] The specific clusters selected for study were those containing stable versus mobile consonants in C_1 and /l/ or /r/ in C_2 positions—the same phonetic environment examined by Diver (1979) and Davis (1984/1987).[10] The data were culled from two standard and popular dictionaries (Even Shoshan 1978; Alcalay 1990).

The number of initial consonant clusters in monosyllabic words with the general structure $C_1C_2VC_3$ was 249. The phonemes in the study include /p, b, t-T, d, k-q, s, ʃ/, which distribute in the following way:

p	b	t	– T	d	k	– q	g	s	ʃ	total
35	25	26	8	14	37	17	25	27	35	249

The number of consonant clusters of the $C_1C_2VC_3$ variety, where C_2 = /l/ or /r/, is seventy-eight, the distribution of which appears in table 4.11.

The Analysis

Stable versus Mobile—Likes Are Favored, Differents Disfavored

If we examine the data in table 4.11, we see that the mobile phonemes of constriction (p, b, d, k-q, g) as well as the mobile + emphatic apical phoneme (T) favor the mobile /r/ and that the stable phoneme /ʃ/ favors the stable /l/. As Davis (1984/1987: 67) stated the basic principle: "M. Mobile-plus-stable and stable-plus-mobile clusters are more disfavored than clusters of like mobility or stability."

The data in table 4.11 reveal that there are fifty words of like mobility and stability (M + M, S + S) and that there are twenty-eight words of unlike mobility and stability (S + M, M + S), for a total of seventy-eight. Two phonemes, however, appear to be exceptions: the mobile phoneme /t/ appears to prefer stable /l/; and the stable phoneme /s/ is equally divided between stable /l/ and mobile /r/. These apparent exceptions will be discussed later.

Table 4.11 Frequency Distributions for Occurrences of *l* and *r* in Initial Clusters in Hebrew

	p	b	t	- T	d	k	- q	g	s	ʃ	Totals	Cross-Totals
l	3	2	5	0	1	5	2	4			22	28
r	6	6	2	3	3	7	5	10			42	50
l									4	4	8	
r									4	2	6	

Additional Articulators Are Disfavored

The data in table 4.11 confirm the principle that additional articulators are disfavored in several ways (cf. nn. 1, 3, 8, this chapter):

1. The number of clusters with C_1 exploiting one set of oral articulators (0) (voiceless) is greater than the number of clusters where C_1 employs both oral articulators and the larynx (+ 1) (L) (voiced).

2. There are twenty-six voiced clusters and fifty-two voiceless-voiced clusters, for a total of seventy-eight.

3. In the larger corpus of all initial consonant clusters, voiceless clusters consistently outnumber voiced clusters:

/p/	35	/b/	25
/t/	26	/d/	14
/k/	37	/g/	25

4. In the larger corpus of all initial consonant clusters, there are only sixteen (of a total of 249) where C_2 employs oral and laryngeal articulators and the uvula (+ 2) (V) (nasal).

5. /q/, a phoneme of constriction that employs two sets of active oral articulators (lips + posterodorsum), appears less frequently in initial consonant clusters than /k/, a phoneme of constriction employing one oral articulator (posterodorsum) with which it is in a simple pairwise opposition.

6. There are seven /qr-, ql-/ clusters and twelve /kr-, kl-/ clusters.

7. In the larger corpus of all initial consonant clusters, there are only seventeen instances of /q/ and thirty-seven instances of /k/ in C_1 position.

8. /T/, a voiceless emphatic phoneme of constriction—the articulation of which entails pushing the tongue further back (i.e., raising the back of the tongue demanding more control over the tongue accompanied by pharyngeal constriction resulting in increased tension in the organs)—appears less frequently in initial consonant clusters than its opposed nonemphatic phoneme of constriction /t/.

9. There are three /Tr- Tl-/ clusters and seven /tr-, tl-/ clusters.

10. In the larger corpus of all initial consonant clusters, there are only eight instances of /T/ and twenty-six instances of /t/ in C_1 position.

11. The more complex the phoneme, the more articulators there are to employ, the more difficult it is to control, and the less frequently it will appear, as can be

seen in the following ascending hierarchy of difficulty taken from the larger corpus (cf. point 3 above): voiceless, voiced, additional oral articulators/emphatic:

/t/	26	/d/	14	/T/	8
/k/	37	/g/	25	/q/	17

The Disfavoring of the Same Articulators in Adjacent Phonetic Environments

As Diver (1979: 173) has stated: "The strongest disfavorings, the [*tl, dl*] zeros, occur where it is exactly the same musculature that has to be brought under control." Although neither the Italian nor the Hebrew data reached the same extreme in the strongest (zero) disfavorings of the same musculature that the English data did, the principle is still maintained: in the disfavored, different, or unlike (S+M, M+S) clusters, there were eighteen examples where the articulators were different (lip + apex, antero/posterodorsum + apex); and there were only ten examples where the same articulators (apex + apex) were involved.

The Disfavoring of the Same Phoneme in Adjacent Phonetic Environments

Diver (1979: 176–77) has also noted a strong disfavoring when the same articulators are being reused in word-final position after appearing in an initial cluster. This disfavoring is even stronger when the same phoneme is repeated. These principles are confirmed by the data found in the larger corpus composed of initial consonant clusters of the $C_1C_2VC_3$ variety of Hebrew monosyllables: there are 183 instances where C_1, C_2, and C_3 are made by different active articulators; there are fifty-one instances where C_3 is made by the same active articulators as either C_1 or C_2, but not the same phoneme; and there are only fifteen instances where C_3 repeats the same phoneme as either C_1 or C_2.

/sl-, sr-/ Clusters

As previously stated, the stable phoneme /s/ is equally divided between stable /l/ and mobile /r/, with four instances of each. This includes examples from the two different historical phonemes represented as different letters in the alphabet Hebrew from which the modern phoneme is derived:

samekh (ס) and *sin* (שׂ). The latter, with its historical-orthographic partner *shin* (שׁ), has long been known as a subject of linguistic awareness and is designated in the Bible (Judg. 12:4–6) as a way in which the Gileadites distinguished the fleeing Ephraimites, who could not pronounce the *sh* in the word *shibboleth.*

It is very possible that there are various diachronic reasons for the seemingly random distribution of /s/ with stable /l/ and mobile /r/. The collocation of stable apical or anterodorsal /s/ with mobile /r/ may also be related to the pronunciation of a more distant posterodorsal stable ɤ (most common today and attested to in earlier periods as well), which might support the stability and mobility factor. Differences in stricture and airflow may also be a factor particularly since both phonemes of constriction were believed to have originated as apicals. However, the number of examples of /sl-, sr-/ clusters is so small that far-reaching conclusions probably cannot be drawn from the data at hand.

Miron also chose to examine the lexical accessibility and the frequency of the eight words in question (two of which are Aramaic in origin) by presenting them to six university-educated, native speakers between the ages of twenty-five and thirty-five (four male, two female). The subjects were asked to rate each lexical item as known/unknown and frequent/infrequent. The following results were obtained: Two words from each cluster were rated as known/infrequent: (*a*) *slik,* "end, conclusion," "arms cache" (Alcalay 1975: 1779) (only the second dictionary entry was recognized by the speakers); *slav,* "quail" (bird) (Alcalay 1975: 2634); (*b*) *srak* (Aramaic), "emptiness, barrenness" (Alcalay 1975: 1825); *srad,* "service" (as in an official uniform, apartment) (Alcalay 1975: 2717). One word from each cluster was rated as known/frequent: (*a*) *slil,* "coil, bobbin, spool, reel; groove screw; trochlea (med.)" (followed by thirty-two subentries) (Alcalay 1975: 1778–79); (*b*) *srox,* "lace" (shoe) (Alcalay 1975: 2718). One word from each cluster was rated as unknown: (*a*) *slek* (not found in Alcalay [1975]); (*b*) *srik* (Aramaic), "empty idler, vagabond" (Alcalay 1975: 1823). It should also be noted that, if the principle that likes are favored and differents disfavored is not necessarily working here for these clusters (which also may have blocked the principle), the disfavoring of the same articulators in adjacent phonetic environments (depending on which apical or posterodorsal /ɤ/ is being used; the principle that additional articulators are disfavored is clearly at work here since there are no /zl-, zr-/ clusters in the language.

/tl, t-Tr-/ Clusters

I have previously compared and contrasted the emphatic apical mobile phoneme /T/ with /t/ and /d/ and have stated the following: /T/ conforms to the principle that likes are favored and differents disfavored: there are three /Tr-/ clusters and no /Tl-/ clusters. /T/ also conforms to the principle that additional sets of articulators are disfavored: the more complex emphatic /T/ appears less frequently than its nonemphatic voiceless counterpart /t/ and the voiced /d/ in the larger corpus (/t/ 26, /d/ 14, /T/ 8). I would like to add that, in the general lexicon of the language, the emphatic /T/ is also the least frequent of the three according to the number of dictionary entries assigned to each phoneme.

The question, then, still remains as to why /t/ does not conform to the principle that likes are favored and differents disfavored. Not unsurprisingly, /T/ and /d/—which do support the principle—appear much less frequently in these specific consonant clusters: /t/ 7, /d/ 4, /T/ 3. It may very well be that speakers of the language who are confronted with a triad of apical stops—voiceless/voiceless + emphatic/voiced—exert the most energy in producing the least complex member of the triad the most frequently. This commonsense strategy supporting the human factor may also have further consequences in their strategies of communication.

For example, speakers will avoid the more complex voiced and emphatic members of the triad in word-medial and word-final positions, where the force of communication is lowest: (/t/ > /d/ > /T/). Speakers will also avoid the more complex members of the triad in word-initial position, as evinced by the size of the dictionary entries for each: (/t/ > /d/ > /T/). This is especially true in the even more difficult word-initial position with a consonant cluster in general: the simplest member of the triad that is most easily controlled is the most frequently exploited: (/t/ > /d/ > /T/). This is also true in initial consonant clusters of the type being studied: /tl-, tr-/ > /dl-, dr-/ > /Tr-/. Speakers may compensate in initial consonant clusters by preferring to neutralize the principle that likes are favored and differents disfavored in order to avoid the more difficult articulations inherent in the production of the more difficult members of the triad.

Once again, we can see that the same principles are interacting in similar ways in the initial consonant clusters of Hebrew as they were for Italian and English. Let us now briefly examine the same phenomenon for another language, Yiddish.

Table 4.12 Frequency Distributions for Occurrences of *l* and *r* in Initial Clusters in Yiddish

	p	b	t	d	k	g	f	v	s	z	ʃ	x	t͡s	m	Totals	Cross-Totals
l	21	23	1	1	33	12									92	135
r	12	32	41	24	46	34									189	252
l							32	0	11	0	20	0			63	
r							27	1	2	2	11	1			43	
l													1	0		
r													0	2		

Consonant Clusters in Yiddish

The Data

Bernholtz-Priner (1993) collected all the initial consonant clusters found in monosyllabic words in Yiddish of the $C_1C_2VC_3$ variety, including those containing stable versus mobile consonants in C_1 and /l/ or /r/ in C_2 positions—the same phonetic environment examined by Diver (1979), Davis (1984/1987), and Miron (1990). The data were culled from two dictionaries (Harkave 1988; Levinsky 1972). Bernholtz-Priner (1993) found 1,503 monosyllabic words in Yiddish of which 390 are of the type where C_2 is either /l/ or /r/.

The number of consonant clusters of the $C_1C_2VC_3$ type where C_1 is a simple obstruent and C_2 is either /l/ or /r/ is 387, the distribution of which appears in table 4.12.[11]

The Analysis

Stable versus Mobile—Likes Are Favored, Differents Disfavored

Diver (1979: 171) stated the first basic principle for consonant clusters in the following way: "Returning now to the skewings in terms of stable versus mobile, we can make a single statement that combinations of sames are favored and combinations of differents are disfavored." If we examine the data in table 4.12, we see that the mobile phonemes of constriction (b, t, d, k, g) favor the mobile /r/ and that the stable phonemes /f, v, s, z, ʃ, x/ favor the stable /l/.

The data in table 4.12 further reveal that there are 252 words of like mobility and stability (M + M, S + S) and 135 words of unlike mobility and stability (S + M, M + S), for a total of 387. Two phonemes, however, appear to be exceptions: the mobile phoneme /p/ appears to prefer stable /l/; and the stable phonemes /v/ and /z/ appear to prefer mobile /r/.

It is very hard to find a clear-cut explanation for these exceptional skewings. It should be remembered that Yiddish is a language consisting of a group of closely related High German dialects with a lexicon composed of a mixture of large Hebrew, Slavic, and other elements. It may be that the /pl-/ clusters came from /fl-/ clusters and that the single /vr-/ cluster came from a /br-/ cluster, or, alternatively, there may have been an influence of the occlussive-spirant alternation (*BeGeDKeFeT*) in Hebrew (see nn. 1, 4, 10, this chapter, and also chap. 5 below). The rare /zr-/ cluster is also very limited in number. Furthermore, the posterodorsal stable phoneme /ɣ/ (or a similar "back r") may have influenced the results here as well. Once again, far-reaching conclusions probably cannot be drawn from the data at hand.

Number of Articulators

The second principle postulated by Diver dealt with the moving from one articulator per gesture (both shaping and exciting) to two articulators per gesture. Diver (1979: 175–76) states the following: "Comparison of the favored and disfavored combinations, the sames and differents, in terms of voiced versus voiceless, reveals that the voiced member of the pair drops much further in frequency than does the voiceless." This principle is supported by the English, Italian, Hebrew, and Yiddish data for all voiced-voiceless pairs of explosive mobile consonants in general, following Davis's (1984/1987: 52) principle E: "E. Explosive phonemes are favored in initial position."

For English, Italian, and Hebrew, principle E was also supported by the fact that there were no voiced-voiceless oppositions for the stable clusters. In Yiddish, however, if we look at the respective drops between paired mobile voiced and voiceless clusters representing sames (M + M, S + S) and differents (M + S> S + M), we find that this principle is supported only by the /k/-/g/ opposition:

	r	l	
p	12	21	+9
b	32	23	–9
t	41	1	+40
d	24	1	+23
k	46	33	–13
g	34	12	–22

The problem of the failure of /p/ to support the first principle that likes are favored and dislikes disfavored has already been discussed; this may carry over here, where both /p/ and /b/ are equal. Although the drop for /dr-, dl-/ clusters is smaller than that for /tl-, tr-/ clusters, there are almost twice as many of the latter, which, in itself, supports the disfavoring of additional articulators.

However, in Yiddish, unlike English, Italian, and Hebrew, we find that principle E is slightly less strong and that there are a small number of initial stable consonant clusters carrying the voiced-voiceless opposition: /fl-, fr- vs. vr-/ and /sl-, sr- vs. zr-/:

	l	r	
f	32	27	–5
v	0	1	+1
s	11	2	–9
z	0	2	–2

It is interesting to note, however, that this very small number of voiced stable consonant clusters may represent exceptions to the first principle that likes are favored and differents disfavored as well. All the work with consonant clusters in the theory of phonology as human behavior has shown that all the principles and factors are working for the vast majority of cases, and the small residue of exceptions illustrates how these factors and principles interact with each other in slightly different ways across languages. Different languages may weigh these possibly universal factors in diverse language-specific ways, on the basis of the human factor—human behavior, physiology, cognition, and perception—and the communication factor.

The Disfavoring of the Same Articulators in Adjacent Phonetic Environments

It should first be noted that this principle works in all the languages in slightly different ways. Yiddish—like English and Italian—has the most extreme skewing—(1) rather than zero—for the disfavored /tl-, dl-/ combinations, where the same musculature is being exploited in an adjacent phonetic environment. The situation in Hebrew is more complex because of the additional opposition between the voiceless /t/ and the voiceless-emphatic /T/, phonemes previously discussed. In these cases, the disfavoring of additional articulators appears to outweigh the disfavoring of the same musculature in adjacent phonetic environments. The disfavoring of the same articulators in adjacent phonetic environments, however, holds for the voiced /dl-/ combination in Hebrew.

Davis (1984/1987: 42) referred to this principle as principle Q (after the phoneme /q/-/k^w/), which he stated as follows: "Q. Co-articulation by near articulators is disfavored." Diver (1979: 176) found that the strongest disfavoring for the English data was the reuse of the same articulator: "In the case of *dl* all three disfavorings are at work, but it is to be noted that *tl* drops to zero, with only two disfavorings, not being voiced. This, of course, suggests that the third disfavoring is stronger than the second, since *bl* and *gl,* also with two, do not drop nearly as far. In fact, the reuse of the same articulator—i.e., the same musculature—seems itself to be disfavored, even in instances where the reuse is delayed sufficiently so that considerations of abrupt transition cannot be involved. Examples follow, and it will be seen that here, too, the amount of disfavoring is correlated with the degree of additional disfavoring and the consequent piling up of difficulties."

I will repeat Diver's examples and his explanation of them for the reader's convenience before presenting Bernholtz-Priner's parallel data:

> The first two examples, containing a relatively strong additional disfavoring, show an articulator being reused in word-final [position] after appearing in an ini-

tial cluster (as will be seen in a moment, it is the cluster that constitutes the extra disfavoring).

ClVC	189	*slip*	CNVC	60	*snip*
CCVl	40	*spill*	CCVN	98	*spin*
ClVl	1	*flail*	CNVN	0	*smin*

First with *l* there are 189 of the type *slip,* with *l* in the initial cluster, and 40 words of the type *spill,* with *l* in final position, in the presence of an initial cluster. But there is only one word, *flail,* with *l* in both the initial cluster and final position.

So also with nasals—i.e., with reuse of the musculature that opens and closes the nasal passage. There are 60 words of the type *snip,* with *any* nasal in the initial cluster, and 98 of the type *spin,* with any nasal in final position, but no words of the type *smin,* with any nasal in the initial cluster and any nasal in final position. (Diver 1979: 177)

Applying the same principles to the same kinds of examples, Bernholtz-Priner obtained very similar results:

ClCC	134	(*ʃlep*)	"schlep"	CNVC	134	(*ʃnel*)	"fast"
CCVl	19	(*ʃpil*)	"game"	CCVN	22	(*ʃpan*)	"span/spread"
ClVl	0			CNVN	0		

Her results, as well as similar results obtained for Italian and Hebrew, support the disfavoring of the same musculature in adjacent phonetic environments and the even stronger disfavoring of the repetition of the same phoneme in adjacent phonetic environments.

The Human and the Communication Factors

Diver (1979: 177–80) then examined the distribution of initial and final phonemes of constriction in monosyllabic words in English of the CVC pattern with reference to active articulators and the number of sets of articulators. As we have seen, similar work has been done for monosyllabic stems in Italian and for the triconsonantal (CCC) root system and initial consonant clusters of monosyllabic words in Hebrew. In all cases, similar results have been obtained. These results reveal the synergetic role of the human and communication factors in motivating the phontactic distribution of phonemes in each language. The following basic principles have been established for these languages:

1. In word/stem/root-initial position—where the burden of communication is highest and the speaker has to invest the most energy—there is an almost random distribution of phonemes of constriction, sometimes with a slight favoring of apicals (the Hebrew triconsonantal [CCC] root system), but always with a slightly higher favoring for visible phonemes that are both seen and heard.

2. In word/stem/root-final position—where the burden of communication is lowest and the speaker does not have to invest much energy—there is a clear-cut favoring of phonemes of constriction made by the apex (the most adroit active articulator) and of voiceless phonemes of constriction that require only one set of articulators.

3. The same active articulators or musculature is disfavored in word/stem/root-initial position and in word/stem/root-final position.

Not unsurprisingly, similar results have been obtained for Yiddish in support of these principles. In a corpus of 195 monosyllabic words of the CVC pattern, Bernholtz-Priner uncovered the following distribution: For the slight favoring of visual phonemes in word-initial position versus the strong favoring of apical phonemes in word-final position: word initial: 71 labials, 63 apicals, and 61 dorsals, for a total of 195; word final: 38 labials, 93 apicals, and 64 dorsals, for a total of 195. For the number of articulators, it has been established that in word-final position phonemes of constriction employing only one set of articulators will be favored over phonemes of constriction employing more than one set of articulators, as we see in Yiddish: one articulator (p t k): 391 initial, 506 final; two articulators (b d g): 274 initial, 190 final. For the disfavoring of the same active articulators in adjacent phonetic environments, the calculated and the observed co-occurrences of initial and final stops were compared and contrasted in the following ways (L = labial, A = apical, D = dorsal): 37 L + A, 23 L + D, 16 A + L, 26 A + D, 11 D + L, 35 D + A, 11 L + L, 21 A + A, and 15 D + D, for a total of 195. The calculated values are of course obtained by taking, for example, the proportion of initial labials (71/195) and multiplying that by the proportion of final apicals (93/195), giving the proportion of labial plus apical that could be expected to occur if all initials and finals combined freely with each other: 71/195 (.364) × 93/195 (.476) = .173; .173 × 229 = 39. The comparison of the calculated co-occurrences with the actual numbers is as follows:

	L+A	L+D	A+L	A+D	D+L	D+A	:	L+L	A+A	D+D	total
Calc.	37	23	16	26	11	35		11	21	15	195
Obs.	34	23	12	21	11	30		14	30	20	195
Diff.	+3	0	+4	+5	0	+5		−3	−9	−5	

Bernholtz-Priner's results show a slight departure from those obtained by Diver (see chap. 2). That is, almost all combinations with different articulators increase a little, and all those combinations with the same articulators drop. If this hypothesis were in fact entirely ungrounded, we would expect that in each category there would be a 50-50 chance of departing from the calculated amount either in the direction predicted by the hypothesis or in the opposite direction, just as in a single toss of a coin we have a 50-50 chance for heads and for tails. In the case of Yiddish, this was the case for L + D and D + L, which did not occur in English. But with every other individual category departing in the same direction—that is, in the direction predicted by the hypothesis—we have the equivalent of throwing heads nine times in a row. It would appear that, even in the absence of other disfavorings, there is a significant avoidance of reuse of the same musculature from one end of the word to the other.

Once again, it becomes clear that the principles of phonology as human behavior established by Diver for English, which were later extended and expanded for Italian and Latin by Davis and then reapplied to Hebrew and Yiddish here, all seem to be working together for every language, but in slightly different ways for each language. These same basic principles have also been further supported by the consonant cluster data that are being collected for Indo-European: German (Middle High/Modern), Yiddish, Dutch, Afrikaans, Swedish, Norwegian, Danish, (Germanic); Latin (Vulgar/Classical), French, Spanish, Portuguese, Catalan, Romansch, Sardinian, Romanian, (Romance); Russian, Ukrainian, Polish, Czech, Slovak, Serbo-Croatian, Bulgarian, (Slavic); Greek (Classical/Modern), (Hellenic); Lithuanian, (Baltic); Bukharian (Judaeo-Persian)(Indo-Iranian); Semitic: Hebrew, Arabic (Classical/Moroccan), Aramaic; Finno-Ugric: Finnish, Estonian, Hungarian; Caucasian: Georgian (Grusinski); Esperanto and Klingon for most of the clusters with different degrees of skewings across languages, as mentioned in the postscript to chapter 2.

Summary and Conclusions

In this chapter, I have extended previous research in the combinatory phonology of English, Italian, and Latin to the Hebrew triconsonantal (CCC) root system and to initial consonant clusters in Hebrew and Yiddish. All the research presented above has followed a specific approach to phonology inspired by the definition of language as a system of systems used by human beings to communicate. In short, I have attempted statistically to examine the synergetic connection between the human and the communication factors of language as they are reflected in the combinatory phonology of all the languages under study here.

Throughout this chapter, a direct connection was observed between the effort invested by speakers in learning to control the active articulators involved in the production of phonemes of constriction and the observed favorings and disfavorings of these phonemes of constriction. In particular, I discovered certain general tendencies for the triconsonantal (CCC) root system in Hebrew that showed

1. the disfavoring of additional articulators in the phonemic system of Hebrew in general, in C-I and C-III root positions in particular, and in the phonemic oppositions of individual active articulators;
2. the favoring of phonemes with complete stricture in C-I and C-III root positions as well the relation between stricture and the number of active articulators;
3. the avoidance of the use of the same articulators and the repetition of the same phoneme in all triconsonantal (CCC) root positions; and
4. the general favoring of phonemes of constriction made by the apex in all the above environments with an additional favoring of visible phonemes in C-I and C-I = C-II positions.

I have also shown how these tendencies and others may be applied to describe and explain the nonrandom distribution of phonemes of constriction in initial consonant clusters in Hebrew and Yiddish. Some of these additional principles are the following:

5. stable versus mobile (likes are favored, differents disfavored);
6. additional articulators are disfavored;
7. the same articulators in adjacent phonetic environments are disfavored;
8. the same phoneme in adjacent phonetic environments is disfavored;
9. explosive phonemes are favored in initial position;

10. visible phonemes are favored in initial position;
11. apical phonemes are favored in final position; and
12. additional articulators are disfavored in final position.

I have not claimed to have solved all the problems related to the Hebrew triconsonantal (CCC) root system or to the initial consonant clusters of Hebrew and Yiddish. I have merely presented a preliminary set of basic criteria that may serve as a first step toward a better understanding of some of the most fundamental data related to the combinatory phonology of these languages.

In the present part of this volume, the following specific phonological and phonotactic parameters explicitly derived from the theory of phonology as human behavior have been established:

1. the identification of active articulators (vs. the traditional category of place of articulation, which is often a label for passive receptors) and the relative difficulty of learning how to control them;
2. the identification of relative degrees of stricture and turbulent and nonturbulent airflow (vs. the traditional category of manner of articulation) that require different articulatory control (mobile vs. stable) and produce different acoustic patterns for individual sounds and phonation processes (labialization, apicalization, velarization, nasalization, glottalization);
3. the identification of the number of sets of articulators to be controlled (vs. the traditional categories of voicing, the fortis-lenis distinction, and nasality) that require different articulatory control and produce different acoustic patterns; and
4. the identification of phonemes of constriction and phonemes of aperture (vs. the traditional concepts of consonants and vowels) that require different articulatory control and produce different acoustic patterns.

The quantitative results that have been obtained from the theory when applied to all the languages studied and that will be applied further to clinical and nonclinical settings include the following:

1. additional articulators are disfavored;
2. coarticulation by near articulators is disfavored;
3. coarticulation by the same articulators/phoneme is even more highly disfavored (particularly in the roots of Semitic languages);
4. different word, stem, or root positions have different communicative force and thus affect the favoring and disfavoring of different articulatory and acoustic features and phonemes;

5. visual articulators are favored (particularly in word/stem/root-initial position;

6. explosive (mobile) phonemes are favored in initial position;

7. turbulent (stable) phonemes are favored in final position (Hebrew);

8. transitions from one distinct constriction to another within a single phoneme are disfavored;

9. consonant clusters are restricted as far as different articulatory and acoustic features are concerned (e.g., mobility/stability);

10. among constrictions, maximal constriction is favored, and, among apertures, maximal aperture is favored;

11. sequences of phonemes with the same articulators are disfavored unless their juxtaposition is, by virtue of some other factor, mutually beneficial; and

12. apical consonants are favored.

The basic motto underlying all the research in this volume is that language in general—and phonology in particular—can be seen as a mini-max struggle between the desire to create maximum communication with minimal effort.

In next part of this volume, I will apply the theory of phonology as human behavior to the following nonclinical tasks: addressing the problem of the historical occlusive-spirant alternation (*BeGeDKeFeT*) discussed in this chapter; recommending how phonetics may be taught from the point of view of the interface of the human and communication factors (i.e., phonetics as human behavior); and analyzing a specific poetic text. In the final part of this volume, I will also apply the theory of phonology as human behavior to first language acquisition and to the speech and hearing clinic.

III

Phonology as Human Behavior. *Panchronic, Pedagogical, and Textual Applications*

It must be repeated that the question of what speakers know about the sound patterns in their language, how they represent them, and how they use them, cannot be determined by purely armchair speculations however plausible they may sound. Evidence based on the behavior of speakers solving the real phonological problems they encounter is necessary. The essence of science is, first, the recognition that our beliefs may be faulty because appearances of things in the universe can be deceiving and, second, to take measures to refine our observations in such a way as to overcome these potential distortions. . . . We should certainly mistrust our subjective judgements about relationships between words in our language, especially phonological relationships. For this task linguists have the misfortune of being literate, highly educated, and, most dangerous, explicitly schooled in the history of languages. This is bound to bias them in their speculations about mental representations of the lexicon and grammar.
—J. J. Ohala (1988: 32)

'Twas brillig and the slithy toves
Did gyre and gimble in the wabe:
All mimsy were the borogroves,
And the mome raths outgrabe.
—Lewis Carroll ([1871] 1965: 191)

5 Panchronic Applications in Hebrew Phonology

Formalism makes theories explicit. Formally stated theories are easier to test than informally stated ones. Beyond this, formalism has no further function. The formal statement of the theory is the *first* step of the many needed to properly test a theory. —J. J. Ohala and J. J. Jaeger (1986b: 4)

Synchrony is one man's crony, and diachrony is another man's crony.
—H. Matthews

The Stop/Spirant Alternation in Hebrew

The History of the Hebrew Language

Before entering into a discussion of what was referred to as a panchronic view of Hebrew, the special problems of separating synchrony from diachrony for the Hebrew language in general, and the specific phonological problem of the occlusive-spirant alternation (*BeGeDKeFeT*) in particular (see chap. 3, n. 12, and chap. 4, nn. 1, 4), I will first present here a brief history of the Hebrew language.

This chapter deals with modern Hebrew (also known as Israeli Hebrew, contemporary Hebrew, and Ivrit) (Berman 1978: 1–4; Glinert 1989: 1–5; Rosén 1977: 15–24), the national language of the Jewish majority (approximately 4 million) of the State of Israel and a second language for the Jews of the world (as well as the Arab minority residing in Israel). The Hebrew language is usually divided into three or four major historical periods:

1. classical or biblical Hebrew (ca. 1200 B.C.–ca. 200–300 B.C.);
2. mishnaic or rabbinical Hebrew (ca. 300 B.C.–ca. A.D. 400–500);
3. medieval Hebrew (ca. A.D. 500–A.D. 1700); and
4. modern Hebrew (including the period of the Enlightenment and the revival of Hebrew in Israel) (ca. A.D. 1700 to the present).

Despite the wide spread of Jews throughout the world and the ingathering of the exiles in Israel with the multitude of mother tongues that they speak, modern Hebrew is strikingly uniform in its dialects and varieties of usage including both ethnic dialects used by Jews of African-Asian origin (known as Sepharadim) and European-American origin (known as Ashkenazim) as well as sociolinguistic and regional dialects. The generic term *Hebrew* includes all the historical variations of the language, which form a fairly comprehensible continuum of a single, basically synthetic language rather than what might be considered to be different languages such as a more synthetic Old English as opposed to a more analytic modern English (Tobin 1981a, 1981b).

Like other Semitic languages, Hebrew has a fundamentally different structure from the Indo-European languages. In the Semitic languages, the isomorphic connections between phonology, morphology, syntax, and semantics are much more overt. The vast majority of the words of the language can be analyzed into consonantal roots signaling broad semantic fields; these roots are combined with fixed morphophonemic patterns for what are traditionally called nominal, verbal, and adjectival forms. More often than not, the connections and relations between the root and these fixed morphophonemic patterns are transparent—certainly much more so than in English (Tobin 1994: chaps. 2, 8).

The Extralinguistic Implications of the Phonological Problem

As has been established in the previous chapter, what has traditionally been called the occlusive-spirant alternation of biblical Hebrew (*BeGeD-KeFeT*) has been and remains one of the thorniest problems of Hebrew phonology to this very day. There are many reasons for the special status of this particular problem, reasons related to various anthropological and sociological linguistic issues surrounding the Hebrew language itself.

1. Modern Hebrew is unique in that it is a language that has been successfully revived as a national vernacular, although most scholars agree that, as a language of scholarship, liturgy, business, correspondence, and other needs, it never suffered a real demise.[1]

2. As may be expected with a language that—whether revived or not—is under constant linguistic scrutiny regarding its rich written legacy and its concurrent use

as an everyday vernacular for a vibrant, multiethnic society, standardization, in the form of normative prescriptivism advocated by the fairly powerful Hebrew Language Academy, is very rampant.[2]

3. Modern Hebrew has been referred to as a fusion language because it draws simultaneously on a number of linguistic sources, including biblical, mishnaic, medieval, and later literary sources, each of which contributed individually to the language prior to its revival.[3]

4. The strongest or most obvious influence that points 1–3 have had on the language is in the lexicon. Scholars have done much work on the phenomenon that has been referred to as the large-scale relexification of the language through extensive borrowings from both Jewish and contemporary European languages as well as from earlier Hebrew and Aramaic sources.[4]

5. Modern Hebrew has also been referred to as an immigrants' language because it was revived in the context of intense exposure to the other languages that were spoken by Jewish immigrants who originally returned to prestate Israel. This original immigrants' language became the source for the language acquisition of subsequent generations born in Israel, whose own language has subsequently become a standard for new waves of massive immigration to the state of Israel up to and even today.[5]

6. Modern Hebrew, therefore, has contributed to the sociological complexity of what has been called the languages in contact situation, which is simultaneously accompanied by the prescriptive process of consolidating the norms of a revived language that is serving as a colloquial everyday vernacular.[6]

7. It may be inferred from point 6 above that modern Hebrew has been revived in extralinguistic circumstances resembling the birth of a creole language: that is, one can identify the first generation of native speakers who had no other native speakers from whom to acquire their language.

8. The fact that we are discussing a problem of a certain kind of phonological alternation in an earlier form of a language that has been revived in these unique and extreme circumstances of languages in contact as well as creolization under the influence of strong normative consolidation means that this problem has serious implications for the study of language change.

The revival of the Hebrew language has been considered both as a great achievement and as a strong necessity in Israeli society, for the reasons stated above. Therefore, it is not surprising that this particular phonological problem has been of particular interest to linguists.

The Linguistic Implications of the Phonological Problem

The linguistic implications of the occlusive-spirant alternation in Hebrew can be summed up as follows.

1. In biblical Hebrew, there were six phonemes (hence the acronym *BeGeD-KeFeT*) that had a largely allophonic occlusive-spirant alternation in fixed phonetic environments (Garbell 1959; Tur-Sinai 1954).

2. The phonological system of postbiblical, prerevival Hebrew changed from the biblical phonological system, and only three (*BeKeF*) of the original six phonemes retained the occlusive-spirant alternation (Faber 1983).

3. The phonological system of Israeli Hebrew quite naturally differs from phonological systems that prevailed during the previous centuries, particularly in the light of the extralinguistic circumstances mentioned in points 1–8 of the previous section.

4. Therefore, the status—or even the existence—of a *BeGeDKeFeT* or *BeKeF* alternation rule in Hebrew today is the major question and the crux of the problem.

The prescriptive attitude that prevails in the Israeli school system and the media adheres to the principle that speaking with the *BeGeDKeFeT* or *BeKeF* rule belongs to proper Hebrew and is therefore the correct way to speak. This is particularly interesting since the phonological system of Israeli Hebrew differs from that of biblical and postbiblical, prerevival Hebrew and these former allophonic alternations are no longer acquired naturally. Indeed, most native speakers learn of the *BeGeDKeFeT* rule in school and memorize its intricacies for matriculation and other examinations without necessarily implementing it in their own everyday speech. Therefore, the question of "to be or not to be *BeGeDKeFeT?*" clearly divides the prescriptive and descriptive attitudes toward language and has inspired much controversy and research.

Defining the Phonological Problem

It is not surprising that the fundamental phonological status of *BeGeDKeFeT* and the intricate extralinguistic aspects associated with it have concerned various scholars in different ways: Schwarzwald (1981: vii) defines the problem in the following way: "Hebrew grammar as taught in Israeli schools sets the Biblical phonological and morphological rules as norms for Contemporary Hebrew. However, since the phonological system of Contemporary Hebrew is different from the Biblical, deviations from these norms are to be expected. This book describes an empirical study conducted to demonstrate the discrepancies between normative grammar and actual pronunciation especially as found in the verb system, and to account for them in accordance to up-to-date linguistic approaches." Alternatively, Ravid (in press)[7] defines the problem from a slightly different perspective:

> The principle factor worth recalling here relates to the fact that M[odern] H[ebrew] was revived in a linguistic situation typologically akin to the birth of a creole. Thus, in the absence of native speakers of the language, the first generation of Hebrew speakers had necessarily to fall back on innate phonological strategies in order to bridge the discrepancy between the original sound system underlying the B[iblical] H[ebrew] orthography (as transmitted by the Masoretes of the 1st millenium) and the diachronically restructured system available to speakers of the language (all nonnative) at the time of the revival (Bar-Adon 1959; Izre'el 1986; Rabin 1974, 1977; Rosén 1953; Sivan 1970; Téné 1985).
>
> . . . For untutored native speakers and children—especially those "recreating" M[odern] H[ebrew] with no native input available, however, many morphophonemic processes in the language represent opaque linguistic domains . . . , i.e. ones for which rules cannot be elicited from the input because they are no longer directly accessible.

The discrepancy between the *BeGeDKeFeT* alternation rule and the phonology and morphophonology of Israeli Hebrew has been the focus of much research from Chomsky (1951) on. Ravid, Schwarzwald, and others have recently dealt with the problem from the point of view of rule opacity.

Rule Opacity: Description or Explanation?

Ravid (in press) presents a brief definition of rule opacity and a table (reproduced here as table 5.1) illustrating rule opacity (cf. Kiparsky 1982; Lightfoot 1981, 1982): "A rule of the form $A \rightarrow B \,/\, C$ ____ D is opaque to the extent that there are surface representations of the form [shown in table 5.1]." One such area marked by structural opacity is the historical rule of stop/spirant alternation (traditionally known as the *BeGeDKeFeT* rule), which is at present undergoing a process of restructuring.

Just as Schwarzwald linked the level of explanation of the concrete approach to the problem to morphology (the verb system), so do Ravid (in

Table 5.1 Rule Opacity

1. *A* in the environment of *C* ____ *D*, or
2. *B* in the environments other than *C* ____ *D*

Source: Kiparsky (1982: 75).

press) and others link it to the morphophonemic level. Ravid presents lexical examples containing the alternation accompanied by the triconsonantal (CCC) root from which they are derived: "Stop/spirant alternation is a central feature of Hebrew morphophonemics, since it relates consonants to vowels, word-structure to phonology, and classical to more recent periods of the language (Ben-Asher 1969; Barkai 1972; Ben Horin and Bolozky 1972; Ephrat 1980; Faber 1986; Fischler 1975; Morag 1960; Ornan 1973; Ravid 1978, 1988; Rosén 1953; Schwarzwald 1976). This process yields the alternation of the stops *bkp* with their corresponding spirants *vxf* respectively: *ma'aboret* / *avar* 'ferry / passed' (< *'-b-r*); *hiskir* / *saxar* 'let / rented' (< *s-k-r*); *pesel* / *mefasel* 'sculpture / is sculpting' (< *p-s-l*). Historically, this rule assimilated the three pairs of stops (*pb, td, kg*) into their corresponding fricatives (*fv, θð, xχ*) after vowels: *katav* / *mixtav* 'he wrote / letter' (< *k-t-b*). In O[ld] H[ebrew] this alternation was essentially allophonic and unrelated to word structure (Garbell 1959; Tur-Sinai 1954)."

It is clear from the last example that the voiceless apical /t/ alternation of the *BeGeDKeFeT* rule has been lost. Indeed, so has the voiced apical /d/ alternation as well as the voiced dorsal /g/ alternation. Ravid (in press) describes these losses in the system as a collapse of a natural phonological class, which is listed as the first reason why stop spirantization is a typical example of an opaque rule:

In M[odern] H[ebrew], stop spirantization constitutes a typical example of an opaque rule (Kiparsky 1982; Lightfoot 1981, 1982; Schwarzwald 1980, 1981) for the following reasons:

(i) Collapse of a natural phonological class:

Historically, all six stops become spirantized after long vowels, thus forming a distinct and coherent phonological subsystem: two anterior, two coronal, and two velar stops, with a voiced and voiceless stop in each pair. Today, by contrast, only three stops alternate, two voiceless stops and a voiced one. As already noted in Faber

(1983), the other alternations were lost before the revival of M[odern] H[ebrew]. No single phonological feature sets *pbk* apart from the remaining stops that do not spirantize. In other words, the M[odern] H[ebrew] stops that undergo spirantization do not form a natural class, as do, for instance the stridents. This makes it hard for native speakers to characterize formally the class of segments liable to spirantization.

It may appear from the above that the loss of the /t-d/ and the /g/ alternations just happened arbitrarily, that is, at least for no apparent reason that can be explained by a single formal phonological feature. In one fell swoop, *BeGeDKeFeT* has been transformed to *BeKeF,* and none of the formal analyses has even thought of asking why or explaining whether the loss is motivated.[8]

If, on the other hand, we examine the system from the point of view of the principles and factors of phonology as human behavior, we may find a reasonable explanation that could provide a motivation as to why the apicals /t, d/ and the voiced posterodorsal /g/ were the ones that were dropped.

We have learned in the previous chapter that Hebrew had a three-way opposition for apical stops: voiceless /t/, voiceless-emphatic /T/, and voiced /d/. This more complex set of oppositions affected their distribution on the basis of the principle that additional articulators are disfavored. Therefore, it is not very surprising that, of all the members of the original *BeGeDKeFeT* system, the weakest links in the chain were those that have additional articulators involved. It also should be remembered that Hebrew distinguished between front /k/ and back emphatic /q/ as separate phonemes and that the latter also involved the exploitation of an additional articulator: posterodorsum and the lips. Thus, /g/ was opposed to /k/ and emphatic /q/ as well. The question that naturally arises, then, is, Why did /k/ remain in the system if both /t/ and /d/ were lost? The answer lies in the interaction between the human and the communication factors.

From the point of view of the human factor, the phoneme that is easier to control (i.e., has fewer sets of articulators) should have the greater staying power (i.e., /k/ rather than /g/). From the point of view of the communication factor, the number of communicative oppositions made by the apex, the most adroit of the active articulators, is the greatest. Having too many oppositions produced by the same articulator could prove inefficient and overtax the auditory perception of hearers. The number of oppositions at the posterodorsum is much less. Therefore, eliminating additional api-

Table 5.2 Opacity of Phonetic Motivation

A → B / C ____ D	
stp spr V X,	but
A occurs in C ____ D	
stp V ____ X	e.g., *sapar,* "barber"; *hitgabeʃ,* "consolidated"; *sika,* "pin"

cal oppositions—albeit allophonic alternations—and maintaining another—relatively easy to control—posterodorsal opposition makes sense.

We shall see later on that these and other principles of phonology as human behavior can be used to explain other issues related to the original problem of *BeGeDKeFeT,* which now has been reduced to *BeKeF* as well.

Ravid (in press) presents other reasons why stop spirantization is a typical example of rule opacity:

> (ii) Loss of the phonetic motivation of the spirantization rule
>
> Spirantization is no longer phonologically conditioned, since the phonetic environment that characterized it in B[iblical] H[ebrew] has been lost. Since stops become spirantized after long vowels, the phonetic environment for spirantization was unique. In M[odern] H[ebrew], stops do not automatically become spirantized after vowels: *ibdu* / *avdu* "cultivated / worked"; *yesaper* / *yisafer* "will tell / will be counted"; *maka* / *naxe* "(a) blow / crippled". This arises from the circumstance that *stop / spirant alternation* reflects *two* historical phenomena: (i) lenition of stops to spirants after (historically long) vowels, e.g. *saval* "suffered" (<*s-b-l*); and (ii) gemination of stops following a vowel (usually short), with the historical geminate currently reflected as a simplex stop rather than a fricative only in the *bkp* set (e.g. */sabbal/* → *sabal* "porter", same root). While gemination historically took place in a different phonetic environment then lenition, both are reflected today in the same phenomenon of stop/spirant alternation. Thus the contemporary Hebrew speaker has to cope with conflicting phonological cues relating to the environment relevant to spirantization.

She then illustrates the conflicting phonological cues relating to the environment relevant to spirantization in her table 3 (reproduced here as table 5.2 as an example of opacity by loss of phonetic motivation).

If we look at all Ravid's examples, the most interesting of all is, of course, the new modern Hebrew minimal pair derived from the same root: *saval/sabal,* "suffered/porter" (<*s-b-l*), which, in addition to indicating rule opacity by loss of phonetic motivation, further indicates that at least the former allophones [b] and [v] of the phoneme /b/ are separate and distinct phonemes in Israeli Hebrew.

The Phonemic Status of /b, k, p, v, x, f/

We have just seen that minimal pairs for the former allophones [b] and [v] can be found independently within the system: that is, without any other influence from other phonemes within the larger phonological system. The new status of /b/ and /v/ as separate phonemes is even further supported diachronically within the system. The historical phoneme /w/ has unconditionally been changed to /v/, or, as Davis (1984/1987: 56) described the same situation for Latin and Italian, "/w/ has become /v/, wholesale." Therefore, the former allophone [v], which appeared only in specific phonetic environments, ones that were complementary to those of the allophone [b], is now a phoneme in its own right and can appear freely in all environments (e.g., *vav,* "hook") and create new communicative oppositions (*biter,* "carved," vs. *viter,* "gave in").

If we turn now to the [k-x] alternation, we see that each historical allophone now shares the phonetic value of an earlier phoneme (such as /v/ and /w/ above) and can therefore freely appear in all phonetic environments and create minimal pairs with its former allophone and that—like /b/ and /v/ above—each is now a separate and independent phoneme.

We already have established that the phonetic distinction between the historical phonemes /k/ and /q/ has been lost in Israeli Hebrew and that former minimal pairs (e.g., *kol,* "all," vs. *qol,* "voice") are now homophonous. Therefore, /k/ can and does appear in all phonetic environments, thus losing its complementary distribution with its former allophone (now phoneme) /x/, which allows it to create new minimal pairs (e.g., *nimex,* "lowered," vs. *nimek* [historically *nimeq*], "gave reasons"). The phonetic distinction between the former allophone (now phoneme) /x/ and the historical laryngeal voiceless fricative phoneme /ħ/ has also been lost in Israeli Hebrew, and former minimal pairs (e.g., ʔ*ax,* "but, only," vs. ʔaħ, "brother") are now homophonous. Therefore, /x/ can and does appear in all phonetic environments, thus losing its complementary distribution with its former allophone (now phoneme) /k/, which allows it to create new minimal pairs (e.g., *xaf,* "innocent," vs. *kaf,* "spoon").

The situation is slightly different with the historical [p-f] alternation. Their phonetic values have remained intact and have not merged with any historical phonemes. However, they, too, can be considered to be separate and independent phonemes as well.

Owing to other changes in the phonological system previously discussed (/s/ [orthographic *samekh*]) vs. the now homophonous /s/ [orthographic *sin*]), new minimal pairs have been created (e.g., *safa,* "lip, language," vs. *sapa,* "sofa").[9] The Prague school also established alternative ways of defining phonemes—particularly new phonemes resulting from language change—not based on minimal pairs such as free variation. The distribution of phonemes is open and free—as it should be for maximum and efficient communication—and therefore unpredictable, which is why minimal pairs can be determined in word-initial, word-medial, or word-final positions.[10] The distribution of allophones, however, is closed and limited—as it should be since allophones do not change meaning—and therefore predictable because each allophone has a unique phonetic environment and is in a relation of complementary distribution with the other allophones of the same phoneme. There are certain words—both foreign and native—where both /p/ and /f/ appear in the same environment and one cannot predict which of the two could appear (e.g., *festival/pestival; september/seftember; tilfen/tilpen,* "he phoned"; *safarti/saparti,* "I counted").[11] However, in situations where objectively one cannot predict which phoneme *could* appear, educated people claim to know which phoneme *should* appear (usually the old allophone for Hebrew words), and the other alternative is considered to represent uneducated or substandard speech (the new phoneme for Hebrew words).

Ravid (in press) presents similar data as "parasites" on the system that aggravate rule opacity, presented schematically in her table 4 (reproduced here as table 5.3):

(iii) *"Parasites" on the system*

Historical circumstances are responsible for two additional phenomena that have aggravated the opacity of the historical spirantization rule: (i) the introduction of nonnative consonant segments into Hebrew via integrated loan words displaying *p, f, b, v, k* in positions violating historical spirantization. Note how [p, b, k] are retained without change after vowels in *mikroscop* "microscope", *ʒlob* "big person",

Table 5.3 Opacity by Parasites

1. A occurs in environment C ____ D
2. B occurs in environment other than C ____ D

and *bok* "stupid" respectively (case i). Similarly, [f, v] can occur anywhere, e.g. word-initially in *festival* "festival" or in *vakum* 'vacuum' (case ii).

Moreover, obstruents in loans never display Stop-Spirant Alternation, e.g. *fintez/ mefantez* "fantasized / s" (cf. *pirsem / mefarsem* "published / s").

Language-internally, segments have merged . . . : The glide *w* (historical/ orthographic *waw*) merged with the fricative allophone of *b,* to yield *v;* historical emphatic *q* (orthographic *qof*) merged with *k* (orthographic *kaf*), yielding Modern Hebrew *k;* Guttural *H* (orthographic *Het*) coalesced with the spirant allophone of *k,* into *x.* As a result, opacity pervades the system, since the "parasites" that have merged with the allophonic alternants of the original spirantizing class fail to conform to *Stop / Spirant Alternation.* On the other hand, *k* deriving from *qof* never spirantizes, so we get both *sakar / soker / yiskor/* "surveyed / s / will survey", root *s-q-r,* and *saxar / soxer / yiskor* "rented / s / will rent", root *s-k-r,* in the same environment; while on the other hand, *Het*-derived *x* always shows up as a spirant: *saxar / soxer / yisxar* "traded / s / will trade", root *s-H-r,* in the identical environment (note also the low vowel entailed in future tense by the underlying *H*). In the same way, while *b*-derived *v* alternates with the corresponding stop (e.g. *biter / mevater* "carved / is carving", root *b-t-r, w*-derived *v* never does (cf. *viter / mevater* "gave up / gives up", root *w-t-r*) so the same kind of opacity is entailed.

Spirantization thus operates only on historically inherited *stop / spirant* alternants, not on the foreign or merged "parasites" (Fischler 1975; Ravid 1988; Schwarzwald 1980, 1981). What the untutored native speaker observes is seemingly sporadic behavior of *bkp / vxf* segments.

The phonemic status of the stops *bkp* and the fricatives *vxf* can be summarized in the following way. The biblical *BeGeDKeFeT* allophonic alternation and the reduced postbiblical, prerevival *BeKeF* allophonic alternation have given way to a series of separate pairs of independent mobile and stable phonemes, /b-v/, /k-x/, and /p-f/, in Israeli Hebrew that can be established by minimal pairs and at least one other criterion of free variation or nonpredictability. However, the distribution of the old allophonic pairs is still present in the lexicon (e.g., the stops generally do not appear in word-final position, and the fricatives generally do not appear in word-initial position). The old allophonic distinctions are also present in the orthography. As was mentioned previously, alphabets and syllabaries are usually phonemic analyses of the phonological systems of the languages at the time they were created for or adapted to them. Therefore, for /p/ and /f/ at least, the same letter represents both sounds.[12] Often, when both phonemes can appear in the same environment, the historical allophone is considered to be more formal and correct, and the new phoneme is considered to be less formal and is labeled with the anathema *lo tikni,* "nonstandard." [13] Therefore, the choice of one phoneme over the other has far-reaching extralinguistic implications as well.

The Role of Morphology and Lexical Roots

Hebrew is well known as a synthetic language with a lexicon and grammar that revolve around the concept of basically triconsonantal (CCC) roots that are placed in a complex system of fixed verb conjugations (*binyanim*), nominal inflections (*mishkalim*), and other morphological patterns.[14] Therefore, it is not surprising that researchers investigating the acquisition and use of the *BeGeDKeFeT* alternation in Israeli Hebrew have incorporated specific lexical root and morphological patterns in their studies to uncover whether the phonological alternation is acquired naturally or learned normatively by diverse populations chosen according to differences in age, education, and social level.

Schwarzwald (1981: vii) describes the goals of her study in the following way:

> Chapter 2 presents the theoretical framework for the spirantization rule problem. Two linguistic methods deal with *p-f, b-v, k-x* alternations in Hebrew: abstract and concrete: According to the concrete method, *p, f, b, v, k, x* are phonemes and their alternations can be explained only on the morphological level of the grammar. The abstract method argues that the alternations are phonologically motivated and are still productive in Contemporary Hebrew.
>
> Based on the latter method, an empirical study was conducted in order to test whether the "*p-b-k*" rule is naturally phonological or normative. It was assumed that if the rule was naturally phonological, the speakers would use it properly both in familiar as well as in unfamiliar words. Furthermore, there would be no differ-

ences between age groups and social classes: children and adults, disadvantaged and advantaged speakers would use the rule in exactly the same manner. However, if the rule were a normative one, it would apply correctly only to familiar words, and formal education would determine its productivity. Therefore, differences between age groups and social classes would be expected.

Schwarzwald recorded 320 elementary school, middle school, high school, and university students who were equally divided into four age groups and advantaged and disadvantaged social classes and who read a list of 120 sentences, each of which contained either a common or an uncommon verb with *p, b,* or *k* in CI or CII position. Schwarzwald's results strongly support the normative assumption as well as a marked tendency to maintain morphological rather than phonological regularity. The few exceptions in her data to this tendency may be attributed to analogy to frequent nominal or to verbal forms that contain an opposite stop/fricative value or to phonetic assimilation and dissimilation. Her study of different populations showed that only formal study of the normative rules and acquaintance with a large vocabulary enables the speaker to use the historically accurate forms.

Ravid's study was based on previous research in new-word formation in Hebrew that employs roots exclusively in the derivation of new verbs and verb-related nominals (Aronoff 1976; Berman 1978; Bolozky 1982; Ravid 1991). These studies postulate a base form from which all the new words maintain the same consonantal root skeleton and derive their meaning. This morphologization of root segments further contributes to rule opacity when stops and fricatives appear in conflicting environments. Therefore, it is not surprising that Ravid also found that the historical stop/spirant alternation is constantly violated in Israeli Hebrew, especially by less literate speakers, and is a source of difficulty for children acquiring the language as well as for adults.

Ravid defines her study as a cross-sectional experiment testing strategies employed by speakers to alleviate opacity in the stop/spirant alternation. The subjects were asked to perform various grammatical operations on given test items that required responses containing certain stops or fricatives. The 188 subjects were divided into ten groups from six age clusters and two socioeconomic backgrounds. The results of the experimental study were augmented by spontaneous data from a diary study of two children, spontaneous speech samples from the test subjects, and observational data.

Ravid found that the *bkp* alternate found in a basic form was maintained in derived forms, often in violation of the normative rule (Barkai 1972; Berman 1985; Fischler 1975). A similar strategy was found for new words constructed from existing words and their root form, which serves as a go-between linking two lexical entries. This, of course, enhances both the human and the communication factors by connecting semantically related words with similar phonological patterns that can be easily recognized and classified. Speakers of all sociolinguistic backgrounds tend to phonematicize root *bkp* across lexical entries, thus maintaining what Ravid refers to as the principle of semantic transparency, which requires a one-to-one relation between meaning and form (Bates and MacWhinney 1982; Clark 1981, 1982; Hooper 1979; Naro 1978; Lightfoot 1981; Slobin 1977, 1985a). (This principle gives further affirmation to the concept of the linguistic sign, although none of the above necessarily argue for this.)

Ravid's study also shows that the phonematicization of *bkp* radicals sharply delineates child speech and the nonstandard sociolect from the established sociolect. Ravid maintains that unsophisticated speakers maintain the phonematicization of *pbk* in both inflectional and derivational morphology while educated speakers tend to restrict the invariant base to lexical derivation but maintain the historical stop/spirant alternation within grammatical paradigms.

Ravid's data also show that neither group is totally consistent in its choices. The data indicate that all children acquire and exploit /b, k, p, v, x, f/ as separate and independent phonemes. Therefore, the extralinguistic consequence of this fact is that Israeli children's language reflects the nonstandard, naive, or less-educated sociolect. Speakers of the educated sociolect eventually learn to incorporate certain aspects of the *BeKeF* alternation in their speech and use it in the more limited area of inflectional morphology. In other words, the independent phonemic status for *bkp/vxf* is maintained by everyone, but remnants of the historical allophonic variation is partially maintained by literate speakers for inflection.

This sociolinguistic distinction requires Ravid to introduce the concept of *basic word,* which is believed to determine which *BeKeF* alternate will be chosen. However, the notion of basic word (usually the unmarked free masculine singular) may differ across word classes in general and is particularly problematic in the morphologically complex verb system. The data indicate that naive speakers will choose the phoneme in the basic form and usually maintain it in the more complex forms containing additional affixes in accordance to the psycholinguistic principle of formal simplicity

(Clark 1981; Clark and Berman 1984; Ravid 1988). Thus, for example, naive speakers will pluralize *daf,* "page," and *tsahov,* "yellow," as *dafim* and *tsehuvim,* while educated speakers will use the normative *dapim* and *tsehubim,* respectively. However, this is not an absolute, across-the-board phenomenon for either group, and other factors such as word frequency and various pragmatic factors will influence the stop/spirant choice as well.

In other words, all speakers acquire *bkp/vxf* naturally as separate phonemes and exploit them as such in their language. Educated speakers, however, also tend to maintain what appears to be the *BeKeF* allophonic alternation for grammatical inflection only. The question then arises, Can both the historical and the contemporary phonological systems simultaneously and panchronically exist—albeit in a very limited domain—for one segment of the population only? The data seem to indicate this. However, should these six sounds paradoxically be considered both as phonemes and as allophones simultaneously, or can this supposed distinct allophonic status be explained in a simpler, more meaningful manner?

Phonology as Human Behavior

In chapter 1, it was maintained that people generally are aware of the phonemes and unaware of the allophones in the phonological systems of their language. The reason for this lies in the interaction between the communication factor and the human factor. Phonemes create distinctive oppositions and differences in meaning that make them worthwhile to remember. Allophones do not build or change meaning, and being aware of them is therefore less essential.

It was also shown in chapter 1 that one of the reasons that people can be unaware of allophones is that they are restricted to specific phonetic environments. It is also not by chance that each allophone appears in the precise environment for which it is most suited, that is, the environment in which it is the easiest to produce naturally. Therefore, it should not be surprising that educated Israeli speakers who have been formally taught historical allophonic distributions and have also learned that their use is a mark of correct and prestigious language would have an incentive to use them. It is also not surprising that their use is restricted to the limited realm of fixed morphological inflections. Once again, the use of the stop/spirant alternation is clearly learned rather than acquired linguistic behavior and is motivated by clear-cut extralinguistic and pragmatic reasons. But let us go beyond that.

The original *BeGeDKeFeT* allophonic alternation was based on vowel length and gemination, neither of which is part of the new phonological system. Therefore, the former phonetic environments that were so naturally distributed in biblical Hebrew cannot be so today in the absence of phonemic distinctions between short and long vowels and geminate and nongeminate consonants. Therefore, if the remnants of a historical allophonic distribution are going to be even partially displayed by an educated segment of the population, that display should not deviate from certain basic principles of human linguistic and extralinguistic behavior. I will limit myself here to those principles of human behavior that are reflected in phonology and are based on the inherent features found in sounds and sound classes.

Ravid (in press) came close to discovering the importance of the inherent features of sounds and their role in phonotactic distribution, but she credited it to morphology rather than phonology:

> There is one more relevant structural factor here which may override pragmatic considerations. This involves cases where a stop or spirant in a certain morphological environment is retained on account of its inherent features. For instance, *bkp* in initial root position in the *Hif'il* [verb conjugation] scheme follows a consonant and is consequently more likely to yield a spirant throughout the *binyan,* e.g. *Hifrid* "separated", *maxtim* "is staining", *le-havxin* "to notice"; while *bpk* in middle root position in the *Pi'el* scheme is more likely to yield a stop throughout the *binyan,* e.g. *siben* "soaped", *memaker* "addictive", *le-sapek* "to supply", since the middle root position here reflects a historical geminate.
>
> In such cases the invariant character of the morphological structure acts as another significant factor determining the *bkp* alternant selected by the speaker.

With all due respect for inflectional and derivational morphology, morphological and syntactic structure, base forms, principles of semantic transparency and formal simplicity, etc., the answer may be much simpler and directly linked to phonology and human behavior.

If we look at the vast majority of Ravid's examples where the historical allophonic variation is maintained, we find that the stops or mobile phonemes (historical allophones) tend to appear in word/syllable-initial positions more than the fricatives or stable phonemes (historical allophones). Davis (1984/1987: 52) referred to this as principle E: explosive phonemes are favored in initial position (which might imply that nonexplosive phonemes are favored in noninitial position). We also find that the fricatives or stable phonemes (historical allophones) appear in postvocalic position (more than the stops or mobile phonemes, which appear only as geminates, usually after short vowels), which means that they were clearly favored in word/syllable-final positions, particularly in word-final position.

Indeed, these preferences for stops and fricatives in initial and final positions, respectively (particularly voiceless stops and fricatives, which are easier to make), are supported independently by the literature in developmental and clinical phonology. Compton (1975: 88) determined the priority of voiceless stops in initial position and the priority of voiceless fricatives in final position as developmental generalizations in the earliest stages of normal development. By the same token, according to Crystal (1987 [1981]: 35), "fricatives in final position are easier than those in initial position." Therefore, if a certain morphological structure consistently places stops in initial positions and fricatives in final positions, then it is only natural that the correct historical allophone will appear in that morphological structure. However, these individual sounds should not be ambiguously classified as two sounds in the system—one a phoneme and one an allophone. Rather, they should be classified as one single sound—acquired in Israeli Hebrew as a separate and independent phoneme—that inherently favors those phonetic environments in which it most naturally appears both within and across languages. This is clearly not a case of allophonic variation because no stop/spirant allophones have been acquired naturally by any speaker of Israeli Hebrew, for all of whom /b, k, p, v, x, f/ are independent and separate phonemes. Therefore, those instances in which the current phoneme matches the historical allophone should be viewed as another case of the phonotactic or combinatory phonological favorings of distinct phonemes based on the human and the communication factors, which have been verified in and across languages at various word, stem, and root levels.

Davis (1984/1987: 52–53) gives an explanation for the favoring of explosive phonemes in initial position:

> Explosive phonemes have a sudden and drastic release of pressure created by, in this case, pulmonic initiation. Catford [1977] explains "initiation":
>
> By *initiation* we mean a bellows-like or piston-like movement of an organ or organ-group (an initiator) which generates positive or negative pressure in the part of the vocal tract adjacent to it, that is, between the initiator and the place of articulation. The term "initiation" is used for this component of speech production [as

opposed to "articulation" and "phonation"] since it is the activity that "initiates" the flow of air essential for the production of almost all sounds (p. 63). [Notice that the term has nothing to do with *initial* position in the word.]

Initiation may be either "compressive" (positive pressure) or rarefactive (negative pressure, or suction), and it may be pulmonic, glottalic, or velaric in origin. Velaric pressure and pulmonic suction are almost unknown (pp. 64–64), but pulmonic compression occurs in all languages. The rate of lung-volume decreases in pulmonic pressure initiation ranges from 0 cm^3/sec for voiceless stops to 1000 cm^3/sec for [h] (pp. 66–67), with 1°, 2°, and 3° Airflow in between. The explosive release of [p, t, k], and to a lesser extent [b, d, g], maximizes the role of compressive initiation at the beginning of the stem. /f, v/ are consistent with compressive initiation, but as stem-initial constrictions, they take less than full advantage of the power.

. . . By transitivity Factor E accounts for one more comparison: p > f > v [which can be seen in *BeGeDKeFeT*].

Therefore, it is not surprising that we get the following correct forms in what Ravid (in press) refers to as inflectional categories with closely related members (in the sense of Bybee 1985), such as number (*tsahov/tsehubim,* "yellow m/s," and *tof/tupim,* "drum/s" and gender (*rax/raka,* "soft m/f") or verb tense (*barax/tivrax,* "escaped/(you) will escape"). In all these examples, mobile phonemes of constriction favor word/syllable-initial position, and stable phonemes of constriction favor word/syllable-final position.[15]

By following the basic principles of phonology as human behavior, we can look at the *BeGeDKeFeT* problem in a different way from the more formal theories discussed in this chapter. This difference in approach has various theoretical and methodological consequences.

1. We can maintain the integrity of the naturally acquired phonemic system and justify the phonotactic distribution of these phonemes in their favored and disfavored environments rather than postulating the dual contradictory status of phoneme and historical allophone for the same sounds.

2. However, we must always bear in mind that these favorings are gradient rather than physiological absolutes and are influenced by linguistic and extralinguistic factors and that the same principles may therefore function slightly differently in various languages (as we have seen in this volume for English, Italian, Latin, Hebrew, and Yiddish; for Urdu, see Azim [1989, 1993, 1995]) and Jabeen (1993).

3. Earlier in this chapter, I attempted to provide a reasonable motivation to explain why the apicals /t, d/ and the voiced dorsal /g/ were dropped from the biblical

BeGeDKeFeT alternation by appealing to the principle that additional articulators are disfavored, a question that was not even asked by other theories.

4. It should also be noted that maintaining this stop/spirant alternation as a distinct *phonemic* opposition based on easily perceived acoustic differences in degrees of stricture and airflow for the optimal set of labial, apical, and posterodorsal active articulators leads to more efficient communication than the earlier *BeGeD-KeFeT allophonic* alternation did in biblical Hebrew, which kept the stop-fricative (mobile-stable) distinction *phonemic* only for laryngeal consonants.[16]

5. It may also be that those instances in the speech of educated Israeli speakers in the limited realm of inflectional morphology where there is a match between the two phonological systems (e.g., *tof/tupim,* "drum/drums") are specifically learned as separate lexical items in a way similar exceptional or "irregular" singular-plural oppositions marking educated speech are learned in other languages for archaic or borrowed lexical items (e.g., *brother/bretheren, ox/oxen, octopus/octopi, criterion/criteria, phenomenon/phenomena, stratum/strata, kibbutz/kibbutzim, cherub/cherubim, sputnik/sputniki, paparazzo/paparazzi,* etc. in English).[17]

In all the above, however, the interaction between the human and the communication factors is always taken into account as part of the definition of language as a system of systems used by human beings to communicate. This definition of language also leads the analyst to abide by the synergetic motto that language represents a striving toward maximum communication with minimal effort.

This chapter has raised many issues concerning what constitutes a native speaker's knowledge of language. It has also highlighted the many differences that occur in language production and performance within a language community. The data discussed by all researchers dealing with the *BeGeD-KeFeT* problem deal directly with the question of how linguists should analyze the knowledge that native speakers appear to absorb. Research of this kind should always bear in mind the following statements made by John Ohala (1988: 22, 23):

> No doubt whether a native speaker imagines a relationship between two words is a probabilistic thing, the probability being a function of the speaker and the words involved.

> One thing we can probably take for granted: the mere fact that a person is exposed to experiences (things observed) does not mean that person will abstract all possible generalizations from them.

It may be safe to assume, however, that whatever knowledge is acquired and whatever generalizations are abstracted by speakers, they will serve a communicative purpose that will reflect at least one of the many multifarious aspects related to the human factor.

Summary and Conclusions

In this chapter, I presented alternative theoretical and methodological approaches to the stop/spirant *BeGeDKeFeT* allophonic alternation of biblical Hebrew and its panchronic implications for the *BeKeF* allophonic alternation in postbiblical, prerevival Hebrew and the phonemicization of /b, k, p, v, x, f/ in Israeli Hebrew. The complex extralinguistic implications of research in the Hebrew language in general and this phonological problem in particular were detailed. The kinds of studies dealing with both the linguistic and the extralinguistic aspects of the problem were outlined. It was seen that each individual approach concentrated on finding a solution to or an explanation of the diverse aspects of the problem according to different criteria.[18]

In chapter 1, I established that every theory defines and deals with linguistic problems in a different way. As we have seen, some theories are more formal than others, but formalism per se does not necessarily entail explanation, or a better explanation, or, as John Ohala (1984: 14) has said, "Some formal accounts may be more elegant than others and, as we know, the competition between purely formal accounts of the same body of data is thus a continuous process. But in the end purely formal analyses are just systematisations of the data, not explanations of it." In the following chapter, I will present some principles for the teaching of phonetics as human behavior. I will then apply the theory of phonology as human behavior, not to another lexical analysis, but rather to a poetic text that has special metalinguistic and psycholinguistic implications.

6 Pedagogical and Textual Applications

The concept of psychological reality and how to discover what is psychologically real has been made out to be a very subtle and/or complicated issue. I think this has been overdone and would like to attempt to simplify it by means of an extended analogy. Many of us are teachers. One of the tasks required of teachers is certification that students know certain academic material in order that they may receive a grade, a diploma, or a degree. In these cases, the teacher must, in effect, assess the psychological reality of students' knowledge or mental ability. How is this done? By obtaining some behavioral evidence, e.g., performance on a test, presentation of an original scholarly paper, etc., which evidence is consistent with the students having the knowledge or ability attributed to them. Conscientious teachers do not usually take the mere fact that the students have been exposed to the academic material as sufficient evidence that they know and understand the material. Of course, it is not easy to devise good tests and most of us therefore spend much time refining our tests. Nevertheless, I am not aware that anyone in academia rejects, in principle, the need for such overt behavioral evidence in assessing students' knowledge and mental ability. The same practice should apply when we seek to verify the psychological reality of posited phonological constructs.
—J. J. Ohala (1981: 373)

Teaching Phonetics as Human Behavior

In chapter 1 especially, the following basic theoretical and methodological assumptions underlying this volume were established:

1. Language is defined in terms of its function as a system of communication that ecologically reflects the characteristics of its users—human beings.

2. This particular definition of language encompasses the synergetic interaction between the communication and the human factors that determines the raison d'être

and dictates the formulation of the specific problems being addressed as well as the source, amount, and manner in which the data are identified, collected, analyzed, and evaluated.

3. One of the aspects of the theory of phonology as human behavior that separates it from other phonological theories is its recognition of the interdependence of the abstract phonological system of *langue* and the concrete distribution of sounds in *parole*.

4. This integral connection between phonetics and phonology is supported by a theoretical and methodological model based on phonemes and allophones, which are defined as linguistic units containing various features that systematically link them together according to their communicative function and reflect the characteristics of human perception, cognition, and behavior relevant to their exploitation.

5. This integral connection between phonetics and phonology further implies an isomorphic and holistic search for basic principles that can account not only for the sounds of language but for all aspects of language as well, on the basis of the interaction between the communication and the human factors.

6. Therefore, it is not surprising that the same principles underlying the theory of phonology as human behavior presented in this volume to explain the nonrandom and asymmetric distribution of phonemes in language can be integrated into the teaching of sounds of language per se: that is, the teaching of articulatory, acoustic, and distributional phonetics as human behavior.

In this chapter, I will present a brief outline on how phonetics might be viewed and taught in the light of the theory of phonology as human behavior. This will be followed by a more detailed exposition of the application of the theory of phonology as human behavior to a specific text. These two initial sections should serve as an introduction to the application of the theory to the areas of developmental and clinical phonology that will be presented in the final sections of this volume.[1]

The Principles of Phonetics as Human Behavior

The following principles underlie the teaching of articulatory and acoustic phonetics together as part of a single course:

1. Articulatory phonetics in general should be viewed as the history of the airstream from the diaphragm to the release of the air from the oral or nasal passages by the encoder.

2. Each of the articulating organs should be viewed from the point of view of its contribution to modifying the airstream to create new acoustic patterns that are perceived as different sounds by the decoder.

3. Acoustic phonetics should be viewed as the history of the airstream from its release by the encoder to its perception by the decoder.

4. The different acoustic patterns produced by the encoder and perceived by the decoder should be analyzed according to the distinctive articulatory features produced by the encoder to each of which there is a parallel distinctive acoustic feature.

5. Both the production and the perception aspects of human speech should be taught together as part of the same integral process referred to as the speech chain (Denes and Pinson 1963).

The following principles underlie the teaching of the classification of sounds or phones into phonemes and allophones:

1. As seen in chapter 1, phones should be classified as phonemes as opposed to allophones on the basis of their contribution to communication (phoneme vs. allophone), or the communication factor; the specific primary distinctive versus secondary nondistinctive articulatory and acoustic features that they convey; and the nonpredictability of the distribution of phonemes in minimal pairs or in free variation in the same phonetic environment versus the predictability of the complementary distribution of allophones.

2. The systematic interchangeability of phonemes and allophones across languages and within the same language in different periods of time should be stressed and illustrated from the points of view of the communication and human factors.

3. The fact that all languages have a similar number of phonemes (usually between twenty and forty) that are acquired in a similar order across languages and their diachronic and synchronic relations to alphabet systems and orthography should be taught from the point of view of the human factor.

4. The asymmetric relation between the number of phonemes and the number of allophones in language systems and our awareness of the former over the latter should be studied from the synergetic point of view of maximum communication with minimal effort.

The following principles underlie the replacement of traditional and neotraditional phonetic categories and labels with new concepts related to phonology as human behavior that illustrate the unity of sounds and sound classes as part of a single hierarchy:

1. Consonants should be referred to as phonemes of constriction.

2. Vowels should be referred to as phonemes of aperture.

3. Voiced versus voiceless, emphatic versus nonemphatic, ejective versus non-ejective, retroflexed versus nonretroflexed, palatalized versus nonpalatalized, etc.; phonemes of constriction and nasal versus oral and labialized versus nonlabialized, etc.; phonemes of constriction and phonemes of aperture—all should be studied in terms of the number of articulators being exploited simultaneously and the degree of the difficulty of their control from the point of view of the human factor.

4. Place of articulation for phonemes of constriction should be replaced with the notions of active articulators and passive receptors.

5. The tongue and the lips should be viewed as active articulators for phonemes of aperture as far as the height and position of the former and the degree of rounding or spreading for the latter are concerned.

6. The division of the tongue into anterodorsum and posterodorsum as active articulators not only serves to distinguish phonemes of constriction but can also replace the traditional categories of front and back vowels, respectively, as the active articulators for phonemes of aperture.

7. Manner of articulation should be replaced by a hierarchical set of degree of stricture, aperture, and type of airflow that is applicable to both phonemes of constriction and phonemes of aperture, which may now be viewed as a single, holistic continuum or cline of sounds.

8. Mobile and stable phonemes can replace former categories of manner of articulation for phonemes of constriction (stops, fricatives, affricates) and could be applied to both phonemes of constriction and phonemes of aperture, replacing such categorizations as obstruents/sonorants and syllabic/nonsyllabic phonemes.

9. Tenseness/laxness and fortis/lenis can be studied from the point of view of the amount of effort needed to control different sets of articulators and musculature for all sounds regardless of their classification as phonemes of constriction or aperture.

10. The difference between simple phonemes and complex phonemes (between stops and fricatives; and affricates and monophthongs; and diphthongs) can be explained from the point of view of the synergetic interaction between the desire for maximum communication and that for minimal effort for both phonemes of constriction and phonemes of aperture in a similar way.

11. Many of the other various traditional categories of consonants and vowels as opposed to semivowels—plosives, trills, flaps, glides, liquids, approximants, etc.—can be replaced by a single, unified hierarchy of sounds based on degree of stricture, aperture, and type of airflow.

The following principles can explain the nonrandom distribution of sounds both within the phonemic inventory of a language system and within meaningful units of language on the basis of the principles of phonology as human behavior as a means to include distributional phonetics in a basic course on phonetics as human behavior:

1. For both phonemes of constriction and phonemes of aperture, maximum communication is achieved by investing human effort in the exploitation of the extremities of the oral vocal tract that provide the most distinct acoustic cues (e.g., grave and acute loci) in opposition to a neutralized center: the lips versus the posterodorsum in opposition to the apex (front-back-middle), the most adroit of the articulators for phonemes of constriction; the vowel triangle /i/ versus /u/ in opposition to /a/ (front-back-middle) for phonemes of aperture.

2. When these optimal oral oppositions are exploited, further communicative distinctions are made by exploiting the musculature between the extremes and the middle or by extending their boundaries: by adding additional passive receptors (teeth, hard palate) or new, less adroit active articulators (anterodorsum, uvula, pharynx, glottis) or the vocal folds (for tone, murmur, creakiness, etc. in addition to voicing) for phonemes of constriction and aperture; by exploiting the intermediary tongue positions between the high and the low front and back points of the vowel triangle /e/, /ɛ/, /æ/, /ɔ/, /o/, etc.

3. Additional communicative distinctions can be made by exploiting the adroit active articulators in different ways requiring more effort and thus creating marked sounds such as lateral, retroflex, emphatic, ejective, velarized, nasalized, etc. phonemes of constriction and aperture.

4. More complex sounds requiring greater effort (affricates, diphthongs, etc.) can create further communicative distinctions as well.

5. In all the above processes, there will also be a favoring of adroit active articulators and a preference for the excitation of fewer sets of articulators when possible as a result of the human factor.

6. The differences in the communicative force of utterance-initial, utterance-medial, and utterance-final positions will also affect the choice of more adroit over less adroit, or more visual over less visual, articulators and phonemes requiring one, two, or three sets of articulators.

7. In most, if not all, languages, the relative number and the proportion of marked and unmarked phonemes will be similar, although the features being marked will differ from language to language.

8. In most, if not all, languages, the number and kind of phonemes and their role in syllable structure will be based on the differences of the communicative forces of phonemes of constriction, which impede the airflow, in relation to phonemes of aperture, which provide free movement of air.

The common denominator underlying the teaching of phonetics as human behavior is the analysis of the sound systems of language and the nonrandom distribution of sounds in language from the synergetic point of view of achieving maximum communication with minimal effort, taking into account the different roles of encoder and decoder needed to achieve efficient communication. Efficient communication implies the creation of discourse and texts, which leads to the next application of the theory of phonology of human behavior: a text analysis constructed as part of a course on phonology as human behavior.

A Text Analysis: "Jabberwocky"

The Metalinguistic Connection

> The human urge for essential apprehension and structure, however, needs to be reconciled with the realm of phainomena, or appearances. Since representation always involves something that mediates between things and knowledge of them, an analysis of structure which deals with signs and their values provides the natural means of access to this mediating level. Every sign in its synchronic aspect actually encapsulates a historical dimension as part of its ontological constitution.
>
> —M. Shapiro and M. Shapiro (1988: 1)

> Words! Mere words! How terrible they were! How clear, and vivid and cruel! Once could not escape from them. . . . Mere words! Was there anything so real as words?
>
> —Oscar Wilde ([1891] 1965: 26)

In this section, I have applied the theory of phonology as human behavior to a panchronic problem in Hebrew, involving both the lexicon and the grammar, and I have discussed the pedagogical implications of the theory to the teaching of phonetics. The validations of the theory in individual languages in the previous chapters have been based on lexical analysis only, using dictionaries or the analyst's active vocabulary (Diver 1979, 1955: 71–72). However, the theory has also been applied successfully to a large number of spoken and written texts of various kinds. In this chapter, I shall apply the theory to a special text. Very often in the linguistic literature in general and in the research done in phonetics and phonology in particular, the role of nonsense words in determining, describing, and explaining metalinguistic and psycholinguistic phenomena is central. Furthermore, poetry and the language of poetry are usually singled out as being more phonologically determined than other styles, registers, and genres. For these reasons, I thought of illustrating the theory here in a discourse or text analysis of a specific text. And I did not choose just any text, but probably the most famous nonsense or near-nonsense poem in the English language—"Jabberwocky" by Lewis Carroll (1965 [1871]: 191). An additional short poem by Carroll, "The Crocodile," was added in order to have a corpus comprising one hundred words, for which "Jabberwocky" provides most of the data.[2] The complete texts of both poems follow:

Jabberwocky

'Twas brillig and the slithy toves
 Did gyre and gimble in the wabe:
All mimsy were the borogroves,
 And the mome raths outgrabe.

"Beware the Jabberwock, my son!
 The jaws that bite, the claws that catch
Beware the Jubjub bird, and shun
 The frumious bandersnatch!"

He took his vorpal sword in hand:
 Long time the manxome foe he sought—
So rested he by the Tumtum tree,
 And stood awhile in thought.

And, as in uffish thought he stood,
 The Jabberwock, with eyes of flame,
Came whiffling through the tulgey wood,
 And burbled as it came!

One, two! One, two! And through and through
The vorpal blade went snicker-snack!
He left it dead, and with its head
He went galumphing back.

And hast thou slain the Jabberwock?
Come to my arms, my beamish boy!
O frabjous day! Callooh! Callay!
He chortled in his joy.

'Twas brillig and the slithy toves
Did gyre and gimble in the wabe:
All mimsy were the borogroves,
And the mome raths outgrabe.

The Little Crocodile

How doth the little crocodile
Improve his shining tail,
And pour the waters of the Nile
On every golden scale!

How cheerfully he seems to grin,
How neatly spreads his claws,
And welcome little fishes in
With gently smiling jaws.

"Jabberwocky" has been chosen because it contains twenty-nine words created by the poet. Each of these words looks, sounds, and functions grammatically as an English word and is dispersed freely within the larger text composed of real English words. Therefore, this study will apply the theory of phonology as human behavior not only to poetry but also to a minilexicon of neologisms in English created by a single man.[3]

The Analysis

The Number of Syllables per Word

The corpus was first divided into monosyllabic, bisyllabic, trisyllabic, and polysyllabic words. The nonrandom skewing is quite apparent, clearly

Table 6.1 Number of Syllables per Word (General Corpus)

Number of Syllables	Number of Words
One	68
Two	24
Three	7
Four	1
Total	100

Table 6.2 Number of Syllables per Word (Neologisms)

Number of Syllables	Number of Words	%
One	6	21
Two	16	55
Three	6	21
Four	1	3
Total	29	100

favoring monosyllables, followed by words with two, three, and four syllables, in a sharply descending order, as seen in table 6.1. The monosyllabic words (sixty-eight) greatly outnumber the bisyllabic (twenty-four), trisyllabic (seven), and polysyllabic (one) words. We see a sharp drop in number in descending order from monosyllabic to polysyllabic words. This indicates a clear-cut synergetic favoring of maximum communication with minimal effort, which is reflected in child language acquisition (one word–one syllable utterances) as well as in human communication in general.

The syllable structure of Carroll's neologisms differs from the syllable structure of the words in the larger corpus, as can be seen in table 6.2, which indicates that twelve of the twenty-nine words (roughly 42 percent) are either monosyllabic (six) or trisyllabic (six); that sixteen of the twenty-nine words (roughly 55 percent) are in the middle of the road, or bisyllabic; and that one word of twenty-nine (roughly 3 percent) is a polysyllabic word of four syllables. If we examine Carroll's neologisms—the special words in the text—we find that the usual favoring of monosyllabic words is not maintained. This is not too surprising. These special words have unique meanings and connotations and are worthy of more attention and effort. Yet the number of monosyllabic and trisyllabic words is about equal, and bisyllabic words are predominant and polysyllabic words highly disfavored.

Stress Skewings

Both the regular English words containing more than one syllable—which usually have initial stress—and the neologisms strongly favor initial stress. The distribution for word-initial, word-medial, and word-final stress for the general corpus may be found in table 6.3, which indicates that twenty-seven of the thirty-two words of more than one syllable (roughly 85 percent) have initial stress; that only one trisyllabic word in the thirty-two-word corpus (roughly 3 percent) has medial stress; and that four bisyllabic words in the thirty-two-word corpus (roughly 12 percent) have final stress. The distribution of word stress per word position for the corpus of Carroll's neologisms appears in table 6.4, which indicates that twenty of the twenty-three neologisms of more than one syllable (roughly 87 percent) have initial stress; that two of the twenty-three neologisms of more than one syllable (roughly 12 percent) have medial stress; and that only one of the twenty-three neologisms of more than one syllable (roughly 3 percent) has final stress.

It has already been established that word-initial position carries the heaviest burden on spoken communication. Word-initial stress may be viewed as catering to the need to put the maximal effort in initial position. A similar strategy can be found in writing classes. Students are taught to write clear and concise opening sentences, a complete introduction, and topic sentences for each paragraph. Indeed, just as hearers may tend to fill in information and therefore pay less attention in utterance-medial and utterance-final positions, the same goes for readers. Readers often skim by reading the opening words and the beginning of each paragraph in order to receive the general message or the basic information of a text.

Table 6.3 Stressed Syllables (General Corpus)

Word Position	Number of Words	%
Initial	27	85
Medial	1[a]	3
Final	4[b]	12
Total	32	100

[a]Trisyllabic.
[b]All bisyllabic.

Table 6.4 Stressed Syllables (Neologisms)

Word Position	Number of Words	%
Initial	20	87
Medial	2	9
Final	1	4
Total	23	100

There is great disfavoring for medial stress, which also reflects human short-term memory. People have been shown to recall initial and final members of series and forget the medial segments. The majority of trisyllabic words and the single polysyllabic word favor initial stress. None of the trisyllabic words or the single polysyllabic word had final stress. This might be connected with the planning and organization of the air. People prefer to save their energy and air and exploit them where it counts to elicit more efficient communication.[4]

The Disfavoring of Additional Articulators in Initial Position

The difficulty of learning to control more than one set of articulators simultaneously has been established for English, Italian, and Hebrew for those phoneme pairs where voicing served as a distinctive feature as well as for nasals. Diver (1979: 174) likened the control of two sets of articulators to the childhood game of trying to pat your stomach and rub your head at the same time.

In word-initial position—the position with the highest communicative load—there is an almost random distribution of phonemes.[5] The reason for this free distribution is that, for initial position, the more oppositions the merrier and therefore the more efficient the communication. However, even in word-initial position, the principle of the disfavoring of additional articulators is still upheld within both the general corpus and the corpus of neologisms. The slight disfavoring of additional articulators in word-initial position for the pairs /p, b; t, d; k, g; f, v; θ, ð; s, z; ʃ, ʒ; t͡ʃ, d͡ʒ) distributes as shown in table 6.5.

Of the sixty-four words in the general corpus beginning with pairs of phonemes of constriction for which voicing serves as a distinctive phonemic feature, phonemes of constriction requiring the activation of only one set of articulators are slightly favored (thirty-four of sixty-one words, roughly 56 percent), and phonemes of constriction requiring the activation of two sets of articulators are slightly disfavored (twenty-seven of sixty-one words, roughly 44 percent). This slight disfavoring of additional articulators is not absolute or across the board: /b/ (twelve) is strongly favored over /p/ (one); /ð/ (three) is slightly favored over /θ/ (two), which may be accounted for by the presence of the function words *the* and *that;* and /d͡ʒ/ (six) is favored over /t͡ʃ/ (one), which may be accounted for by the words *Jabberwocky* and *Jabberwock.* The same tendency for the disfavoring of additional articulators is also evident for nasals: there are only four words in the entire corpus of one hundred words that begin with /m/ and no words that begin with /n/. It should be noted that these disfavorings are similar to the results obtained for the specific languages examined by the theory.

The neologisms also support the principle of a slight disfavoring of additional articulators in word-initial position. Not unsurprisingly, the number of phoneme pairs in the corpus is more limited and includes /p, b; t, d; k, g; f, v; s, z; t͡ʃ, d͡ʒ/ (see table 6.6). Of the eighteen words in the corpus of Carroll's neologisms beginning with pairs of phonemes of constriction for which

Table 6.5 Voicing in Word-Initial Position (General Corpus)

Mobile +/– Pairs						Stable +/– Pairs										Totals	%
p	1	t	9	k	7	f	4	θ	2	s	8	ʃ	2	t͜ʃ	1	34	56
b	12	d	3	g	2	v	1	ð	3	z	0	ʒ	0	d͜ʒ	6	27	44
																61	100

Table 6.6 Voicing in Word-Initial Position (Neologisms)

Mobile +/– Pairs						Stable +/– Pairs						Totals	%
p	0	t	3	k	2	f	2	s	2	t͜ʃ	1	10	56
b	4	d	0	g	2	v	1	z	0	d͜ʒ	1	8	44
												18	100

voicing serves as a distinctive phonemic feature, phonemes of constriction requiring the activation of only one set of articulators are favored (ten), and phonemes of constriction requiring the activation of two sets of articulators are slightly disfavored (eight). This disfavoring of additional articulators is not absolute or across the board: /b/ (four) is favored over /p/ (0); and /k/ (two) and /g/ (two) and t͜ʃ (one) and d͜ʒ (one) are equal. The same tendency for the disfavoring of additional articulators is also evident for nasals: there are only three words in the corpus of twenty-nine neologisms that begin with /m/ and no words that begin with /n/. This is particularly interesting in the light of the fact that three of the four words in the entire corpus beginning with nasals are neologisms. It may be that the lesser extent of the favoring of additional articulators in the "Jabberwocky" corpus is accounted for by the fact that neologisms—which are inherently marked semantically and pragmatically—may be isomorphically marked phonologically as well.

Active Articulators in Word-Initial Position

It has already been clearly established that word-initial position holds the greatest burden of communication and therefore has the most random

Table 6.7 Distribution of Active Articulators in Word-Initial Position (General Corpus)

	Lips (/p, b, f, v, w, m/)	Apex (/t, d, θ, ð, s, l, r/)	A-P-Dorsum (/ʃ, k, g/)	Larynx (/h/)	Total
No.	30	30	11	6	77
%	39	39	14	8	100

distribution of phonemes of constriction with reference to active articulators as well. In other words, in that phonetic environment that demands the most communicative oppositions, speakers exploit as many different active articulators as possible.

This principle is evident in the word-initial position of the following active articulators and phonemes in the general corpus: lips: /p, b, f, v, w, m/; apex: /t, d, θ, ð, s, l, r/; (antero-/postero-) dorsum: /ʃ, k, g/; and larynx: /h/ (see table 6.7). Of the seventy-seven words in the corpus that have phonemes of constriction (excluding affricates employing two active articulators) in word-initial position, there is a random distribution of labial and apical phonemes of constriction (thirty, or roughly 39 percent, for each), followed by a slight favoring of dorsal (both antero- and postero-) phonemes of constriction (eleven, roughly 14 percent) over the laryngeal phoneme of constriction /h/ (six, roughly 8 percent). It should be remembered that similar distributions were obtained for the specific languages examined for this principle as well.

This principle of close to random distribution for active articulators in word-initial position is also supported in the corpus of neologisms consisting of a smaller number of phonemes, including the following: lips: /b, f, v, w, m/; apex: /t, s, l, r/; and posterodorsum: /k, g/ (see table 6.8). Among the twenty-two words in the corpus of neologisms that have phonemes of constriction (excluding affricates) in word-initial position, there appears to be less of a random distribution: there is a favoring of labial phonemes of constriction (twelve, roughly 55 percent), followed by apical (six, roughly 27 percent) and dorsal (both antero- and postero-) (four, roughly 18 percent) phonemes of constriction. This favoring of labials in initial position is not new and leads to the next major principle in the theory of phonology as human behavior: visible phonemes are favored in initial position.

Table 6.8 Distribution of Active Articulators in Word-Initial Position (Neologisms)

	Lips (/b, f, v, w, m/)	Apex (/t, s, l, r/)	A-P-Dorsum (/k, g/)	Total
No.	12	6	4	22
%	55	27	18	100

The Favoring of Visible Phonemes in Word-Initial Position

We have just seen that visible phonemes are favored in word-initial position for the corpus of neologisms, which, of course, makes supreme sense for such new and unique words. We have also seen what appears to be a random and equal distribution between labial and apical phonemes of constriction (thirty each) in word-initial position for the larger corpus. However, the apical fricatives /θ/ and /ð/ have either the upper front teeth or the apex protruding between the upper and lower teeth as their dental passive receptor, thus making them apicodental fricatives. Concerning dentals, Ladefoged (1982: 6–7) has stated: "Some people have the tip of the tongue protruding below the upper front teeth; others have it close behind the upper front teeth. Both these kinds of sounds are normal in English and both may be called dental." And compare Bronstein (1960: 85): "The fricative continuant *th* sounds are tip of tongue-teeth sounds, emitted orally. They are made with the tongue-tip in contact with the inner surface of the upper teeth, or with the tongue-tip between the upper and lower incisors."

If we now include the apicodental phonemes /θ, ð/ among the visible phonemes of constriction—which indeed they are (particularly the interdental ones), according to lip-readers—we may also find evidence for a slight favoring of visible phonemes of constriction in word-initial position in the general corpus as well (see table 6.9). There are thirty-five (roughly 46 percent) visible phonemes of constriction (involving the lips and the teeth), /p, b, f, v, w, m, θ, ð/; twenty-five (roughly 32 percent) less visible or nonvisible phonemes of constriction made by the apex, /t, d, s, l, r/; eleven (roughly 14 percent) less visible or nonvisible phonemes of constriction made by the dorsum (both antero- and postero-), /ʃ, k, g/; and six (roughly 8 percent) instances of the less visible or nonvisible laryngeal phonemes of

Table 6.9 The Favoring of Visible Phonemes in Word-Initial Position (General Corpus)

	Visible: Lips/Teeth (/p, b, f, v, w, m, θ, ð/)	Nonvisible: Apex (/t, d, s, l, r/)	Nonvisible: A-P-Dorsum (/ʃ, k, g/)	Nonvisible: Larynx (/h/)	Total
No.	35	25	11	6	77
%	46	32	14	8	100

constriction, /h/. Similar results were obtained for the specific languages examined for this principle as well. Furthermore, it should always be remembered that most of the phonemes of aperture are also visible because the lips are either spread or rounded in their articulation, thus greatly increasing the number and percentage of visible phonemes in word-initial position.

Explosive Phonemes Are Favored in Word-Initial Position

The favoring of explosive phonemes of constriction in initial position has already been established in the previous chapters, particularly for the *BeGeDKeFeT* alternation in Hebrew. The favoring of the explosive mobile phonemes of constriction /p, b, t, d, k, g/ over the stable nonexplosive phonemes of constriction /f, v, θ, ð, s, z, ʃ, ʒ/ is found in the general corpus. If we examine the data displayed in table 6.10, we find that thirty-four of fifty-four (roughly 63 percent) words have mobile, explosive phonemes in word-initial position and that twenty of fifty-four (roughly 37 percent) words have stable, nonexplosive phonemes in word-initial position.

In the corpus of neologisms, explosive phonemes are also favored for a more limited number of phonemes of constriction: /b, t, k, g/ versus /f, v, s/. If we examine the data contained in table 6.11, we find that eleven of the sixteen (roughly 69 percent) words have mobile, explosive phonemes in word-initial position and that five of the sixteen (roughly 31 percent) words have stable, nonexplosive phonemes in word-initial position. These favored versus disfavored distributions are similar to those obtained in the specific languages examined for the principles of the theory as well.

Table 6.10 The Favoring of Explosive Phonemes in Word-Initial Position (General Corpus)

	Explosive: Mobile (/p, b, t, d, k, g/)	Nonexplosive: Stable (/f, v, θ, ð, s, ʃ/)	Total
No.	34	20	54
%	63	37	100

Table 6.11 The Favoring of Explosive Phonemes in Word-Initial Position (Neologisms)

	Explosive: Mobile (/b, t, k, g/)	Nonexplosive: Stable (/f, v, s/)	Total
No.	11	5	16
%	69	31	100

The number of explosive mobile and nonexplosive stable consonants in word-final position were compared as well. For the general corpus, there was a random distribution of thirty-nine each in both positions. For the neologisms, however, there was a very slight favoring of nonexplosive stable phonemes in word-final position: nine stable and seven mobile phonemes of constriction.

Apical Consonants Are Favored in Word-Final Position

The favoring of phonemes of constriction made by the apex—the most adroit of the active articulators—has already been established for all the languages studied for word/stem/root-final position. It is in final position where the burden of communication is at the lowest and the least amount of effort needs to be expended in the synergetic struggle for maximum communication with minimal effort. The nonrandom favoring of apical phonemes of constriction in word-final position is found in the general corpus containing the following phonemes and active articulators: lips: /b, v, m/;

Table 6.12 The Favoring of Apical Articulators in Word-Final Position (General Corpus)

	Lips (/b, v, m/)	Apex (/t, d, s, z, l, r/)	A-P-Dorsum (/ʃ, k, g, ŋ/)	Total
No.	10	50	7	67
%	15	75	10	100

Table 6.13 Percentage of Active Articulators in Word-Initial and Word-Final Position (General Corpus)

	Word Initial (%)	Word Final (%)
Lips	39	15
Apex	39	75
Antero-/posterodorsum	14	10
Larynx	8	

apex: /t, d, s, z, l, r/; antero-/posterodorsum: /ʃ, k, g, ŋ/. The data displayed in table 6.12 indicate that apicals are highly favored, fifty of sixty-seven (roughly 75 percent) of the phonemes of constriction in word-final position being produced with the apex; that ten of sixty-seven (roughly 15 percent) of the phonemes of constriction in word-final position are produced with the lips; and that seven of sixty-seven (roughly 10 percent) of the phonemes of constriction in word-final position are produced with the antero- or posterodorsum (all of which are found in the neologisms).

If we compare the percentage of the distribution of active articulators in word-initial and word-final positions for the general corpus, we find a sharp increase for the exploitation of the apex and a decrease for all the other articulators (see table 6.13). Similar favorings were found in the specific languages examined for this principle as well, and more extreme favorings have been discussed in Diver (1979, 1993, 1995).

The favoring of apical phonemes of constriction in word-final position is

Table 6.14 The Favoring of Apical Phonemes in Word-Final Position (Neologisms)

	Lips (/b, m/)	Apex (/d, s, z, l, r/)	A-P-Dorsum (/ʃ, k, g, ŋ/)	Total
No.	5	8	7	20
%	25	40	35	100

Table 6.15 Percentage of Active Articulators in Word-Initial and Word-Final Position (Neologisms)

	Word Initial (%)	Word Final (%)
Lips	55	25
Apex	27	40
Antero-/posterodorsum	18	35

so slight that it can be seen as being almost random in the corpus of neologisms for the more limited phonemes: lips: /b, m/; apex: /d, s, z, l, r/; and antero-/posterodorsum: /ʃ, k, g, ŋ/. The data found in table 6.14 indicate that apicals are very slightly favored, in that eight of twenty (roughly 40 percent) of the phonemes of constriction in word-final position are produced with the apex; that seven of twenty (roughly 35 percent) of the phonemes of constriction in word-final position are produced with the antero- or postero-dorsum; and that five of twenty (roughly 25 percent) of the phonemes of constriction in word-final position are produced with the lips.

If we compare the percentage of the distribution of active articulators in word-initial and word-final positions for the corpus of neologisms, we find sharp increases for the apex and antero-/posterodorsum and a decrease for labial phonemes of constriction (see table 6.15). Once again, it may be true that these unique neologisms are more highly marked semantically and pragmatically and therefore may exploit more active articulators even in word-final position, where the communication load is low.

Table 6.16 The Disfavoring of Additional Articulators in Adjacent Phonetic Environments (General Corpus)

	Monosyllabic	Polysyllabic	Polysyllabic Problematic
CC	6	8	20
CVC	15	26	26
	22	34	46

The Disfavoring of Additional Articulators in Adjacent Phonetic Environments

It was found that additional articulators were disfavored in the phonemic inventories of all the languages studied. It was further discovered that additional articulators in adjacent environments were disfavored in the Hebrew triconsonantal (CCC) root system in CI + CII and CI + CIII positions where the disfavoring was the strongest for the former, more adjacent phonetic environment. The disfavoring of additional articulators in adjacent phonetic environments was found to hold for consonant clusters across languages as well.

The number of sets of articulators—voiceless (0), voiced (+1), nasal (+2)—being exploited in adjacent phonetic environments was also examined for the monosyllabic and polysyllabic (two or more syllables) words in the corpora. The polysyllabic words were then divided into syllables, and each syllable was analyzed separately as either containing a consonant cluster (CC) or comprising the consonant-vowel-consonant (CVC) syllable structure. The number of monosyllabic words and the syllables within polysyllabic words in which the number of sets of articulators is repeated in adjacent phonetic environments distribute as shown in table 6.16.

In the monosyllabic words, the repetition of the same sets of articulators occurred twenty-two times. This represents 32 percent of the sixty-eight monosyllabic words in the corpus, indicating a clear disfavoring of this kind of collocation. There is also a sharp drop for the tendency to repeat the same number of articulators in consonant clusters (CC) (six) as opposed to syllables of the consonant-vowel-consonant (CVC) variety (fifteen), indicating

Table 6.17 The Disfavoring of Additional Articulators in Adjacent Phonetic Environments (Neologisms)

	Monosyllabic	Polysyllabic	Polysyllabic Words in Corpus
CC	0	5	8
CVC	2	20	26

that the more adjacent the environment, the less likely that similar sets of articulators will be used. These data are similar to the Hebrew triconsonantal (CCC) root data discussed in chapter 4 as well as to the data for all the consonant clusters studied in all the languages.

After the thirty-two polysyllabic words were divided into syllables, thirty-four occurrences of the repetition of the same set of articulators were found, indicating a tendency for this kind of collocation to occur in words of more than one syllable. However, if we count the number of syllables found in all the polysyllabic words (seventy-three), we see that this tendency constitutes only 44 percent of all the syllables in polysyllabic words. Once again, this disfavoring is stronger for syllables with consonant clusters (CC) (eight) than for syllables of the consonant-vowel-consonant (CVC) type (twenty-six), indicating that the closer the proximity, the more effort and control are necessary to produce these consonant clusters.

Kurtz (1992) attributes the disfavoring of the collocation of consonants that entail the simultaneous excitation of two or more sets of articulators in adjacent environments to the human factor. The simultaneous control of two sets of articulators, particularly the vocal folds, over an extended period of time requires a great deal of effort. She compares the disfavoring of additional articulators in adjacent environments to doing sit-ups. The first sit-up is relatively easy, but, as one continues, the exercise becomes harder because the same set of muscles is being used continuously without enough time to relax.

The corpus of neologisms was also examined for the disfavoring of additional articulators in adjacent phonetic environments. Not unsurprisingly, it was found that the majority of the polysyllabic words in which the same number of sets of articulators occurred in adjacent environments were among the neologisms (see table 6.17).

The neologisms increased the disfavoring of additional articulators in adjacent environments for the general corpus. The twenty-nine neologisms account for 63 percent of all the polysyllabic words containing consonant clusters. The neologisms further constitute 77 percent of all the polysyllabic words of the CVC type as well. However, the principle of the disfavoring of additional articulators in adjacent environments still holds for the neologisms. There are fifty-four syllables in all the polysyllabic neologisms, which indicates that only 37 percent of all the polysyllabic neologisms contain the repetition of the same set of articulators in adjacent environments. The monosyllabic neologisms of the CVC type (two) also show an obvious disfavoring (32 percent). Once again, words or syllables of the CVC type that require less effort and control allow for the repetition of the same set of articulators in adjacent environments more than words or syllables containing consonant clusters.

The Disfavoring of the Same Articulators in Adjacent Phonetic Environments

The principle of the disfavoring of the same articulators in adjacent phonetic environments was found to be the strongest principle for initial consonant clusters in English, and it has also been confirmed in all the other languages studied as well. Not unsurprisingly, the repetition of the same active articulators within monosyllabic words and within the individual syllables of the polysyllabic words was found to be disfavored both in the general corpus and among the neologisms. It is also not surprising that within the general corpus the apex was the active articulator most repeated (see table 6.18).

There are only twenty monosyllables of sixty-eight (roughly 29 percent) that use the same active articulators, of which seventeen (roughly 85 percent) exploit the apex, which has been established as the most adroit of the active articulators. Diver (1979: 19) likened the frequent use of the apex to the preference of right-handed people for using the right hand to perform difficult tasks.

If we examine the number of polysyllabic words that use the same active articulators in the same syllable (fourteen), of the total number of polysyllabic words (thirty-two), the disfavoring is not very strong (roughly 45 percent). However, if we compare the same number of syllables containing

Table 6.18 The Distribution of the Same Articulators in Adjacent Phonetic Environments (General Corpus)

		Apex Used
Monosyllabic words	20	17
Polysyllabic words	14	7
	34	24

the same active articulators (fourteen) with the number of syllables found in all the polysyllabic words (seventy-three), there is a much greater disfavoring (roughly 19 percent). Eight of these fourteen collocations of phonemes of constriction made by the same active articulators within the same syllable are made with the apex (65 percent).

Thirty-five (of one hundred) words employ the same active articulators in adjacent phonetic environments (35 percent), which in itself represents a disfavoring. Once again, this disfavoring is directly linked to the difficulty of controlling the same musculature for an extended period of time. Kurtz (1992) compares this disfavoring to trying to hammer a particularly stubborn nail into a very hard piece of wood. After a few minutes, your arm gives out, and you lose control over the hammer.

Only 22 percent of the words in the corpus were found to use the same articulator in both word-initial and word-final positions, which, in itself, indicates a strong disfavoring. Diver (1979) finds a parallel to this in boxing, where a skilled boxer continuously uses an "educated left jab" to fend off his opponent until the proper moment appears for his right-hand knockout. This kind of skill takes training and control. The unskilled boxer rushes in, alternating between this right and his left, which shows a natural avoidance of using the same musculature. It is particularly interesting to note that, in eighteen of the twenty-two words (82 percent) that employ the same active articulator in word-initial and word-final positions, the apex—the most adroit active articulator—is used.

A similar disfavoring of the same articulators in adjacent environments can be found in the corpus of neologisms as well. Half the monosyllabic neologisms (three of six, or 50 percent) and about a third (eight of twenty-three, or 36 percent) of the polysyllabic neologisms reuse the same active articulators, as can be seen in table 6.19. The skewings of the disfavorings

Table 6.19 The Distribution of the Same Articulators in Adjacent Phonetic Environments (Neologisms)

		Apex Used
Monosyllabic words	3	1
Polysyllabic words	8	4
	11	5

here are similar to those of the entire corpus—twelve words of twenty-nine (roughly 40 percent). The apex accounts for almost half the repetitions, followed by the lips. Five of the twenty-nine neologisms (roughly 17 percent) employ the same articulators in word-initial and word-final positions, indicating an even stronger disfavoring.

The Disfavoring of the Same Phoneme in Adjacent Phonetic Environments

An even greater disfavoring of the use of the same phoneme—exactly the same musculature—in adjacent environments was also found for all the languages examined. This is also the case in both our corpora here. Three monosyllabic words were found to repeat the same phoneme in word-initial and word-final positions (*mome, dead,* and *did*), and one bisyllabic word employed the same phoneme in a single syllable (*mimsy*). Two bisyllabic words were found to repeat the same phoneme in word-initial and word-final positions (*manxome* and *little*). Of the six words that reuse the same phoneme in an adjacent phonetic environment, three are neologisms. The apex is the repeated active articulator for all the established words, and the lips are reused for all the neologisms (supporting the visibility principle previously discussed).

Initial Consonant Clusters

There were five examples of the kind of initial consonant clusters previously examined for English, Italian, Hebrew, and Yiddish: monosyllabic words were C_1 = stop/fricative and C_2 = /l/ or /r/. The examples include two differents—*blade* and *claws* (mobile + stable)—and three sames—*flame* and *slain* (stable + stable) and *tree* (mobile + mobile)—all of which come from the general corpus.

In addition, there were four polysyllabic words containing the same initial clusters, three of which appear in neologisms—two instances of sames, *brillig* and *crocodile* (mobile + mobile), and two instances of differents, *frabjous* and *frumious* (stable + mobile). The data for this phonetic environment are fundamentally random. The limited number of words (one hundred) in our corpus and their random and special nature (neologisms) may have influenced these results.

Summary and Conclusions

In this chapter, I have applied the theory of phonology as human behavior to the teaching of phonetics. These pedagogical applications are based on the fact that one of the underlying theoretical and methodological tenets of this theory is the existence of a strong interdependence between phonetics and phonology.

It must also be remembered that the theory of phonology as human behavior has been applied primarily to lexical analyses using dictionaries or the active vocabulary of the analyst as the database. The theory has also been applied to the analysis of a large number of texts as part of a course in phonology as human behavior at three different universities. In this chapter, I have presented the analysis of a specific text with very special metalinguistic and psycholinguistic implications. In the majority of cases, when the theory was tested in the text—both for the general corpus and for neologisms—the principles of the theory of phonology as human behavior were supported.

I have tried to show that the teaching of phonetics and phonology as well as textual phonological analyses can be described and explained by directly appealing to the principles of the theory of phonology as human behavior. The theory of phonology as human behavior is based on the synergetic principle of maximum communication with minimal effort and the trade-off between the human and the communication factors in language. This synergetic principle reflects the opposing roles and needs of encoders and decoders. This motto has served to explain most of the nonrandom distribution of phoneme systems within and across languages, in the historical development of languages, and in the creation of neologisms in poetic texts. In the final part of this volume, I shall discuss the developmental and clinical applications of the theory of phonology as human behavior.

IV

Phonology as Human Behavior

Developmental and Clinical Applications

The wealth of our experience makes it possible to give a structural analysis of language in its making and to look for general laws, or tendencies, if one prefers a more prudent formulation. At the beginning of this century M. Grammont stated the problem with impressive accuracy: In the child's speech, he said, there is "neither incoherence nor chance occurrences. . . . The child undoubtedly misses the mark, but he always deviates from it in the same fashion. . . . It is the consistency of the deviations which strikes us in his language and which, at the same time, allows us to understand the nature of the MODIFICATION." What, then, is the principle of this DEVIATION in the successive acquisition of phonemes?
—Roman Jakobson (1971: 7–8)

Every phonological system is a STRATIFIED STRUCTURE, that is to say, is formed of superimposed layers. The hierarchy of these layers is practically universal and invariable. It occurs in the synchrony of language; consequently we have to do with a PANCHRONIC ordering. If there exists a relationship of irreversible solidarity between two phonological values, the secondary value cannot exist without the primary and the primary cannot be eliminated without the secondary. This ordering is to be found in any EXISTING phonological system, and it governs all its mutations; the same ordering determines . . . the acquisition of language, a system in the process of build up; and—let us now add—it reappears in language disorders, where we have to do with a system in the process of regression and disintegration.
—Roman Jakobson (1971: 12–13)

7 Developmental Phonology and Functional Clinical Applications

Hearing and producing speech sounds are biological processes that enable the acquisition of spoken language. In its general meaning, phonology is a term that denotes sound pattern. . . .

Although phonology can be isolated to some degree from other components of language or from the overall behavior of humans, phonology is best understood in relation to language in toto and in relation to human biology [and behavior]. Ohala (1990) has argued that phonology should not be regarded as an autonomous area of study but as one that is fully understandable only in relation to other areas, such as phonetics. The same can be said about phonological development. Phonological development in the child occurs in a larger developmental context. —Raymond D. Kent (1992: 67)

The purpose of evidence adduced in support of a theory is not to prove that theory true but to demonstrate that competing theories account for facts less well and thus no longer demand our attention. Evidence, therefore, if it can unambiguously decide between competing theories, helps the discipline to spend its resources on only a few issues at a time. —J. J. Ohala (1986: 3)

Language Acquisition and Phonology as Human Behavior

I will begin this chapter with a brief summary of child phonology (Jakobson 1941/1968), also known as developmental phonology, from the point of view of the theory of phonology as human behavior. I will also discuss the theoretical and methodological implications of developmental phonology for language disorders as they have been discussed in the literature under the new rubric of *clinical phonology* (Crystal 1987 [1981]). Both developmental and clinical phonology have been embraced by a wide assortment of modern descriptive, generative, and what one might perhaps call postgenerative, natural, autosegmental, and nonlinear phonological theories. In the final part of this volume, I will discuss the application of the theory of phonology as human behavior to the clinic in order to explain certain elements of language development and disorders as well. But I shall now begin at the beginning with the important role played by Roman Jakobson, who initially showed the integral connection between developmental and clinical phonology before they were identified as such by later scholars working in these fields.

The Role of Roman Jakobson and Developmental Phonology

The first most fundamental and basic work on phonological development in children is Roman Jakobson's (1941/1968) *Kindersprache Aphasie und allgemeine Lautgesetze* (Child language, aphasia, and phonological universals), on which most, if not all, subsequent research in this area has been based or by which it has been inspired.[1] In an article giving a historical survey of phonological theory and child phonology, Lise Menn (1980: 23) characterizes Roman Jakobson's role in establishing the field of developmental phonology as part of a larger theory of general phonology as follows: "Child phonology is a young field. We occasionally consult sources of data perhaps 100 years old. However, we tend to go no further than Leopold's great work published in the 1930s and 1940s. Child phonology, as a field, whose theory is supposed to be part of a general theory of phonology begins with Jakobson's *Kindersprache, Aphasie und Allgemeine Lautgesetze* (1941). His elegant vision of the successive acquisition of phonemic contrasts became the standard account, cited everywhere, especially after Keiler's translation of *Kindersprache* in 1968."

The volume *Kindersprache* itself and the man who wrote it have a unique history as well. As Menn (1980: 27–29) elaborates:

> *Kindersprache* was published in 1941 in Sweden, where the author's long flight from the Nazis had taken him. He had no reason to believe that this last accessible refuge would remain safe; his book is almost certainly more speculative and daring that it would otherwise have been.
>
> World War II and delays in translation meant that the full work was little studied in this country until 1968, although it was well known in Europe and less detailed versions had been published earlier. Simplified versions of the acquisition theory were included in works in English written during the interim, notably Jakobson, Fant, and Halle (1955) and Jakobson and Halle (1956). These, however, were missing

many of the subtleties, exceptions, cautions, and details present in *Kindersprache*. In these works the reader finds an elegant theory grandly integrated with general linguistics and presented with force and assurance. There seems to have been no competing account that could be called a theory, and the preceding descriptive accounts were few in number.

Velten and Leopold became acquainted with *Kindersprache* shortly after its publication. They found its broad outlines valid and stimulating, admired it greatly, but, speaking from their excellent data bases, each offered some reservations and modifications. In one striking example of such a reservation, Leopold (1953) states clearly that, in the case he studied, babbling overlapped with speech for many months, flatly contradicting Jakobson's notion of a "silent period."

Such reservations, however, were not generally noticed; instead, an overwhelmed *ipse dixit* response to Jakobson's work was found in every general mainstream text, from McNeill's chapter in Mussen (1970) to the phonology section of Dale (1976). Cautions in a general work are not seen until Clark and Clark (1977). (Ingram's 1976[a] text has a critical discussion, but that work is specifically on phonology.) Consequently, those who had difficulties accepting Jakobson felt that they ought to do a great deal of fieldwork before they could publish counterarguments; one might suggest that the entire cautious and meticulous modern tradition of child phonology fieldwork was forged by this necessity. Referring to the framework set up in the introduction, we have Jakobson as a scientist from the center who made a highly economical initial extension from his structuralist phonology to child phonology. In retrospect, we can analyze his extension as having a strong interpolative component. The extremes are the child who makes no contrasts on the one end and the adult who maintains many on the other; the interpolation consists of the postulation of the successive sequence of contrasts, and some intermediate data points are taken into account in deriving the order in which those contrasts are supposedly acquired. The rest of the extension consists of the straightforward transfer of concepts and terminology (contrast, phoneme, minimal pair) and so falls under the heading of parallel projection. Jakobson proceeded from the infant to the adult in the most economical way, and was concerned only with accounting for the development of the behaviors of interest to structuralist phonology: the development of contrast. Though phonetics was discussed, it was not of theoretical concern: Jakobson was not trying to account for all of the acquisition of phonology, but only to show that one major aspect of it could be derived from his sweeping general theory. We must note that his general theory was not based on his acquisition theory, and does not logically depend on it. Unlike generative theory, Jakobson's general theory does not claim that it ought to depend on acquisition either. His account of phonological acquisition, like his account of aphasia, was primarily intended as an illustration of the power of the general theory.

Jakobson's study of child language is based on the acquisition of phonemes and distinctive features as the hypothetical units of child language acquisition, which, of course, has been the subject of much debate (see chap. 1, nn. 6–10).[2] His basic claims regarding phonological development have been summarized by de Villiers and de Villiers (1978: 38–39): "One of the most influential theories of phonological development in the early words is that of Roman Jakobson (1968 [1941]), based on his distinctive feature analysis of the sound systems of many languages. Jakobson made the following claims about phonological development: (1) Babbling is essentially unrestricted and bears no relation to the child's later acquisition of adult phonology. (2) Phonological development is best described in terms of the mastery of distinctive features. (3) The child does not approximate the adult's phonemes one by one, but he develops his own system of phonemic contrasts, not always using the same features as adults to distinguish between words. . . . (4) Finally, the pattern of phonological development in all children is systematic and universal."

From the point of view of phonology as human behavior, we accept Jakobson's choice of the phoneme and distinctive features as legitimate, hypothetical theoretical and methodological units of phonological analysis. It is interesting to note that even those linguists who categorically reject these notions and even summarily dismiss much of Jakobson's approach to development phonology still recognize its value and importance. According to Atkinson, Kilby, and Roca (1988: 329), "One of the best-known discussions of phonological development is offered by Roman Jakobson in his book *Child language, aphasia and phonological universals.* Much of what he says there is now regarded as inaccurate and certainly the data on which he based his generalisations are often anecdotal. Against this, however, his work shows remarkable sophistication in its attempt to explain phonological development and is usually taken as a reference point for any discussion of this topic." De Villiers and de Villiers (1978: 41–42) evaluate and summarize Jakobson's contribution to developmental phonology as follows: "We conclude, therefore, that there appears to be a regular development of correct production of distinctive features, as Jakobson claimed, but his specific predictions about the order of acquisition of phoneme contrasts are difficult to apply to the child's early words and seem to be incorrect in many instances.

There is also a great deal of individual variation among children in their early phonological development. Finally, we shall see . . . that Jakobson's arguments for the strict discontinuity between babbling and speech, and his claim that there is no general order of development in the babbling period, are false. Jakobson's contribution to the study of child phonology was his stress on the orderliness of the child's development and his concentration on the child's own phonological system."

Were I to point out a weakness in Jakobson's theory of child phonology, it would be that the concept of combinatory phonology, central to the theory of phonology as human behavior, was not sufficiently taken into consideration. This can be explained by what has been said in chapter 1: Jakobson and the Prague school concentrated on the teleological-functional-communication approach almost exclusively. Combinatory phonology adds the important role of the human factor as an explanatory device in phonology and phonotactics, and the theory of phonology as human behavior focuses on the interplay between the two.

The absence of a phonotactic level of explanation in Jakobson (1941/1968) was pointed out by Atkinson (1982: 27) in his discussion of several difficulties (to which he refers as "facts") in the interpretation of Jakobson (1941/1968): "Put alongside these facts the additional observations that Jakobson pays hardly any attention to the positions in which sounds appear and that he provides no explicit discussion of what it means to acquire a particular contrast, and it is apparent that his claims face many problems. Nevertheless, the theory has inspired a large number of studies which have assumed his framework (e.g. Velten 1943, Shvachkin 1948 [1973], Garnica 1971, 1973) and has provided the starting point for many less sympathetic treatments. More importantly, however, it retains many interesting features as a developmental theory." Atkinson, Kilby, and Roca (1988: 334) further elaborate on the specific problem of what they view as the inadequacy of Jakobson's theory from the point of view of phonotactics: "An approach which merely emphasises the acquisition of oppositions is going to be inadequate. It simply is not clear that children do acquire oppositions in any straightforward way—rather, they seem to control oppositions in some contexts and not in others—and it appears that we are going to have to take account of the whole of the child's developing phonological system, where this will include specifications of context-sensitive processes . . . if we wish to come to terms with this."

Atkinson and his colleagues, however, do not necessarily view these combinatory, phonotactic, context-sensitive processes as being part and parcel of theoretical phonological explanation from the point of view of the human factor, as I have claimed in this volume. Yet, despite this and all the other weaknesses of Jakobson's theory, it is still among the most highly valued approaches to developmental phonology, even among its harshest critics. Atkinson (1982: 37) adds the following concerning the success of Jakobson's theory and its isomorphic implications: "More worthy of emphasis is its level of success. This level of success, added to the claims Jakobson makes about the relationships between different areas of language study, makes this theory one of the most attractive of those available."

Having established Jakobson's crucial and controversial role in this area of developmental phonology, I will now discuss some of the more accepted tenets of his theory from the point of view of phonology as human behavior.

Jakobson's Claims and Phonology as Human Behavior

It has been established that Jakobson's theory of child phonology made several claims regarding the systematic opposition of phonemes and distinctive features that have been open to theoretical and methodological debate. De Villiers and de Villiers (1978: 39) shed light on one of the most fundamental empirical methodological problems involved in testing Jakobson's theory with the limited data elicited from young children (a topic that has been discussed in Kiparsky and Menn [1977] as well), at least from the point of view of speech production: "Jakobson's theory has proved difficult to test in studies of phoneme development. Part of the problem lies in the difficulty of determining which sound distinctions function to signal differences in meaning in the child's speech. Children simply do not produce enough minimal pairs, for example *pin* versus *bin,* words that differ only in one phoneme yet have different meanings [cf. chap. 1, n. 13, and chap. 2, n. 14]. The linguist therefore has to work a little like a detective, looking for clues that the child distinguishes between different phonemes."

However, Atkinson, Kilby, and Roca (1988: 330–31)—as well as most, if not all, other scholars—have accepted the following of Jakobson's claims for child phonology, which I will analyze according to the precepts of phonology as human behavior:

1. Children acquire back consonants only after they acquire front consonants.
2. Children acquire fricatives only after they acquire homorganic stops.

3. Children acquire affricates only after they acquire homorganic stops and fricatives.

4. Children acquire nasal vowels only after they acquire corresponding oral vowels.

These claims were then expanded by Jakobson to *laws of irreversible solidarity* for the distribution of oppositions across languages, and therefore statements 5–8, which follow, are parallel to or correspond with statements 1–4 above and may be considered to be universal principles:

5. If a language has back consonants, then it has front consonants.
6. If a language has fricatives, then it has homorganic stops.
7. If a language has affricates, then it has homorganic stops and fricatives.
8. If a language has nasal vowels, then it has corresponding oral vowels.

From the point of view of phonology as human behavior these principles are easily supported and explained. First, the front of the vocal tract contains the most adroit active articulators (lips, apex) and the largest number of passive receptors (teeth, alveolar ridge, hard palate), which are both easiest to control and provide the most potential communicative distinctions (bilabial, labial-dental, apical-dental [inter and otherwise] [cf. chap. 6], apical-alveolar, apical [or blade] palatal). The back of the vocal tract has less adroit articulators (antero-posterodorsum) and fewer passive receptors (soft palate, uvula), which are harder to control and provide fewer communicative distinctions. Therefore, Jakobson's tenets 1 and 5 make supreme sense when we view language as a constant struggle for maximum communication with minimal effort. Next, we have already learned in the previous chapters that mobile sounds (i.e., stops with zero [0] stricture, aperture, and airflow) appear more frequently and are easier to make than stable sounds (i.e., fricatives with a very slight [1] degree of stricture, aperture, and [turbulent] airflow), which require greater control of the musculature over time. Therefore, Jakobson's tenets 2 and 6 make supreme sense when we contrast these mobile and stable phonemes of constriction by the amount of control or effort needed to produce them. Then, in chapter 3 we learned that transitions from one distinct constriction to another within a single phoneme are disfavored. As Davis (1984/1987: 59) explained, this principle (factor T) is accounted for by the difficulty of performing two distinct tasks, even consecutively, with one organ in one gesture, a little like trying to open a bottle of champagne gradually. Therefore, Jakobson's tenets 3 and 7 make supreme sense when we contrast the amount of effort and control necessary to make simple sounds (stops and fricatives) and complex sound (affricates). Then again, we have already learned that the simultaneous control of more than one set of articulators increases the difficulty involved in the production of sounds. Nasal sounds, as natural as they may be (cf. chap. 2, n. 9, and chap. 4, n. 11), require the simultaneous control of three sets of articulators. Therefore, Jakobson's tenets 4 and 8 make supreme sense when we contrast the amount of effort and control necessary to make nasal vowels and oral vowels in general. The same principle also explains why so few languages actually have nasal vowels as phonemes (cf. chap. 3, n. 18). Ultimately, if, indeed, these are universal concepts, their universality more probably rests on cognitive and perceptual aspects related to the human factor than on any linguistic or phonological principle per se.

Ingram (1976b: 17–22) also discusses some of the hypotheses postulated by Jakobson (1941/1968) and Jakobson and Halle (1956) concerning the universal order of phoneme acquisition during what he refers to as the holophrastic stage of language acquisition (1–1½ years of age). During this particular period of language acquisition, children have a rather limited or primitive phonology, acquiring about fifty words, and their vocabulary expands rapidly (Nelson 1973). Many of the studies of child phonology reflect this early stage of language development. Some of the particular hypotheses postulated by Jakobson that Ingram discusses include more specific claims than the ones discussed above: the first syllables are CV or CVCV reduplicated; the first consonants are labial, most commonly [p] (or perhaps [m]); these are followed by [t] and [k]; and the first vowel is [a], followed later by [i] and/or [u].

Ingram checked these claims against lists of the first twenty-five forms recorded by diary-keeping parents of four normal children (Velten 1943; Menn 1971; Leopold 1947; Ingram 1974) and arrived at the following conclusions: With regard to syllable structure, CV is common, but VC also appears; there is individual variation in reduplicated syllables; and CVC syllables shortly follow. In terms of consonantal segments, the use of labials agrees with Jakobson's prediction; dentals are also prominent and are acquired quite early; velars are not among the first sounds; and nasals are not among the dominant first sounds of children. The basic vowel triangle is probably established during this period, thus supporting Jakobson's claims.

These results can also be accounted for by the theory of phonology as human behavior. As I have previously stated (chap. 2, n. 10, and chap. 6), syllable structure may be explained by the different communicative roles and relative degrees of strictures and kinds of airflow of phonemes of constriction versus phonemes of aperture. Consonants constrict the airflow and are therefore harder to make, but they provide better communicative oppositions. Therefore, it is not surprising that they are preferred in syllable-initial position, where the need for maximum communication is the greatest. Vowels provide maximal airflow and minimal constriction, which makes them easier to make, but they create communicative distinctions that are less clear-cut than those created by consonants. Therefore, it is not surprising that they usually intermediate between consonants within syllables and regulate the airflow that is constricted by consonants. Thus, vowels are most suitable to serve as the nuclei of syllables allowing for the free flow of air. Vowels also provide the greatest acoustic information in the form of clear-cut acoustic formants. Indeed, we usually identify the active articulators of consonants primarily by their relation to the transitions with the acoustic formants of vowels. The less frequent syllables containing initial vowels often appear in reduplications and might also be studied with regard to the degree of difficulty involved controlling the musculature when making the consonants following the vowels.

In terms of consonantal segments, the favoring of labials (which are both visible and easy to control), followed by dentals (the passive receptor for both the apex and the lips, which are easiest to control), has been discussed and substantiated by the theory in the previous chapters. By the same token, the disfavoring of velars (the passive receptor for the posterodorsum, which is relatively less flexible and more difficult to control than either the lips or the apex) and the nonoccurrence of other active articulators (e.g., the anterodorsum, the pharynx, and the larynx, which are even more difficult to control) have also been discussed and substantiated by the theory in the previous chapters. The strong disfavoring or nonoccurrence of nasals that require the control of three sets of articulators has already been explained as well.

The establishment of the basic vowel triangle in this early period of language acquisition confirms that the effort needed to produce /i/ and /u/, the highest front and back vowel extremes, in opposition to /a/, the lowest, central vowel (the one requiring the least effort), provides the child with the most efficient compromise for establishing maximum communication with a small investment in effort. This same principle of the search for maximum communication (front vs. back extremes vs. middle position in the oral tract) can also be seen in the favoring of the labial-apical-posterodorsal triad of active articulators for the phonemes of constriction.

Crystal (1987 [1981]: 34) presents a sample list of the chronological acquisition of phonemes for English-speaking children based on a synthesis of Ingram (1976b: chap. 2), Olmstead (1971), Sander (1961), and Templin (1957): by age 2 children have acquired /p, b, m, n, w/, by 2½ /t, d, k, g, ŋ, h/, by 3 /f, s, l, j/, by 4 /ʃ, v, z, r, ʧ, ʤ/, by 5 /θ, ð/, and later /ʒ/. Crystal then discusses the theoretical and methodological problems involved in attempting to list the order in which a child acquires the various phonemes of a language: "(i) the simplification of the phonological system and the information which is omitted in such phoneme acquisition lists regarding: (a) the appearance of a specific phoneme in all word/syllable positions, (b) the compatibility of adult versus children's phonological systems, (c) the correct articulation of all the allophones of a phoneme in all word positions for every word; (ii) the question of whether all children achieve the same level of mastery at that age [interpersonal variation]; (iii) the question of individual variation of mastery within the same child [intrapersonal variation]" (Crystal 1987 [1981]: 34).

Once again, if there are universal concepts of language or phonological acquisition, their universality most probably rests on cognitive and perceptual aspects related to the human factor in general rather than on any unique linguistic or phonological principle per se, for any child or in any specific language. It should also be noted, however, that the principles underlying the nonrandom distribution of phonemes can be seen to work in the same way for the acquisition of both consonants and vowels in all languages when we view human language in general, and phonology in particular, as the striving for maximum communication with minimal effort.

Post-1968 Claims and Phonology as Human Behavior

De Villiers and de Villiers also discuss studies published after the 1968 translation of Jakobson (1941) that present additional arguments against the phoneme as the primary unit for the study of child phonology. I would like to relate to this word- and syllable-oriented research, which will also be highly relevant to my clinical material, from the point of view of phonology as human behavior:

> Two other phonological aspects of the child's early words are worth noting. First, children seem to actively avoid producing words containing certain speech sounds and prefer words with other sounds that they have mastered (Ferguson and Farwell, 1975; Menn, 1976; Vihman, 1976; Ferguson, 1977[b]). A child might understand several adult words with nasals, but attempt to produce very few or none of them (Vihman, 1976). Other children might produce many words with bilabial stops or nasals and avoid fricatives or velars (Leopold, 1947). In each case the child seems to perceive the words appropriately in comprehension, but does not try to produce them.
>
> A second basis for selective production seems to be word shape. Some children will almost exclusively attempt CVCV words like *doggie, mommy, pretty,* or *baby;* others will only attempt CV(C) words. Children also frequently impose a specific word shape on their early words regardless of adult models, normalizing all words to CVCV or CV forms. The adult "baby talk" of most language communities typically provides similar phonologically simplified models for the child (Ferguson 1964, 1977[a]). (de Villiers and de Villiers 1978: 40–41)

These developmental phenomena dealing with selective production as well can be explained by the principles of phonology as human behavior:

> (1) The active avoidance of producing words with difficult sounds and substituting for them words containing sounds that have already been mastered (or are easier to produce) is a common phenomenon, one attested to in both children and adults. Such lexical avoidance has been discussed by Davis (1984/1987) regarding the choice of a lexical versus discourse methodology in phonological theory and is illustrated with an amusing note (see chap. 3, n. 2).
>
> (2) Children may perceive nasals, but, because the production of nasals involves the simultaneous excitation and control of three sets of articulators involving three different musculatures, some children may not be able to produce phonetically what they have perceived phonologically.
>
> (3) It has already been established that mobile stops with zero (0) stricture, aperture, and airflow appear more frequently and are easier to produce than stable sounds, that is, than fricatives with a very slight (1) degree of stricture, aperture, and (turbulent) airflow, which require greater control of the musculature over time.
>
> (4) The facts that nasals are among the most articulatory complex phonemes of constriction and that the bilabial nasal stop /m/ may have special status in child phonology has already been discussed in chapter 2, note 9.

(5) It has also been established that (apical and) labial sounds are easier to produce than dorsal sounds.

(6) Therefore, there may be a playoff of relative degrees of difficulty between bilabial stops and nasals versus apical and dorsal fricatives in child language development across languages.

(7) The fact that the CVC syllable and alternations thereof—CV(C) and CVCV—all begin with consonants followed by vowels has been discussed in chapter 2, note 10.

(8) It is also not surprising that children's phonology and adult baby talk represent a simplification of adult phonology since children do not have the fine motor ability and muscular control that are needed to produce the entire phonological system of a language (cf. Kent 1992).

(9) The fact that comprehension exceeds production ability is further support for the theoretical and methodological difference between abstract phonology and concrete phonetics (discussed in chap. 1 and passim).

(10) All the points discussed in (1), (2), (8), and (9) above indicate that many of children's errors or deviations reflect their phonetic ability rather than their phonological knowledge.

This leads us now to the next major step in developmental phonology: the examination of so-called natural phonological processes and the fundamental question of whether these processes are phonological or phonetic in nature. These issues are significant not only to the functional (or normal) processes of first language acquistion but to the pathological or organic processes found in the clinic as well.

Phonological Processes and Phonology as Human Behavior

The next major post-Jakobsonian development in child phonology was the study of generative rules of acquisition and natural phonological processes.[3] The place of phonological processes in child speech research has been defined and summarized by de Villiers and de Villiers (1978: 42) as follows:

We have so far considered two very different approaches to the development of speech sounds. One looks at the successive approximations of the child to the adult speech sounds (phones) and measures accuracy and frequency of production of the various vowels and consonants [Ferguson 1977b]. The other examines the acquisition of phonemic contrasts and distinctive features. This second approach attempts a phonemic analysis of child speech and measures the accuracy and frequency of production of distinctive features.

But there is a third approach that supplies us with information about regularities in the child's phonological development that is not captured by the other two. Neither of the other approaches concerns itself with consistent errors of regular substitutions for adult sounds that children typically make. The third approach attempts to characterize the child's development in terms of regular stages in his own speech sound system, to say why he consistently substitutes certain sounds for the adult sounds, and to characterize systematic strategies that he adopts to simplify his pronunciation of adult words. This is done by writing a set of phonological rules, rules for the combination of distinctive features or phonemes into words, for each stage of development. These rules relate what the child actually produces to what he is aiming at. Some linguists (for example, Smith, 1973) maintain that the child represents the adult word (his target) exactly. This assumes that the child *hears* the adult word correctly, but just cannot *produce* it. But the Garnica (1973) and Edwards (1974) studies of the developing perception of distinctive features demonstrate that the child's perception of the adult form of a word may often be inaccurate. The child is developing the ability to perceive the adult sounds at the same time as he is learning to produce them. Nevertheless, the phonological rules are usually written relating the adult form to the child's form of the word since it is extremely difficult to establish for each child his perception of the adult word at each stage of development.

The concept of phonological processes may be viewed as an attempt to include combinatory, phonotactic, or context-sensitive rules in developmental phonological research. It is not surprising that these natural processes found in normal language acquisition generally have been thought to represent different aspects of the child's simplification of the adult phonological system surrounding it. This is related, of course, to the difference between language perception and production and the fundamental question of whether these processes represent phonetic or phonological phenomena.[4]

Crystal (1987 [1981] 44) distinguishes between phonological and phonetic disability in both developmental and clinical phonology as follows:

> The distinction between the abstract phonological system (however defined) and the phonetic realization of that system is central to the enquiry. There are three main ways in which the relationship between these two levels of language organization can be abnormal:

(i) the phonological system is normal, but its phonetic realization is abnormal (*e.g.* immature or deviant pronunciations of phonemes, but without the range and pattern of phonemic use being affected);
(ii) the phonological system is abnormal, but its phonetic realization is normal (*e.g.* the range of phonemes used may be considerably delayed, but their pronunciation is within normal limits);
(iii) both the phonological system and its phonetic realization are abnormal; delay or deviance affecting both aspects of the analysis.
The notion of "phonological disability" could be applied to all three of these abnormal relationships, but it is more useful to restrict it to categories (ii) and (iii) only—that is, to cases where there has been a failure to learn or retain the underlying system. Category (i) problems would then be referred to as "phonetic disability."

I would like to take a stand on this phonology-phonetics issue. My experience has shown that usually most children in general, and all the subjects discussed in this chapter, perceive all the phonemic contrasts of their native language but may not have sufficient motor control to produce them. Therefore, in my view, most of the phonological processes discussed in the literature on developmental and clinical phonology are phonetic rather than phonological in nature. I believe that phonological processes or errors can be considered to have occurred only when it can be determined by discrimination tests that the phonological system perceived by the child differs from that of the adult language community. In other words, in my experience, most children's perception of the abstract phonological system of their language is usually complete, but their concrete phonetic production is limited. Very often their errors show subtle differences—usually not picked up by others—that indicate their own idiosyncratic phonetic renderings of different phonemes.[5]

As far as what constitutes linguistic competence, Dressler (1988: 5) considers that "competence represents the types, performance represents the respective tokens (Herdan 1966). Thus, if the tokens of a given type, for example, realization of a given phoneme, are never produced, one might assume that the type itself is unavailable. But this is rarely the case, at least for the structuralist concepts of phonemes and phonemic representations, and lack of production does not imply lack of comprehension (cf. Kohn, Schoenle, & Hawkins, 1984), for example, distinguishing and/or identifying a given phoneme."[6]

The following include most of the major and minor natural "phonological" processes found in functional (or normal) language acquisition (adapted from Grunwell 1982, 1987; Ingram 1976a, 1976b, 1989), accompanied by an explanation derived from the principles obtained from the theory of phonology as human behavior in the previous chapters:

Functional Processes Influencing Syllable Structure

1. Final consonant deletion: CVC → CV: *out* [au], *bike* [bai].
Explanation: Word-final position has less communicative force; consonants require more articulatory control (are harder to make) than vowels.

2. Deletion of unstressed syllable (usually in word-initial position): *banana* [næna].
Explanation: Stressed syllables give more communicative, perceptual, and cognitive information than unstressed syllables; the more syllables in the word, the more effort it takes to pronounce it; in noninitially stressed words, there is less information in word-initial position, which usually has the greatest communicative force.

3. Consonant cluster reduction: CC → C: *floor* [fɔr], *step* [tep].
Explanation: A consonant cluster requires greater effort than a consonant-vowel sequence and may be reduced or replaced at the expense of maximum communication; in addition, coarticulation by near articulators is disfavored; phonemes of constriction give clearer communicative distinctions than phonemes of aperture (that is why there are more consonants than vowels in language), but they require more articulatory control (hence the ideal CVC syllable).

4. Reduplication: repetition of a syllable or part of a syllable: *rabbit* [wæwæ], *noodle* [nunu].
Explanation: The reduplication often comes as a means to avoid more difficult sound combinations and/or to maintain the number of syllables in the word: sequences of phonemes with the same articulators are disfavored unless their juxtaposition is, by virtue of some other factor, mutually beneficial. I also found that newly acquired sounds were often reduplicated as a means of practice or of hypercorrection in the clinical situation.

5. Coalescence: characteristics of two consecutive sounds merge into one sound: *swim* [ʍim], *slide* [ɬaid].

Explanation: Fewer articulatory gestures resulting in fewer distinctive units at the expense of maximum communication.

6. Epenthesis: addition of segments, usually an unstressed vowel: *snow* [sənou], *drum* [dərʌm].
Explanation: The additional unstressed vowel often eases the transition to more difficult consonants or clusters.

Examples 5 and 6 above as well as assimilation processes 1 and 2 below may also be explained by the factor that sequences of phonemes with the same or near articulators are disfavored unless their juxtaposition is, by virtue of some other factor, mutually beneficial.

Assimilation Processes (Consonant/Consonant-Vowel Harmony)

1. Velar/nasal/labial etc. assimilation: *duck* [gʌk], *friend* [frɛ̃], *top* [bap].
Explanation: A nonvelar/nasal/labial sound changes to a velar/nasal/labial because of the influence or the domination of a velar/nasal/labial sound, which entails fewer articulatory gestures at the expense of maximum communication.

2. Prevocalic voicing of consonants: *pen* [bɛn], *tea* [di].
Explanation: An unvoiced consonant becomes voiced generally before a vowel: the speaker anticipates the control of two sets of articulators in what is usually a longer acoustic phonological segment.

3. Devoicing of final consonsants: *bed* [bɛt], *big* [bɪk].
Explanation: Additional articulators are disfavored; voiced consonants become unvoiced in word-final position; where the communicative force is least important or crucial, the speaker opts to activate one set of articulators rather than two.

Substitution Processes

Processes Reflecting the Substitution of Active Articulators

1. Fronting: back (nonapical) consonants are substituted for by apical consonants, usually preserving the same manner and voicing values: k → t

book [bʊt], g → d *dug* [dʌd], ʃ → s *shoe* [su], ʒ → z *beige* [beɪ͜ʒ], ŋ → n *sing* [sɪn].
Explanation: The apex is the most flexible and easy to control of all the active articulators: the earliest and most frequent examples of the substitution of active articulators are fronting and apicalization, which sharply reduce the number of communicative distinctions available to the speaker.

2. Backing: the back pronunciation of front sounds (usually consonants): t/d → k/g: *dog* [gɔg], *tiger* [ka͜ɪgə].
Explanation: A (possibly idiosyncratic) later, less frequent process where the dorsum (or other back articulators) replaces the apex (or other front articulators); it is often found in children who have difficulty controlling the musculature of the apex and/or try to reduce the number of communicative distinctions made by the apex (or other front articulators).

Processes Reflecting the Substitution of Turbulence and Airflow

1. Stopping: fricatives/affricates are replaced by stops: s/ts → t: *seat* [tit], *soup* [dup].
Explanation: Maximum constriction is favored particularly when mobile phonemes of constriction are easier to control than stabile phonemes of less constriction, which require greater control of the musculature since a small aperture must be created and maintained in order to produce a stronger turbulent airflow; this is the most frequent manner of substitution for children.

2. Affrication: stops/fricatives are replaced by affricates: t → t͜ʃ: *tree* [t͜ʃi].
Explanation: Maximum constriction precedes and leads into partial constriction and turbulent airflow since mobile phonemes of constriction require less articulatory control than stable phonemes of constriction, which produce greater turbulence; this is a less frequent manner of substitution for children.

3. Gliding of liquids: l/r → j/w: *rock* [wak], *lap* [yæp].
Explanation: This is the substitution of a lower for a higher degree of aperture (from consonants to semivowels), which may also require less articulatory control.

4. Vocalization: nasals and liquids (syllabic consonants) are replaced by vowels: *apple* [æpo], *flower* [fawo].
Explanation: This is the favoring of maximal aperture, particularly when

phonemes of aperture (vowels) require less articulatory control than phonemes of constriction (consonants).

5. Denasalization: m → b, n → d, ŋ → g: *no* [do], *home* [hob], *sung* [sʌg].
Explanation: Additional articulators are disfavored; nasal stops become their equivalent oral stops; two sets of articulators are exploited rather than three.

6. Deaffrication: ʧ → ʃ, ʤ → ʒ: chips [ʃips], *juice* [ʒus].
Explanation: Transitions from one distinct constriction to another within a single phoneme are disfavored; a more complex sound requiring greater effort or control is reduced to a less complex sound after the speaker has acquired the ability to produce the more difficult stable sounds (cf. affrication).

7. Glottal replacement: *butter* [bʌʔər].
Explanation: Additional articulators are disfavored; a glottal stop replaces an intervocalic consonant or a consonant in syllable-final position; articulatory control of one set of articulators rather than two in an appropriate phonetic environment.

8. Gliding of fricatives: /f/ → [w], /s/ → [l,j].
Explanation: A more extreme substitution of a lower for a higher degree of aperture (cf. point 3 above, the gliding of liquids) requiring less articulatory control: this is an idiosyncratic process.

Most of the processes reflecting the substitution of turbulence and airflow listed above confirm the following factors obtained from the theory of phonology as human behavior: among constrictions, maximal constriction is favored, and, among apertures, maximal aperture is favored.

It should be clear from the examples given above that more than one process can appear in the same word and that most of these functional processes can be related to the principles obtained from the theory of phonology as human behavior. It also should be noted that there is a chronology of natural processes that determines and separates normal processes from deviant functional or organic ones.

According to Grunwell (1987: 210), who has applied these processes to the clinic, Stampe (1969, 1979 [1972])—the founder of the theory of natural phonology from which these functional processes were derived—claims that they have "psychological reality," on the one hand, but are actually "articulatory" (i.e., phonetic, not phonological), on the other: "Stampe endows the processes with 'psychological reality' since he refers to them as 'mental operations'. He apparently regards them as reflexes of the natural production restraints which restrict the speech mechanism. In his view they are specifically *articulatory* restrictions, which inhibit the child *producing* sound differences he is well able to perceive auditorily."

The theory of natural phonology and these functional processes, however, have been presented as an explanatory theory of language development. These processes are considered to be universal and innate. I have tried to show here that the labeling, classification, and categorization of these (basically phonetic) processes merely describe the articulatory and phonotactic phenomena without explaining them. I have attempted to explain them by appealing to the principles of phonology as human behavior.

Functional Processes in Hebrew-Speaking Children

Although these natural functional processes are believed to be universal and innate, the clinical data that I will be presenting in this volume are taken from Hebrew speakers. For this reason, I will briefly present some of the data on functional processes culled from Hebrew-speaking children as well. In a very limited study, Shaked (1990) examined the frequency of functional errors of twenty Israeli children (from 1:7–2:7 years of age), with the following results.

The most frequent functional processes found include the following:

1. fronting, particularly of fricatives: ʃ/x → s *ʃalom* → [salom];
2. consonant cluster reduction: *pɣaxim* → [paxim] (flowers) (fricatives deleted, stops maintained);
3. syllable-final consonant deletion/medial consonant cluster reduction: *taxtonim* → [tatonim] (underwear);
4. devoicing of final consonants: *berez* → [beres] (faucet);
5. difficulty producing voiced stops (activating two sets of articulators for mobile consonants) (children 2–4 years);
6. deletion of unstressed syllables: *ambatja* → [batja] (bath);
7. gliding: 1 → j: *lelet* [jedet] (door) (+ metathesis);
8. deletion of syllable/word-initial consonant (in unstressed syllable): *mita* → [ita] (bed); and
9. deaffrication: *tsav* → [tav] (turtle).

The least frequent functional errors and processes found include the following:

10. backing (considered to be idiosyncratic by Grunwell [1982, 1987] and others): *mixtav* → [mitax] (letter) (+ consonant cluster reduction, + metathesis); and

11. stopping: *sus* → [tut] (horse).

Similar findings were also reported in Halperin (1984), Izmailov (1983), and Lavi (1978) for Hebrew-speaking children (aged 1:5–3, 3–4, and 3–5) regarding functional processes as well as norms for the acquisition of consonants.

Zonshain (1974) has studied the early one-word utterances of Hebrew-speaking children (1–1:6 years of age). Berman (1977) has studied the natural phonological processes at the one-word stage of her Hebrew-English bilingual daughter (1:6–1:11.5 years of age). These studies concentrated more on syllable and word structure rather than on the articulation of specific segments.

The processes uncovered in Berman (1977) conform to the previous studies done in natural phonology in general and in Hebrew in particular, including the following:

1. reduplication (discussed by Jakobson [1962a: 542] as a "necessary nursery device");
2. transposition (which may be viewed as metathesis on the syllable level);
3. deletion of consonant clusters in word-initial and word-medial (at syllable-boundary) positions;
4. deletion of individual consonants at word-initial and word-final positions, indicating a marked preference for CV and CVCV syllable structure and the subject's inability to produce #C . . . C# strings in her early speech development; and
5. syllable reduction (usually of nonstressed syllables).

The phonetic data presented in these studies conform to the explanations of natural functional processes according to the theory of phonology as human behavior discussed in the previous section. I have found that the phonetic data presented in other studies dealing with the acquisition of Hebrew from morphological and syntactic points of view (e.g., Bar-Adon 1971; Walden 1982) can be accounted for by the theory as well.

Gan (1994) examined the natural functional processes of six English-Hebrew bilingual children 3–4:5 years of age using English and Hebrew articulatory word tests to examine whether there was evidence of two distinct phonological systems or a single extended system for her bilingual subjects. Her results strongly indicated the existence of two distinct phonological systems, one for each language. It was also shown that both qualitatively and quantitatively there was a strong asymmetry between the functional processes found for both languages, which could be linked directly to the language-specific differences. Similar discrepancies in the processes found for both languages were also found for the data obtained from spontaneous responses when compared to responses elicited from imitation. All these differences were explained by the principles of phonology as human behavior as it was applied to each language (Diver 1979; Tobin 1990a, 1990c). These findings have also appeared in Gan, Ezrati, and Tobin (1995) and Gan (1995).

In addition, the theory of phonology as human behavior specifically has been applied to the language acquisition of a 4–6-month-old Hebrew-speaking and a 4:3-year-old bilingual Hebrew-English child (Segal 1993; Haran 1989). In both of these studies, the general order of acquisition of phonemes and functional processes conforms to that found in studies already discussed in this chapter and includes the following:

1. the systematic order of the exploitation of active articulators (labial-apical-posterodorsal);
2. the systematic favoring of consonants requiring extreme degrees of constriction and minimal airflow (stops preceding fricatives or mobile preceding stable phonemes of constriction); and
3. the disfavoring of phonemes of constriction requiring the excitation of more than one set of articulators (when there are phonemic oppositions based on this factor): voiceless (0) are most frequent, followed by voiced (+1) and the absence or extremely limited use of nasals (+2).

For all the studies involving monolingual Hebrew or bilingual Hebrew/English-speaking children, the simpler Hebrew five-vowel system (i, e, a, o, u) was acquired and produced without apparent error or deviation. The bilingual children showed both a delay in the acquisition and a difficulty in the production of the more complex English vowel system.[7] All these findings conform to the tenets of the theory of phonology as human behavior and clearly indicate the development of phonological systems reflecting a striving for maximum communication with minimal effort. The theory of phonology as human behavior has also been applied to the first language acquisition of a Russian-speaking child (Tsatkin-Pessin 1994).

Functional Processes in a Hearing Child of Deaf Parents

Samet (1993) investigated the functional processes of a hearing child of deaf parents and compared the frequency of the functional processes found in her study with those found for Hebrew speakers. Samet analyzed the speech of Elita (2:8), the daughter of deaf, signing parents who are Russian immigrants with a limited knowledge of Hebrew whose speech is extremely difficult to understand. Elita was brought for therapy because of late language development and a medial level of comprehensibility (possibly due to lack of input). Elita showed the following functional processes in descending order of frequency (according to Shaked 1990):

1. consonant cluster reduction: *bgadim* → [gadim] (clothes);
2. deletion of unstressed syllable: *tsalaxat* → [laxat] (plate);
3. syllable-final consonant deletion/medial consonant cluster reduction: *taxtonim* → [tatonim] (underwear);
4. final consonant deletion: *sipuɣ* → [sipu] (story);
5. initial consonant deletion: *le-ʃam* → [(ʔ)e-ʃam] (to-there);
6. stopping: *xatula* → [katula] (kitty); and
7. deaffrication: *ɣotsa* → [ɣota] (want).

Samet then applied the theory of phonology as human behavior to explain the processes. All these processes save for (5) initial consonant deletion clearly conform to the principles of phonology as human behavior. Example 5 indicating a possible initial consonant deletion appears in an unstressed function word *le,* "to," in the phrase *le-ʃam* → [(ʔ)e-ʃam] (to-there), which, from the point of view of communication, is less crucial than the stressed lexical item *ʃam,* "there," to which it is attached, making this example similar to the deletion of unstressed initial syllables previously mentioned. Elita also has functional processes not found in Shaked (1990):

1. assimilation: *beged* → [geged] (garment), *jeled* → [leled] (boy); and
2. epenthesis (very limited and including the addition of both consonants and vowels).

In the case of Elita, we have a situation where the number and the degree of functional processes require clinical intervention.

Functional processes in general have served as a basis for the evaluation of child language development both in and out of the clinic for at least two decades in English-speaking countries (e.g., Ingram 1976a, 1976b, 1979, 1981; Grunwell 1982, 1985, 1987; Smith 1973). Future studies in the functional processes of Hebrew-speaking children might also serve as a norm for the evaluation of the language development of children acquiring Hebrew as a native language. The underlying assumption that these functional processes represent norms in language acquisition has formed the basis for comparing and contrasting both adult and child language, on the one hand, and so-called normal and disordered language development in children, on the other. Much of the research done in first language acquisition and child language disorders generally has been based on the principles of Jakobsonian, generative, or natural phonological frameworks. One of the most crucial and disputed theoretical and methodological issues in this particular area of developmental phonology is whether children's phonological systems should be viewed as a mere simplification of adult systems or as independent and autonomous systems in their own right.[8]

Functional Clinical Applications

Throughout this book, I have stressed that the theory of phonology as human behavior is based on the synergetic principle of striving for maximum communication with minimal effort and the trade-off between the human and the communication factors in language related to the opposing roles and needs of encoders and decoders. This motto has served to explain the nonrandom distribution of phoneme systems within and across languages as well as the historical development of phonological systems within languages. This motto has also served as the pedagogical basis for a model of teaching phonetics and phonology and as a way of analyzing the phonological distribution of neologisms in a poetic text.

In this chapter, I have viewed child phonology as a more extreme example of this mini-max principle because of the developmental limitations on the child's control over the articulatory musculature. These limitations are exemplified by the natural functional processes that have been postulated for child phonology in English, Hebrew, and other languages.

As we have previously stated, functional processes have been assigned chronological values and may serve as norms for child language acquisition. If deviations from these chronological values and norms are discovered in a child's speech, that child may be sent for speech therapy. Children who are labeled as having functional disorders in their speech will usually reach the clinic when

1. early processes continue past their normal period,
2. early processes coexist with later errors and processes, or
3. normal functional processes are accompanied by idiosyncratic processes (such as backing, gliding of fricatives, or affrication).

Grunwell (1987: 232, 278) summarizes the analysis of disordered child speech according to the following criteria and classifications of developmental disorders:

1. *delayed development:* persisting normal processes;
2. *uneven development:* chronological mismatch; and
3. *deviant development:* systematic sound preference, unusual/idiosyncratic processes, and variable use of processes.

Functional processes that reach the speech clinic clearly reflect an even more extreme case of the struggle for maximum communication with minimal effort, usually under the following circumstances: The simultaneous coexistence of several functional and/or idiosyncratic processes of simplification (the human factor) reduce the number of communicative distinctions (the communication factor) exploited by the child. Only if and when the child becomes or is made aware that his or her communication is impaired will further effort be exerted to produce more communicative distinctions in the quest for maximum communication with minimal effort. In other words, the child will usually exert effort only in order to enhance communication.

Defining Language Disorders

Functional versus Organic Disorders

In the previous sections introducing the speech clinic, I have used such terms as *functional processes, disorders,* and *delayed* or *deviant language development* interchangeably. In clinical phonology—like all other kinds of phonological and linguistic theories—terminology and technical terms often become the source of much debate over whether "that which we call a rose by any other name would smell as sweet." I would like briefly to present some of the major issues and problems dealing with the nomenclature involved in clinical phonology as they have appeared in the literature in a roughly chronological order.

Ingram (1976b: 98) raises the issue of the interchangeability of terms and devotes almost two chapters in his book to the classification of different kinds of deviant phonology: "So far, several terms have been used interchangeably to refer to the phonological problems of these children [studied in the previous chapter]—dysfunction, disorder, deviance, disability, delay. These have been used simply to refer to a child whose speech requires attention. In this chapter I will group all these under the term 'deviance' and try to specify what is meant by each use."

Grunwell (1981: 4) considers children with phonological disabilities who are referred to speech therapists as having *severe functional articulation disorders:*

> The term "severe" refers to the tendency for the child's speech to be unintelligible, as a result of the large number of sounds mispronounced. "Functional" is the term used in both general medical science and speech pathology to imply that the disorder has no readily detectable organic basis and no other known aetiology. "Articulation disorder" indicates that there are specific pronunciation difficulties. The speech pathologist's view of this disorder can be deduced from the following typical quotation:
>
>> The term FUNCTIONAL ARTICULATION DISORDERS encompasses a wide variety of deviate speech patterns. These can all be described in terms of four possible types of acoustic deviations in the individual speech sounds: omissions, substitutions, distortions and additions. An individual may show one or any of these combinations. (Powers 1959, p. 711)
>
> It is evident from the above that though it is asserted, by the inclusion of the term "functional" that the disorder does not result from any structural or organic defect, the traditional approach entails the treatment of disordered articulation.

She implies and specifies the following as the structural or organic requirements necessary for a disorder to be classified as a functional rather than an organic disorder:

1. normal hearing for speech;
2. no anatomical or physiological abnormalities of the speech-producing mechanisms;
3. no detectable neurological dysfunction relevant to speech production;

4. intellectual abilities adequate for the development of spoken language; and
5. comprehension of spoken language appropriate to mental age.

It may be assumed that a lack of, or the presence of, one or more of the negatively defined criteria listed above would classify articulatory disorders as being organic rather than functional.

I shall follow this fundamental, dichotomous classification contrasting functional and organic disorders in this volume. I am aware, however, of the fact that many apparently functional disorders may be a result of slight organic or minor motor difficulties. Furthermore, there are additional ways of defining and classifying organic disorders as well. For example, according to Grunwell (1987: 287–88) (whose categorizations of articulatory, phonetic, and phonological disorders may also be open to disagreement), there are "confusable conditions of dysarthria—an articulation disorder; dyspraxia—a phonetic disorder; and dysphasia—a phonological disorder."

In short, many articulatory disorders may span the opposition between an extreme and rigid functional and an organic dichotomy. Speech therapists themselves may differ in their definition of what constitutes a functional or organic speech disorder or even disagree about whether a client has a particular organic disorder. In this volume, I will maintain a very broad distinction between functional articulatory disorders (discussed in this chapter) and organic ones (discussed in the following chapters). The reader should be aware that these classifications are being used in an informal way and are based on the original nomenclature, classifications, and diagnoses of the individual speech therapists who worked with each subject or client.

Common versus Individual or Idiosyncratic Processes

There is a further subcategorization of functional processes that has been made in the literature and that has already been mentioned: common, frequent, or primary functional processes as opposed to less common, individual, or idiosyncratic functional processes. Crystal (1987 [1981]: 38) introduces this distinction after presenting a list of the three basic kinds of processes previously discussed: substitution, assimilatory, and syllable-structure processes: "Several other individual processes have been suggested in the literature, some of fairly general applicability, some that seem to be idiosyncratic (*e.g.* Priestley 1977). In addition, there have been several proposals arguing for a hierarchical organization of these processes, *e.g.* Smith (1973, 1974) where harmony and cluster reduction are seen to be primary."

The determination of what is more general, frequent, common, or primary is not always as clear-cut or self-evident as may be imagined, particularly in such relatively new fields as developmental and clinical phonology, where the role of interpersonal and intrapersonal variation is so great and the number of statistical investigations rather limited. The important but problematic theoretical and methodological roles of individual differences are described by Crystal (1987 [1981]: 42) in the following way: "*Individual differences* are often cited usually as an escape-route by the analyst, but in the case of phonological acquisition there does seem to be plenty of justification for the notion. Authors repeatedly cite it: Ferguson and Farwell (1975: 438) talk of the 'idiosyncratic paths which particular children follow in learning to produce their languages,' and the point is echoed by several others. . . . For example, Shibamato and Olmstead (1978: 454) talk about individual 'phonological preferences' for particular articulatory patterns; and then there is Priestley's detailed study (1977). See also the discussion in Menyuk and Menn (1979: 52)."

Grunwell (1981: 32–33) discusses the issue of "unusual phonological rules" as defined by Compton (1975, 1976), bringing further light to the theoretical and methodological difficulties of determining, defining, and assigning a role to these idiosyncratic processes:

> Compton in both his 1975 and 1976 papers presents the same account between normal phonological development and phonological disability. He lists the following "developmental generalizations" (1975, pp. 88–89) which occur in the earliest stages of normal development:
>
> the predominance of the open syllable;
>
> the priority of voiceless stops in initial position; the priority of voiceless fricatives in final position [cf. chap. 5];
>
> the tendency for fronted place of articulation substitutions;
>
> the tendency for errors in manner features only to occur with place of articulation held constant;
>
> the occurrence of "exceptions" which are residues from the child's previous patterns.
>
> These patterns, he claims, are also observed in phonological disability. However, there are also patterns in phonological disability, which Compton designates "un-

usual phonological rules" (1976, p. 93). His explanation of these is as follows: ". . . children with defective speech may also develop various idiosyncratic phonological patterns—often bizarre, but nonetheless quite innovative—perhaps as an attempt to compensate for a phonological system that is failing to meet their communicative needs by rendering them unintelligible" (1975, p. 90; 1976, p. 88). This tentative explanation is, however, directly contradicted by a later observation on the nature of these rules: "In general, there appears to be an inverse relationship between the degree of commonality of phonological rules and the extent to which they disrupt intelligibility, i.e. the less common the rule is, the greater the communicative impairment (1976, p. 93). This latter observation suggests that the unusual rules make a significant contribution to the result of this disorder—unintelligible speech. They are also probably crucial in defining the nature of the disability, since as Compton points out they do not occur in the speech of children developing speech normally and "consequently . . . may be an important diagnostic sign for detecting potential phonological disorders in young children (1976, p. 94). Compton's second explanation of the unusual rules would appear to be more plausible.

Grunwell (1987: 238) also cautions us about the classification of "normal" as opposed to idiosyncratic, unusual, or "abnormal" processes: "As has been indicated in the discussion of systematic sound preference, processes have been observed in the pronunciation patterns of children with developmental phonological disorders which have been described as 'unusual' or 'idiosyncratic'." It is, however, advisable to adopt a rather cautious interpretation of what is alleged to be 'normal' and even more what is designated to be 'abnormal' in phonological development." I shall not deal with the thorny issue of common, frequent, primary, or normal as opposed to individual, unusual, unique, idiosyncratic, or abnormal processes here; in the remaining clinical discussions I shall instead use the designations assigned by the clinicians who provided the data.

The Aims of Clinical Linguistics

The rest of this volume may be viewed as an exercise in applying the theory of phonology as human behavior to the field of clinical linguistics. Crystal (1987 [1981]: 2) defines clinical linguistics as "the application of linguistic science to the study of communication disability, as encountered in clinical situations." He (1987 [1981]: 2) then identifies seven specific aims for the subject, which constitute the linguist's interpretation of the clinical demands made upon him. These aims, easy to state, more difficult to achieve, are as follows:

(i) the clarification of areas of confusion arising out of the traditional metalanguage and classification of speech pathology;
(ii) the description of the linguistic behaviour of patients, and of the clinicians and others who interact with them;
(iii) the analysis of these descriptions, with a view to demonstrating the systematic nature of the disabilities involved;
(iv) the classification of patient behaviours, as part of the process of differential diagnosis;
(v) the assessment of these behaviours, by demonstrating their place on scales of increasing approximation to linguistic norms;
(vi) the formulation of hypotheses for the remediation of these behaviours, insofar as the therapy and management of patients require reference to linguistic variables, and evaluating the outcome of these hypotheses, as treatment proceeds;
(vii) the evaluation of the remedial strategies used in intervention, insofar as linguistic variables are involved.

In this volume, I will not attempt to fulfill all the aims of clinical linguistics as listed above. I shall limit myself simply to the presentation and description of the phonetic output of the patients involved and try to provide an explanation for this phonetic output that is based on the principles of the theory of phonology as human behavior. In the rest of this chapter, I will present some general and idiosyncratic functional processes found in children who have been brought for treatment to speech clinics in Israel.[9]

Phonology as Human Behavior and Functional Clinical Applications

The most comprehensive studies applying the theory of phonology as human behavior to functional disorders in the clinic are Katz (1993, 1995). Katz describes and explains a sample of 250 utterances obtained from eight 4:6– 5:6-year-old children. The results of this analysis were compared with an analysis based on natural phonology (Stampe 1969, 1979 [1972]), which has been used routinely in the speech clinic in Israel for several years, an analysis originally based on the work of Ingram (1976b) and Grunwell (1982, 1987).

Katz found that most of the parameters that were examined in attempts to explain the nonrandom distribution of phonemes in the various languages analyzed according to the theory of phonology as human behavior were also relevant to the speech disorders of the subjects being studied. All the disorders were of the phonetic type previously discussed, that is, the child had acquired the normal phonological system of the language but was unable to produce phonetically all the phonemes of the system.

The following are the most common functional processes found in Katz (and the other clinical studies listed in n. 9, this chapter), which I will explain according to the theory of phonology as human behavior. This list of functional processes appears in the order in which they were previously presented in this chapter rather than in the order of their relative frequency in the clinical studies mentioned.

Functional Processes Influencing Syllable Structure

The most common functional processes influencing syllable structure, which appeared in almost every case, are the following:

1. Final consonant deletion.

Explanation: Word-final position has less communicative force; consonants require more articulatory control (are harder to make) than vowels.

2. Deletion of unstressed syllables (usually in word-initial position).

Explanation: Stressed syllables give more communicative, perceptual, and cognitive information than unstressed syllables; the more syllables in the word, the more effort it takes to pronounce it; in non–initially stressed words, there is less information in word-initial position, which usually has the greatest communicative force.

3. Consonant cluster reduction.

Explanation: A consonant cluster requires greater effort than a consonant-vowel sequence and may be reduced or replaced at the expense of maximum communication.

There also were several cases of the following:

4. Reduplication.

Explanation: The reduplication often comes as a means to avoid more difficult sound combinations and/or to maintain the number of syllables in the word: sequences of phonemes with the same articulators are disfavored unless their juxtaposition is, by virtue of some other factor, mutually beneficial. It was also found that newly acquired sounds were often reduplicated as a means of practice or of hypercorrection in the clinical situation.

There were very few individual cases of the following:

5. Coalescence.
Explanation: Fewer articulatory gestures result in fewer distinctive units at the expense of maximum communication.
6. Epenthesis.
Explanation: The additional unstressed vowels often ease the transition to more difficult consonants or clusters.

Processes 4–6 above may be related to the principle of phonology as human behavior that sequences of phonemes with the same or near articulators are disfavored unless their juxtaposition is, by virtue of some other factor, mutually beneficial.

Assimilation Processes (Consonant/Consonant-Vowel Harmony)

All the assimilation processes found in the literature appeared in various ways for most of the cases. The most frequent assimilation process was devoicing in general and devoicing of final consonants in particular:

1. Velar/Nasal/Labial, etc. Assimilation.
Explanation: A nonvelar/nonnasal/nonlabial sound changes to a velar/nasal/labial because of the influence of or the domination of a velar/nasal/labial sound, which entails fewer articulatory gestures at the expense of maximum communication.
2. Prevocalic voicing of consonants.
Explanation: An unvoiced consonant becomes voiced generally before a vowel: the speaker anticipates the control of two sets of articulators in what is usually a longer acoustic phonological segment.
3. Devoicing of final consonants.
Explanation: Additional articulators are disfavored; voiced consonants become unvoiced in word-final position; where the communicative force is least important or crucial, the speaker opts to activate one set of articulators rather than two.

Examples 1 and 2 are also directly related to the factor that sequences of phonemes with the same or near articulators are disfavored unless their juxtaposition is, by virtue of some other factor, mutually beneficial.

Substitution Processes

Processes Reflecting the Substitution of Active Articulators

The most frequent and prevalent substitution process of active articulators was fronting in general and apicalization in particular. In addition to all the reasons previously discussed regarding the favoring of the apex across languages and in child language development, Katz further points out that, according to Daniloff and Adams (1985), the apex contains more sensory receptors than the other active articulators, facilitating greater articulatory precision (see chap. 2, n. 6). There was a more limited number of cases containing backing, which may be why it has been considered to be an idiosyncratic process. It is interesting to note, however, that in most of the cases of backing there were also indications of either delayed language development, possible sensorimotor difficulties, possible sensori-tactile problems, or a prolonged use of a pacifier with the child, which may have indicated a weakening of the musculature involved in the excitation of the apex.

1. Fronting.

Explanation: The apex is the most flexible and easy to control of all the active articulators; the earliest and most frequent examples of the substitution of active articulators are fronting and apicalization, which sharply reduces the number of communicative distinctions available to the speaker.

2. Backing.

Explanation: A (possibly idiosyncratic) later, less frequent process where the dorsum (or other back articulators) replaces the apex (or other front articulators); it is often found in children who have difficulty controlling the musculature of the apex and/or try to reduce the number of communicative distinctions made by the apex (or other front articulators).

Processes Reflecting the Substitution of Turbulence and Airflow

Stopping and deaffrication were among the more prevalent processes reflecting the substitution of turbulence and airflow. A phenomenon similar to vocalization often appeared when the consonants of syllables were deleted and only the vowels remained maintaining the number of syllables per word. There were also some sporadic cases of gliding (of both liquids and fricatives) and glottal replacement, which may indicate why these have often been considered idiosyncratic processes.

1. Stopping.
Explanation: Maximum constriction is favored particularly when mobile phonemes of constriction are easier to control than stabile phonemes of less constriction, which require greater control of the musculature to create and maintain a small aperture for a stronger turbulent airflow; this is the most frequent manner of substitution for children.

2. Deaffrication.
Explanation: Transitions from one distinct constriction to another within a single phoneme are disfavored; a more complex sound requiring greater effort or control is reduced to a less complex sound after the speaker has acquired the ability to produce the more difficult stable sounds.

3. Vocalization.
Explanation: The favoring of maximal aperture particularly when phonemes of aperture (vowels) require less articulatory control than phonemes of constriction (consonants).

4. Glottal replacement.
Explanation: Additional articulators are disfavored; a glottal stop replaces an intervocalic consonant or a consonant in syllable-final position; there is articulatory control of one set of articulators rather than two in an appropriate phonetic environment.

5. Gliding of liquids.
Explanation: There is substitution of a lower for a higher degree of aperture (from consonants to semivowels), which may also require less articulatory control.

6. Gliding of fricatives.
Explanation: This is a more extreme substitution of a lower for a higher degree of aperture (cf. point 5, the gliding of liquids, above), requiring less articulatory control; this is considered an idiosyncratic process.

The processes reflecting the substitution of turbulence and airflow listed above confirm the following factors obtained from the theory of phonology as human behavior: among constrictions, maximal constriction is favored, and, among apertures, maximal aperture is favored.

There were also a few individual cases of what I will call nasalization + backing: /l/ → /ŋ/ (not a Hebrew phoneme). These cases showed extreme apicalization (for phonemes made both by the anterodorsum and by the posterodorsum), and therefore the number of phonemic distinctions being made by the apex was larger than usual. There were also several examples of devoicing, which indicated that the number of phonemic distinctions was even more limited in their phonetic realizations than usual. Therefore, as a compromise gesture between the human and the communication factors, these children invested a little more effort to add an additional phonetic realization of a phonemic contrast in their limited repertoire of sounds.

On the basis of the functional processes that she observed in the clinic, which are directly related to the synergetic interaction of the human and communication factors underlying the theory, Katz has added the following factors to the theory of phonology as human behavior:

1. The preservation of as many distinctive features as possible (usually two out of three features per phoneme) in substitution processes, which require more effort than deletion processes;
2. The preservation of as many communicative oppositions as possible in the original word (e.g., the number of phonemes per word) in substitution processes, which require more effort than deletion processes;
3. The use of a readily available phoneme already found in the speaker's repertoire in accordance with the immediate phonetic environment in substitution processes, which require more effort than deletion processes;
4. The preservation of the original phonetic structure of the word in deletion processes not involving syllable reduction and in reduplication;
5. The preservation of the stressed syllable bearing the most communicative information if the original structure of the word is reduced by the deletion of syllables; and
6. The use of epenthesis, even when the original structure of the word is enlarged, if the epenthesis makes the transition to or between more difficult sounds easier.

In all the studies of general and idiosyncratic functional processes in the clinic where the theory of phonology as human behavior was applied, we found that all exemplified extreme cases of the striving for maximal communication with minimal effort wherein the human factor clearly dominated the communication factor.

Description versus Explanation in the Clinic

One of Katz's major theses was that the theory of phonology as human behavior can *explain* rather than merely *describe* the functional processes of the children with whom she worked. In chapter 1, I claimed that description answers the questions of how, what, and where while explanation represents the answer to the fundamental question of why. (In the present chapter dealing with child phonology, and in the following chapters dealing with the processes and errors of clients with organic disorders, we can see that that explanation may also be directly related to the question of who.) This issue of explanation versus description is tied in, of course, with the basic problems that have been previously discussed concerning the difference between abstract phonology and concrete phonetics in general and whether the functional processes dealt with in the clinic are phonological or phonetic in nature in particular. Once again, I would like to take a stand on these fundamental issues. Bernthal and Bankson (1988: 279) reflect my own ideas derived from the theory of phonology as human behavior:

> Some speech-language clinicians have suggested that the presence of phonological processes in their clients is evidence of a cognitive-linguistic deficit, thereby providing an *explanation* of the phonological errors. This may not be an appropriate interpretation since phonological process analysis procedures are only *descriptive* devices and do not reveal cause or provide explanations of the error patterns. Smith (1981) warned that when studying phonological development with a linguistic-based pattern analysis, ". . . one must avoid falling into the trap of believing that a child's behavior has been *explained* by having written a series of formal rules or a list of processes relating to particular phonological observations." . . .
>
> An example demonstrating the inherent difficulty in arriving at an explanatory statement for a given phonological process was provided by Hoffman and Schuckers (1984) with respect to final consonant deletion. One explanation for that process might be that the child misperceives the adult word, e.g., perceives [dɔg] as [dɔ]. A second explanation might be that the child's underlying lexical representation for dog is [dɔ]. A third possible explanation is that the child's perceptual system functions appropriately and the lexical match between what the child perceives and what he or she has stored is consistent with the adult standard, but she or he has a phonological production rule that calls for the deletion of word-final stops. A fourth possibility is that the child has a motor production problem; in this case the child may have the appropriate perception but does not possess the necessary motor skill to make the physiological gesture to produce the sound.
>
> This discussion is not intended to minimize the value of the information provided from a phonological process analysis, but rather to emphasize that when such procedures are used to analyze a child's speech, they serve to describe, not explain, behavior. In other words, when doing an analysis one cannot assume that because a phonological process (e.g., final consonant deletion) has been identified, . . . such

patterns can be attributed to specific cognitive-linguistic, perceptual or motor explanations. Pattern analyses are only descriptive devices, not explanations. Explanations or identification of phonological errors demand additional supporting data.

I believe that the kind of additional supporting data necessary to provide explanations mentioned by Bernthal and Bankson may be found in the previous work done for the analyses of the nonrandom distribution of phonemes of constriction across languages according to the theory of phonology as human behavior. The principles postulated for the explanation of this nonrandom linguistic or phonotactic distribution have always been supported by extralinguistic evidence culled from other human activities requiring fine motor musculature control as well, which I have called the human factor. Furthermore, the human factor has always been connected intrinsically to the communication factor in the theory of phonology as human behavior as a means to explain and not merely describe the phenomena being studied.

Katz (1993, 1995) was able to describe and explain speech disorders as representing favorings and disfavorings of certain allophones in different phonetic environments. These favorings were similar to the favorings and disfavorings of certain collocations of phonemes in different phonetic environments that were found in the various languages examined by the theory of phonology as human behavior. In both cases, the nonrandom distribution of the sounds reflects specific aspects of the interaction of the human and communication factors underlying the theory. For the subjects of her studies, a marked preference for the human factor over the communication factor was found.

Katz found that the theory of natural phonology facilitates description of the data and that the theory of phonology as human behavior promulgates an explanation of the data. Katz concluded that the implicit parameters gained by natural phonology are made more explicit by the theory of phonology as human behavior. According to Katz, the theory of natural phonology provides a much needed developmental dimension to the data.

The analysis according to the theory of phonology as human behavior represents the communication disorders and natural processes as a functional phonetic deviance and explains them by appealing to the synergetic principle of striving for maximum communication with minimal effort and the trade-off between the human and the communication factors in language related to the opposing roles and needs of encoders and decoders. Katz's results indicate the benefits of the routine use of the theory of phonology as human behavior in clinical practice as a means to describe and explain speech disorders and possibly even develop a plan or program for speech therapy.[10]

Summary and Conclusions

In this chapter, we have seen that the theory of phonology as human behavior can account for the various hypotheses and claims made for the acquisition of sounds both in so-called normal and in disordered first language acquisition made by a wide variety of theoretical phonological approaches. In every case, the theory of phonology as human behavior was guided by the mini-max principle of establishing a system providing maximum communication with minimal effort. In the final chapters of this volume, I will discuss the clinical applications of the theory of phonology as human behavior in the most extreme cases of the search for maximum communication with a highly restricted or limited human factor, that is, the processes produced by individuals with organic disorders.

8 Clinical Applications to Organic Disorders

> Mr. Grave's way of speaking did not displease Watt. Mr. Graves pronounced his *th* charmingly. Turd and fart, he said, for third and fourth. Watts liked these venerable Saxon words. —Samuel Beckett

> Moreover, for teachers and all those whose work calls for an exact knowledge of the child's mind, facts take precedence over theory. I am convinced that the mark of theoretical fertility in a science is its capacity for practical application. —Jean Piaget

Phonological Theory and the Speech Clinic

Many of the major phonological theories from descriptivist phonemics to nonlinear phonology have been applied to the speech clinic, with various degrees of interest and success across a highly diverse set of populations.[1] The problems incurred by the first attempts to apply phonological theory to the clinic (many of which are still relevant today) have been described and summarized by Ingram (1976b: 9–10), one of the early leaders and innovators in the field, in the following way: "The goals and interests of phonological theory differ in many ways from those of the clinician. The clinician who turns to it to acquire information for his or her practice will be confronted with numerous issues that are of no interest. For example, there are various phonological theories, and much of phonological study is devoted to theoretical arguments for or against each other. Also, there is usually a strong concern for formalism. The emphasis on theory and formal issues are [*sic*] often obscure exercises for the clinician who has to deal daily with very practical matters. In addition, phonology concerns itself with all languages, not just English."

Not surprisingly, much of the impetus for applying theoretical phonology to the clinic came as part of the early optimism of generative grammarians and phonologists concerning the psychological reality of their theories to the human mind in general. This premature theoretical cum psychological confidence was reflected in their version of distinctive feature analysis as it was applied to first language acquisition in particular. In his earlier work, Ingram (1976b: 2) voiced some skepticism about what might be viewed as this forced marriage between generative phonologists and clinicians and their resultant progeny, skepticism that may still be relevant today: "In the last few years there have been several articles discussing the value of generative (or transformational) approaches to phonological disability. The authors usually claim that they are providing an effective means to describe the phonological patterns of deviant children. Also, they claim that these descriptive devices, e.g. recent suggestions for the use of distinctive features, have therapeutic value. However, because of the assumptions made about the reader's linguistic background, these articles are often not understood by those concerned primarily with a clinical application. So, too, the conclusions drawn by the authors are often more theoretical than practical in scope. The result has been a rather negligible influence on most clinical practice."

As was stated in the previous chapter, the theory of natural phonological processes (Stampe 1969, 1979 [1972]) has been adopted by several researchers in the field of developmental phonology and subsequently has served as the basis for a new theory of clinical phonology for both children and adults (e.g., Crary and Fokes 1980; Hodson and Paden 1983; Grunwell 1982, 1985, 1987; Ingram 1976a, 1976b, 1981, 1989). Over the years, the theory of natural phonology has become one of the most predominantly used theories in the speech clinic, especially in Great Britain and the United States as well as in many other countries that have followed their lead, such as Israel. In this chapter, I will discuss the application of the theory of phonology as human behavior to the speech clinic in Israel for organic rather than developmental or functional disorders.

Phonology as Human Behavior and the Speech Clinic

I will begin by summarizing the major principles of and the results obtained from the theory of phonology as human behavior and add to them, in parentheses, their theoretical implications and methodological applications to the speech clinic. The four orientations underlying the theory of phonology as human behavior are

1. the communicative orientation (difficulties or breakdowns in communication),
2. the physiology of the vocal tract (functional or organic),
3. the acoustic medium (audiology), and
4. the human factor (in the client and the clinician).

The fundamental analytic position of the theory of phonology as human behavior is as follows:

1. Users of a language behave as though they have learned certain distinctive units, the phonemes, which they deploy for communicative purposes (analyzing and distinguishing between speech errors that are phonetic and those that are phonemic/phonological).
2. We cannot observe directly what it is that they behave as though they have learned (analyzing and comparing the speech of clients with the norm).
3. We can, however, observe the phonotactic skewing, a skewing that has been built up over the centuries and millenia in the very mouths of the speakers (and that should be the same for all speakers).
4. We can infer that these long-range skewings represent favorings and disfavorings on the part of users of the language. It is to be observed that the skewings are not idiosyncratic to particular languages; their general characteristics recur from language to language. (The skewings of clients are idiosyncratic and may differ from those of other speakers within and across languages.)
5. We can then examine the favorings and disfavorings against the background of the orientation—which means with independent knowledge of the kinds of favorings and disfavorings to which humans are prone in areas other than the use of language (control of fine motor movement in clients with other possibly related motor problems: apraxia/dyspraxia, Down's syndrome, etc.).
6. We can infer that a disfavoring, for example, represents a difficulty in a learning process, and, by a close examination of what it is that constitutes a difficulty in the way of a particular learning process, we can infer what it is that is being learned (analyzing the difficulties of clients).
7. We may identify what it is that is being learned as a characteristic of the distinctive units (and analyze and compare the units of clients and other speakers).

The following include the specific phonological and phonotactic parameters explicitly derived from the theory, as opposed to traditional categories:

1. the identification of active articulators, as opposed to the traditional category of place of articulation, which is often a label for passive receptors, and the relative difficulty of learning how to control them (for clients versus other speakers);

2. the identification of relative degrees of stricture, aperture, and turbulent and nonturbulent airflow, as opposed to the traditional category of manner of articulation, that require different articulatory control, such as mobile and stable, and produce different acoustic patterns for individual sounds and phonation processes, such as labialization, apicalization, velarization, nasalization, and glottalization (which may differ among clients and other speakers);

3. the identification of the number of sets of articulators to be controlled, as opposed to the traditional categories of voicing, the fortis-lenis distinction, and nasality, that require different articulatory control and produce different acoustic patterns (which may differ among clients and other speakers); and

4. the identification of phonemes of constriction and phonemes of aperture, as opposed to the traditional concepts of consonants and vowels, that require different articultory control and produce different acoustic patterns (which may differ among clients and other speakers).

The theory has obtained the following quantitative results within and across languages, including the establishment of the following factors, which have been used as a means of explaining the functional processes dealt with in the clinic:

1. Additional articulators are disfavored (devoicing, denasalization, glottal replacement).

2. Coarticulation by near articulators is disfavored (consonant cluster reduction, deletions, and substitutions).

3. Coarticulation by the same articulators/phoneme is even more highly disfavored, in monosyllabic words, in stems, as well as in the triconsonantal (CCC) roots of Semitic languages (unless their juxtaposition is, by virtue of some other factor, mutually beneficial [see point 13 below]: reduplication, coalescence, assimilatory processes, deletions, substitutions).

4. Different word, stem, and root positions have different communicative force and thus affect the favoring and disfavoring of different articulatory gestures, the number of articulators, the number and type of acoustic features, and the distribution of phonemes (devoicing of final consonants, deletion of final consonants, deletion of unstressed initial syllables, initial epenthesis).

5. Apical articulations are favored in general and in final position in particular (fronting, apicalization).

6. Visual articulations are favored particularly in word/stem/root-initial position (labialization).

7. Explosive (mobile) phonemes are favored in initial position (affrication).

8. Turbulent (stable) phonemes are favored in final position (deletions, substitutions).

9. Transitions from one distinct constriction to another within a single phoneme are disfavored (deaffrication).

10. Consonant clusters are restricted concerning different articulatory and acoustic features, for example, mobility/stability (stricture, aperture, airflow substitutions, and deletions).

11. Among constrictions, maximal constriction is favored (stopping).

12. Among apertures, maximal aperture is favored (vocalization, gliding).

13. Sequences of phonemes with the same articulators are disfavored (unless their juxtaposition is, by virtue of some other factor, mutually beneficial (see point 3 above): reduplication, coalescence, assimilation processes, velarization, nasalization, labialization, prevocalic voicing).

As was stated in the previous chapter, Katz (1993, 1995) has added the following factors to the theory of phonology as human behavior on the basis of the functional processes that she observed in the clinic that are directly related to the synergetic interaction of the human and communication factors underlying the theory:

1. the preservation of as many distinctive features as possible (usually two of three features per phoneme) in substitution processes, which require more effort than deletion processes;

2. the preservation of as many communicative oppositions as possible in the original word, for example, the number of phonemes per word, in substitution processes, which require more effort than deletion processes;

3. the use of a readily available phoneme already found in the speaker's repertoire in accordance with the immediate phonetic environment in substitution processes, which require more effort than deletion processes;

4. the preservation of the original phonetic structure of the word in deletion processes not involving syllable reduction and in reduplication;

5. the preservation of the stressed syllable bearing the most communicative information if the original structure of the word is reduced by the deletion of syllables; and

6. the use of epenthesis, even when the original structure of the word is enlarged, if the epenthesis makes the transition to or between more difficult sounds easier.

The theory of phonology as human behavior supports the following conclusion regarding language synergy in general:

Conclusion 1: Language in general—and phonology in particular—can be seen as a synergetic mini-max struggle: the desire to create maximum communication with minimal effort (see Tobin 1990c: chap. 3).

The theory of phonology as human behavior as it has been applied to developmental phonology and functional processes or errors in the clinic in the previous chapter supports the hypothesis that both developmental and functional clinical phonology are more extreme versions of conclusion 1, where the human factor very often overrides the communication factor and clinical intervention serves as an attempt to balance the two:

Conclusion 2: Developmental and functional clinical speech processes or errors may be viewed as an extreme version of this synergetic mini-max struggle: there is less than maximum communication because of either extreme minimal effort or a lack of control over the articulatory tract or mechanisms. Greater effort will be exerted in order to achieve more efficient or better communication through clinical intervention.

In this chapter, I will deal with a set of even more severe processes or errors collected from individuals with organic clinical disorders. The data will show that in these cases we have the most extreme version of this synergetic mini-max struggle:

Conclusion 3: The clinical speech processes and errors of individuals with organic disorders may be viewed as the most extreme version of the synergetic mini-max struggle: there is an extremely minimal or even a severe breakdown in communication because of organic difficulties, usually in the central nervous system and in the control of the musculature of the articulatory tract or mechanisms. Even greater effort will be exerted in order to compensate wherever possible for these organic disorders in order to achieve better communication through clinical intervention.

Clinical Applications to Organic Disorders

Apraxia and Dysarthria

One of the more common neurological disorders found in the speech clinic is apraxia, which has been defined as "a neurologically based motor speech disorder that adversely affects the abilities to execute purposeful speech movements. Muscle weakness is not associated with apraxia" (Shipley and McAfee 1992: 387). More specifically, the background of apraxia as a motor speech disorder has been summarized as follows:

At the highest level of the nervous motor system are those circuits laid down through learning for the arousal and control of the muscular responses through which we use language expressively in speaking (and writing). Consideration of this matter would lead to the whole question of the neurophysiological basis for motor learning, which we cannot explore. Certain hypotheses, however, help to explain normal function and some of the acquired and developmental disorders in the articulation process. Essentially, learning a pattern of articulation movements depends on a kind of *programming* of the brain in such a way that *engrams* [traces] are laid down, through learning, for the expressive speech movements. Where there is a dysfunction of the central nervous system, a child may, apart from mental retardation, be physiologically incapable of forming these memory traces; also brain damage acquired by older individuals who have learned language normally may cause them to lose the ability to execute the movements for the expressive use of language in speaking or writing. The terms *developmental apraxia* and *acquired apraxia* may be applied to these conditions, or they may be referred to generally as forms of *central dysarthria*. (Carrell 1968: 6)

Various kinds of apraxia have been defined, discussed, and categorized, with particular regard to the difference between apraxia and dysarthria, the latter term comprising motor disorders that affect verbal expression in both children and adults.[2] The latter has been classified as a phonetic problem (Crystal 1987 [1981]: 195) and defined in a resource manual of speech pathology as follows: "a group of motor speech disorders associated with muscle paralysis, weakness, or incoordination. It is associated with central or peripheral nervous system damage" (Shipley and McAfee 1992: 390). More specifically, the background of dysarthria as a motor speech disorder has been summarized as follows:

Articulation movements are mediated by a flow of nerve impulses to those muscles which produce and modulate the sounds of speech. These impulses arrive at the muscles through a *lower motor neuron* network composed of branches from certain cranial nerves whose nuclei (or point of origin) lies in the *bulbar* portion of the brain-stem, and whose peripheral fibers insert into the articulation musculature. This portion of the system is, so to speak, the final common pathway over which are routed the nerve impulses which excite the speech movements. A pathology at this point can impair articulation movements in two possible ways: (1) complete destruction of the nucleus or peripheral fibers of any nerve will result in complete loss of movement and tone in the muscles that nerve serves; or (2) partial destruction of the nucleus or peripheral fibers will result in weakness of motion and a reduction of muscle tone. The effect on speech may range from complete loss of articulation movements to weakness of motion. The term *lower motor neuron dysarthria* can be used for conditions of this kind. (Carrell 1968: 5)

Grunwell (1987: 276–77) also defines dysarthria as a phonetic problem: "For the sake of completeness, mention must be made here of the acquired speech disorders which are classified neurologically as *dysarthrias*. These disorders result from clearly observable neuromuscular impairments involving breakdowns in the accuracy, mobility, general control, timing and coordination of movements of the speech musculature (for details see Darley et al. 1975; see also Grunwell & Huskins 1979). The impairments are consistently present in both speech and non-speech contexts, though fatigue and other factors may exacerbate the condition in certain circumstances for individual clients. It will therefore be evident that dysarthric impairments entail a phonetic disability in speech production."

As was previously mentioned, apraxia has been further divided into adult (acquired) and developmental apraxia, which have been defined and characterized as follows: Adult verbal apraxia is a central nervous system disability in the planning and control of voluntary muscles without problems of weakness, coordination, and automatic actions of the muscles characterized by inconsistent speech errors: substitutions, additions, repetitions, lengthenings, as well as other voluntary oral activities not connected to speech usually brought on by brain trauma. Developmental apraxia of speech (DAS) is seen in children with articulatory problems in imitation and spontaneous speech production and is believed to be of neurological cause; children so afflicted lack the necessary mobile control for speech but have the necessary muscular functions for speech production.

Characteristics of Developmental Apraxia of Speech

The characteristics of developmental apraxia of speech (adapted from Bernthal and Bankson 1988) are as follows:

1. distinction between voluntary and involuntary muscle control;
2. blatant difficulty in imitation;

3. difficulty maintaining fluent phonological coordination;
4. normal speech comprehension;
5. problems in acquiring reading and writing skills;
6. very slow progress in traditional speech therapy;
7. unfocused neurological signs (motor problems);
8. often accompanied by oral apraxia;
9. mixed right-left hand dominance;
10. greater occurrence in boys; and a
11. history of language and speech problems in the family.

It is generally agreed that apraxic children have an abnormal phonological system and that their articulatory behavior is based on a systematic attempt to simplify the complexity of speech sounds. There is very little agreement, however, concerning the substance of their speech errors because of what has been assumed to be their inconsistency.

Characteristics of Apraxic Children's Speech Patterns

Apraxic children show the following characteristic speech patterns: They tend to make more errors in consonants than in vowels. They are more likely to make errors in fricatives, affricates, and consonant clusters. The degree of error rises as a function of the length, complexity, and frequency of the word. And it is easier for the child to express visible phonemes, usually bilabial consonants.

Error Types of Apraxic Children

Apraxic children show the following error types (adapted from Marquardth and Reinhart (1979): phoneme substitutions; word simplification through phoneme deletion; phoneme addition; and substitution of closely related phonemes with a word.

Case Study (Adopted from Segev 1993)

Tal (male, 4:3) is one of seven children, at least two of whom showed delayed language development. His language comprehension is normal, and he shows no overt signs of motor difficulties. He does, however, have problems concentrating. He is being treated because of the extremely low degree of intelligibility in his speech. T. speaks in phrases and short sentences without a single word complete or free of error. It is extremely difficult to find any consistent pattern to T.'s errors other than that he preserves the original vowel pattern of words, that he consistently deletes the /r/ phoneme: /ʁ/,[3] and that, while he can produce all the other phonemes, his substitutions and deletions appear to be inconsistent and random.

Analysis of T.'s Speech According to Phonology as Human Behavior

1. *The problem:* The production of dorsal (back) consonants.
   The strategy: Fronting-apicalization.
   Examples: xatul → [satul] (cat), *kova* → [tova] (hat), *oxel* → [osel] (eats), *bokeʁ* → [bote] (morning), and *dag* → [dad] (fish).
2. *The problem:* Control over three sets of articulators in word-medial position for the nonvisible apical nasal /n/.
   The strategy: Control over one to two sets of articulators only (denasalization and/or devoicing).
   Examples: balonim → [balosim] (baloons) and *anavim* → [alavim] (grapes).
3. *The problem:* Transition from mobile-stable, stabile-mobile.
   The strategy: Substituting mobile-mobile, stable-stable (apical).
   Examples: sigaʁiot → [silalot] (cigarettes), *mispaʁayim* → [mitaiyim] (scissors), and *sipuʁ* → [silu] (story).
4. *The problem:* Coarticulation by the same articulators in adjacent phonetic environments.
   The strategy: Replace second articulator (usually to apical).
   Examples: pamutim → [palutim] (candlesticks), *mapit* → [maθit] (napkin), and *mimʁax* → [ʃiʔax] (chocolate spread).
5. *The problem: /ʁ/*
   The strategy: Deletion or substitution of the /r/ phoneme /ʁ/:
   Examples: vaʁod → [vaʔod] (pink), *ʁamzor* → [mazo] (traffic light), and *ʃavuʁ* → [ʃavu] (broken).

Conclusions Based on the Theory of Phonology as Human Behavior

The following conclusions can be derived:

1. T. preserves the vowel patterns of the original word (phonemes of aperture are easier to make than phonemes of constriction and provide more acoustic information [formants-transitions]).

2. He prefers to maintain or substitute phonemes of constriction in word-initial position (where the demands of communication are the highest), while he usually deletes phonemes of constriction in word-final position (where the demands of communication are lowest).

3. He prefers to substitute dorsal sounds with apical sounds, which are easier to control.

4. However, in a later stage of therapy, when T. started producing dorsal consonants in word-initial position, he would reduplicate them in word-medial or word-final position even at the expense of apical consonants: *katom* → [kakom] (orange), *kubiyot* → [kubiyok] (dice), and *gamad* → [gamag] (dwarf). This reduplication may have been beneficial to his practicing of the new sound at the expense of losing a communicative distinction in word-medial or the less adjacent and least important word-final position.

5. Also, T. prefers to exploit one or two sets of articulators, which are easier to control, rather than three sets of articulators when visibility and communication factors of word position do not play a major role.

6. He prefers to avoid sharp transitions that cross mobile-stable distinctions and thus maintain similar kinds of articulatory gestures in adjacent phonetic environments.

7. He presents an even more extreme version of the mini-max struggle for maximum communication with minimal effort: because of developmental apraxia, the human factor perforce outweighs and overcomes the communication factor, thus considerably reducing the intelligibility of his speech and therefore (ideally) motivating him to try to achieve better planning and more control over his articulatory musculature.

Other case studies involving acquired apraxia and/or dysarthria have been analyzed according to the theory of phonology as human behavior. Kopold (1991) analyzed the speech of R.S. (female 42), who was diagnosed as apraxic (including elements of dysarthria?) as a result of a cerebral vascular accident (CVA), that is, a stroke where there is damage to the brain because of a disturbance in the blood supply (Shipley and McAfee 1992: 388). R.S. suffers from paralysis of the right side of her body and has been in speech therapy for over a year and a half. Most of her problems are articulatory (e.g., voicing, placement of the tongue for stable phonemes of constriction). Her speaking voice is very weak, which may be an acquired habit. R.S. was originally analyzed as having inconsistent articulations and is now capable of correcting most of her misarticulations. She also has an occasional problem with naming (lexical retrieval), which she usually overcomes either with or without linguistic and extralinguistic cues. Her ability for abstraction is low. (It is not clear what it was prior to the stroke, although R.S. was an art teacher in a religious girls' school). She has difficulty forming syntactically well-organized sentences and cannot abstract the central points in reading comprehension.

Isan (Weinreb) (1994) has analyzed the speech of children of various ages diagnosed as apraxic, dysarthric, and spastic. The following processes (explained by the principles of phonology as human behavior in parentheses) were discovered to be prevalent in these cases (adapted from Kopold 1991; Isan [Weinreb] 1991, 1994):

1. stopping (stable phonemes replaced by mobile phonemes);
2. devoicing (control of fewer sets of articulators);
3. denasalization (control of fewer sets of articulators);
4. fronting (favoring of easier active articulators to control);
5. apicalization (labials to apicals: preference for most flexible and sensitive active articulator);
6. epenthesis before the posterodorsal voiced fricative /ɣ/ (more effort to allow for an easier transition);
7. consonant cluster reduction (preference for less complex sound units with either maximum constriction or aperture);
8. assimilatory vowel substitution (sequences of phonemes with the same articulators are disfavored unless their juxtaposition is, by virtue of some other factor, mutually beneficial);
9. backing (lack of control of musculature);
10. nonstressed syllable reduction (communication factor); and
11. final consonant deletion and/or devoicing (communication factor).

Dyspraxia and Dysphasia

Another organic pathology found in the speech clinic is dyspraxia, which is often related to, or considered to be at least partially or totally synonymous with, apraxia and which has been contrasted with acquired dysphasia.[4] Grunwell (1987: 272–74) defines and contrasts these disorders with regard to her view of phonological as opposed to phonetic errors as follows:

> The distinction between phonetic and phonological speech disorders is particularly important in the differential diagnosis of acquired speech disorders. . . .
>
> *Acquired dysphasia* is traditionally defined as a language disorder. Phonetic and phonological analysis and classification of the speech errors produced by dyspha-

sic clients demonstrate this to be so; they indicate a phonological disability. . . . Dysphasic mispronunciations—often called literal or phonemic paraphasias in the traditional speech pathology terminology—tend to be phonologically similar to the target pronunciations. . . .

The diagnostic characteristic of all pronunciation errors in dysphasic speech is that they result in phonemically and phonotactically permissible phonological units. . . . They are therefore evidence of a *phonological* disability in which the *system is disorganised,* but not necessarily inadequate. This explanation is based on the observation that on occasions many dysphasic clients will produce correct pronunciations of words which previously and subsequently they might mispronounce. This suggests that in some clients the phonological system is not destroyed by the cerebral lesion, but that its functioning is impaired. The speech difficulties of the dysphasic client usually appear to involve an intermittent access and incongruent organisation of the phonological constituents and sequential structure of the linguistic units.

In contrast to the purely phonological errors in dysphasic speech, both phonological and phonetic difficulties are evidenced in *acquired articulatory dyspraxia* (often referred to as *apraxia of speech*). Clients with this disability tend to exhibit great difficulties in achieving *their* intended pronunciations; they "struggle" to control and direct their articulatory gestures. On many occasions they appear unable to locate and execute the target articulatory movement and placement; articulation is almost always effortful and frequently visibly so. The control and co-ordination of sequences of articulatory gestures present major difficulties. There is, however, no evidence of paralysis of the organs of articulation and the movements that may be presenting difficulties on one occasion may be adequately performed at another time, in speech and/or in non-speech oral activities. Nevertheless, in most attempts at speaking there is evidence of a disordered speech production mechanism, that is a *phonetic* disability.

Crystal (1987 [1981])—who does not have a separate entry for or discussion of apraxia—says the following about dyspraxia and its potential importance to linguistic analysis as far as the systemicness of the data is concerned: "[Dyspraxia] is [a condition] which offers most scope for linguistic investigation, given the limited analysis it has received within traditional paradigms of enquiry. In particular, the extent of the systemicness of the data referred to as dyspraxic needs to be established."

Dyspraxia is an impairment in the control of the motor system. Verbal dyspraxia connected to speech can be accompanied by oral dyspraxia, a severe impairment of the individual's ability to produce voluntary movements involving the muscles of the throat, jaw, tongue, lips, palate, and cheeks, although the automatic movements of the same muscles are not impaired. Adult dyspraxia is brought on by brain trauma.

Developmental dyspraxia affects children who can understand spoken language but have difficulties acquiring language despite normal intelligence and hearing abilities and relatively good comprehension. Children so afflicted have difficulty planning and organizing the movements necessary for the production of specific phonemes or a series of phonemes. The origin of the condition is unclear: it may be genetic, it may occur during the development of the fetus, or it may occur after birth.

Characteristics and Results of Verbal Dyspraxia

Children afflicted with verbal dyspraxia show a reduction in the number of phonemes and distinctive features, "inconsistent" deletions and substitutions of phonemes/syllables, and difficulty producing series of syllables necessary for units of discourse. Degrees of difficulty vary individually, from the inability to imitate a single syllable to the ability to reproduce one syllable or a series of connected syllables. Speech production significantly diminishes as the demand for rapid speech increases, causing deletions, substitutions, and repetitions. At the age of three to four, when normal children have acquired the rudiments of syntax and the lexicon, the orally dyspraxic child may have to fight to produce a meaningful two- to three-syllable utterance. The dyspraxic child succeeds the most producing combinations of visible phonemes and usually controls the vowels. Verbal dyspraxia is often accompanied by symptoms of general dyspraxia: late walking, lack of precision in movements, and slowness and strangeness in general motor production.

Characteristics of the Expressive Language of Dyspraxic Children

The expressive language of dyspraxic children shows the following characteristics: The acquisition of expressive language is slower. The majority of the lexicon is composed of nouns and verbs, with the deletion of function words. Syntax develops slowly. Comprehension is much greater than expression. The child builds up a large supply of one-word expressions before he or she advances to two-word utterances. Two-word utterances remain asyntactic long after normal children begin producing three- or four-word sentences. At a later stage, when the lexicon has developed further, there are difficulties in word retrieval—dysnomia—accompanied by hesitations and repetitions.

Error Types of Dyspraxic Children

Dyspraxic children show the following error types (adapted from Eisenson 1972; Segal Friedenreich 1992):

Speech errors are held to be inconsistent and random.

The same words are produced differently.

There is a reduction in the number of phonemes and distinctive features and a deletion of syllables.

Researchers disagree whether the problem is in the planning on the phonetic motor level or in the planning on the phonological level.

Case Study (Adapted from Segal Friedenreich 1992)

Y. (male, 3:6), diagnosed six months earlier for developmental dyspraxia, suffers from general motor difficulties ("awkwardness") and receives treatment in occupational therapy. He shows normal intelligence. His speech sample was taken from spontaneous speech recorded in a free-play session.

Analysis of Y.'s Speech According to Phonology as Human Behavior

The speech sample contained fifty words with substitutions and/or deletions out of a total of sixty-five words. Substitutions appeared in twenty-eight words (of twenty-nine instances), deletions in thirty-eight words (of forty-seven instances). Instances of substitution appeared in only eleven words, instances of deletion in only twenty-one words, and instances of substitution and deletion in eighteen words. Sixty-four percent of the words had one error only.

As far as the number of syllables containing errors is concerned, the larger the number of syllables per word, the more errors: thirteen of nineteen monosyllabic words contained errors (68 percent), twenty-nine of thirty-eight bisyllabic words (76 percent), and eight of eight trisyllabic words (100 percent). As for the location of the error (word stress and word position), there are more errors in nonstressed syllables than stressed: twenty-eight errors appeared in stressed syllables, thirty-three in nonstressed syllables, thirty-four in word-initial position, fifteen in word-medial position, and nineteen in word-final position. When connections are made between error type and word stress (polysyllabic words), we see that substitutions were preferred in stressed syllables and deletions in unstressed syllables and that nineteen substitutions and nine deletions appeared in stressed syllables and thirty deletions and three substitutions appeared in nonstressed syllables.

Errors in word-initial position can be characterized as follows: Of seven monosyllabic words, five showed substitutions, and two showed deletions (more substitutions than deletions for monosyllabic words). Of twenty-seven polysyllabic words, four showed substitutions, eighteen showed deletions, and five showed both substitutions and deletions (more deletions than substitutions for polysyllabic words). Twenty-five of twenty-seven polysyllabic words were unstressed in word-initial position. Twenty-one of the twenty-five polysyllabic words without word-initial stress had additional errors in the stressed syllable. Of those twenty-one errors, fifteen were errors of substitution, six errors of deletion. Finally, errors of substitution are preferred in contexts with the highest communication load: word-initial position and stressed syllables.

Of the errors in word-medial position, four were deletions, and eleven were substitutions. Three of the four deletions appeared in unstressed syllables; ten of the eleven substitutions appeared in stressed syllables. Hence, we see a preference for substitutions in stressed syllables.

Of the errors in word-final position, sixteen were deletions, and three were substitutions. Hence, we see that deletions are preferred in word-final position; as expected, deletions appeared in the three unstressed final syllables.

Conclusions Based on the Theory of Phonology as Human Behavior

Fifty of sixty-five words (75 percent) have errors (the human factor). There is a preference (64 percent) for single errors in words: the human factor is regulated by the communication factor (more than one error per word leads to a possible total breakdown in communication). The larger the number of syllables per word, the more errors; this is a result of the interaction of the human and the communication factors: the more syllables, the greater the difficulty in planning/organization (the human factor), the more redundant the information, and the greater the role of stress (the communication factor).

Deletions (forty-seven) are favored over substitutions (twenty-nine) (the human factor): deletions require less effort than substitutions but present greater communicative difficulty. Deletions of consonants and vowels are favored in contexts with the lowest communication load: word-final or syllable-final position and unstressed syllables (the communication factor). Some examples are *nafal* → [nafa] (he fell), *batsek* → [axe] (dough), *ani* → [ni] (I), *yixtov* → [itof] (he will write), and *parpar* → [papa] (butterfly). Deletions are not limited to phonemes; unstressed syllables and even function words (which have a low communicative value) are deleted: *le-haxin* → [axin] (to prepare), *ose kaxa* → [θaxa] (do like this), *la-ʃevet al ha-kise* → [aʃevet iθe] (to-sit [on] [the-] chair), and *sim et ze po* → [θim θe po] (put [object marker] it here). Substitutions—which require more effort (the human factor)—appear in those contexts where the communication load is the highest: word/syllable-initial position, monosyllabic words, and stressed syllables (the communication factor).

There is a tendency for simplication in general, even for apical sounds. All apical affricates and sibilants (both voiced and voiceless) are reduced to a voiceless apical-interdental fricative (θ) (not a Hebrew phoneme) rather than an apical-alveolar (s, z, t͜s) or an anterodorsum (ʃ) (all Hebrew phonemes), which are more difficult to plan and control: s → θ, *sim* → [θim] (put!); z → θ, *ze* → [θe] (this) (+ devoicing); t͜s → θ, *rotse* → [θe] (want) (deaffrication); and ʃ → θ, *ʃev* → [θev] (sit!). As for gliding, the stable apical lateral consonant /l/, which requires more articulatory control, is replaced by the semivowel /y/, which requires less articulatory control or is deleted entirely: l → y, *lo* → [yo] (no); l → o, *t͜salaxat* → [θaaxat] (plate); and l → o, *laʃevet* → [aʃevet] (to sit).

As for the influence of the phonetic environment, the difficulties of planning and organizing motor activities in the production of individual sounds and sequences of sounds are reflected by simplifications in both deletions and substitutions for consonants and vowels. There is a preference to favor the same or adjacent articulators rather than exploit more distant active articulators, regardless of degree of stricture and airflow for consonants: t͜s → k/back vowel, *le-hotsi* → [oki] (to take out); and s → ʃ/back vowel, *kos* → [koʃ] (cup). Front vowels are replaced by back (lip-rounded) vowels with labial consonants, and back vowels are replaced by neutral /a/ in apical and front vowel environments: e → o, *eifo* → [ofo] (where); and o → a, *ose* → [ase] (does). When stable and mobile consonants appear in the same word, there is a tendency to eliminate one of them (in an unstressed syllable) and thus maintain one kind of articulatory gesture (in a stressed syllable) rather than two different articulatory gestures in adjacent phonetic environments of differing communication loads: k → o/stable consonant, *kise* → iθe (chair); and t → o/stable consonant, *tavi* → [afi] (bring) (+ devoicing). There is a tendency to exploit fewer sets of articulators (devoicing): v → f, *kova* → [(k)ofa] (hat); and d → t, *od* → [ot] (more).

Inconsistency is found among apraxic and dyspraxic children, the same word appearing in different ways by the same speaker in the same speech sample: (*a*) *od batsek* → [od aθek] (more dough), (*b*) *hine od* → [hine ot] (here [behold!] more), (*c*) *od exad* → [od exad] (another) (more + one), (*d*) *od pa'am* → [o pa] (again) (more + time), (*e*) *ose od pa'am* → [aθe o pa] (do again), (*f*) *od pa'am te* → [o pam te] (again tea), and (*g*) *od batsek* → [o baθek] (more dough). This may be explained by the theory: the final consonant (*od*) is maintained before vowels to avoid potential consonant clusters across syllables or to maintain the phonetic structure of the utterance (*a, c*); the final consonant is deleted (*od* → [o]) before consonants to avoid potential consonant clusters across syllables (*d–g*); and the final consonant is devoiced (d → t) in word-final position where the communication load is lowest (*b*). Context, therefore, explains the inconsistency. In all the cases listed above, simplification of fine motor movement planning and organization is maintained (the human factor)—often at the expense of the number of distinctive features, phonemes, and syllables in the word (the communication factor). Developmental dyspraxia presents an even more extreme version of the mini-max struggle for maximum communication with minimal effort found in normal functional errors in language acquisition.

In a case of developmental dysphasia that Grunwell (1987: 273–74) defined as a phonological rather than a phonetic problem, the errors in the selection of phonemes indicate processes such as apicalization (in both fronting and backing), affrication, and deaffrication. The errors that she classifies as involving the structure and sequence of phonemes include initial consonant cluster reduction (omission) and epenthesis, that is, the placing of a schwa/ə/ before /l/ (insertion) (both previously discussed), as well as an example of /l/ = /r/ metathesis. Grunwell (1987: 276) also shows a connection between dyspraxia and dysphasia: "It must be appreciated that many of the errors in acquired dyspraxia are in fact similar to the phonological errors in dysphasia. Indeed, the majority of clients with dyspraxia also have some degree of dysphasic impairment."

Seltzer (1992) applied the theory of phonology as human behavior to the clinic and found an extremely high concentration of varied functional processes in a corpus of twenty-three utterances with thirty-six words containing one or more errors in a client (R., male, 4:11) diagnosed with dysphasia. The corpus was culled from a thirty-minute tape-recorded session of spontaneous speech when R. was describing pictures in a family album.

R. was originally brought for therapy at the age of 2:8 because of an almost total lack of speech: his verbal repertoire included a small number of extremely unintelligible "words" that were almost meaningless. R. would cut himself off from his surroundings, roll up in a corner, and make circular movements with his hands or any other object he could find. He generally did not respond to being addressed verbally and would demonstrate great anger and cry when he heard music. Despite this lack of connection to his environment, he had "moments of contact" and a relatively stable relationship with his parents, which helped in his not being diagnosed as autistic.

After two years of therapy, R. acquired a basic vocabulary and began to communicate verbally. The development of his speech included stages parallel to normal language development: that is, one word, two words, meaningful word combinations, and simple sentence formation. With the development of speech and communication skills, several functional processes and other language disorders appeared. R.'s ability for verbal abstraction remained extremely low and below that of his age group. He demonstrated a strong problem with naming, which remains with him today despite a marked improvement. R. describes things that he cannot name by means of similar words or functions. Syntactic phenomena such as the omission of function words (e.g., *and,* prepositions) and the maintenance of the simplest grammatical constructions characterize his speech.

R. has trouble preserving the phonemic structure of words, and his functional processes include substitutions, changes in the syllable structure of words, and deletions. His production appears to be sporadic and random regarding certain sounds that he can produce in certain environments and substitute and delete in others (e.g., in word/syllable-final position). This indicates a nondysarthric disorder. The phonemes that he could not produce, /ɤ/ and /l/, are consistent with delayed language development.

The specific functional processes (explained by the principles of phonology as human behavior in parentheses) found in R.'s spontaneous speech include the following:

1. stopping (stable phonemes are replaced by mobile phonemes);
2. gliding (among apertures, maximal aperture is favored);

3. nasalization (sequences of phonemes with the same articulators are disfavored unless their juxtaposition is, by virtue of some other factor, mutually beneficial);

4. glottalization (additional articulators are disfavored and sequences of phonemes with the same articulators disfavored unless their juxtaposition is, by virtue of some other factor, mutually beneficial);

5. devoicing (additional articulators are disfavored);

6. fronting (apical or labial articulations are favored in general and in final or initial position in particular);

7. apicalization (apical articulations are favored in general and in final position in particular);

8. backing (there is a lack of control of musculature); and

9. consonant deletion in all positions but over 50 percent in word-final position (this is evidence of the human and communication factors).

Most of these processes, which have been labeled or described as natural functional processes and explained by the theory of phonology as human behavior, seem to recur fairly consistently from client to client.

It is becoming increasingly clear that clients diagnosed as having organic disabilities have a much larger number, frequency, and concentration of the most highly diverse functional processes, which have been analyzed in the previous chapter. This larger concentration of diverse errors makes their speech unintelligible. However, children with nonorganic developmental disorders can also be found to have unintelligible speech. It may very well be possible that a scale of intelligibility can be causatively linked with the number, frequency, concentration, and kind of functional processes as an evaluative device. Grunwell (1987: 245) says the following regarding evaluative factors and general versus idiosyncratic kinds of errors, using her definition of phonological and phonetic processes:

> Phonological process analysis has also been used as a basis for other approaches to the evaluation of the speech of children with developmental phonological disorders. For example Norris & Harden (1981) compared the phonological processes occurring in the pronunciation patterns of children rated as having a high error rate with those with a lower error rate. Their findings indicated that there were no processes unique to children with high error rates, but that these children either used more processes in *unusual* ways or overused a few processes, especially deletion processes. These findings conform to the characteristic patterns outlined above; the first observation being predicted from the occurrence of unusual/idiosyncratic

processes, the second from the characteristics of persisting normal processes and systematic sound preference.

Hodson & Paden (1981) address a similar question from a slightly different standpoint. They analysed the phonological processes in the speech of unintelligible children (i.e., children with developmental phonological disorders) by comparison with those used in the speech of normal intelligible children at age 4:0. They found that the unintelligible children's speech evidenced one or more of the following processes: final consonant deletion; fronting; backing; weak syllable deletion; prevocalic voicing; glottal replacement. The intelligible children rarely gave evidence of these patterns, but used post-vocalic voicing, fricative simplifications of (θ, ð) (i.e. realisations of either [f;v] or [s;z] and vocalisation. Once again, these findings are predictable from the characteristics already described; their intelligible children evidenced the patterns of maturing phonologies, while their unintelligible children evidenced persisting normal early processes and some unusual processes.

It would be very interesting to pursue this line of research to see whether a nonrandom distribution of functional and idiosyncratic processes can be found that might be directly related to language intelligibility. Furthermore, this avenue of research might be used as a basis for applying phonological theories in general and the theory of phonology as human behavior in particular to the evaluation procedures in the clinic.

Down's Syndrome

Down's syndrome (or Trisomy 21) has been defined as follows:

Down['s] syndrome is the most common and well-known disorder resulting from a chromosome abnormality. Its name *Trisomy 21* refers to a triplicate (rather than the normal duplicate) of chromosome 21, which results in a total of 47 rather than the usual 46 chromosomes. This chromosomal distinction is present in about 95% of all patients with Down['s] syndrome. Its major characteristics include general hypotonia, open-mouth posture with tongue protrusion, a flat facial profile, brachycephaly (shortened anterior to posterior diameter of the skull), mental retardation or developmental delay, abnormal auricles, and cardiac malformations (in about 40% of the patients).

Approximately 75% of all children with Down['s] syndrome have unilateral or bilateral hearing loss, most commonly a mild-moderate conductive impairment. Associated hearing loss is also common among adults, with an increase in the number of sensorineural losses when compared to the normal population. Speech development is typically delayed and complicated by oral-facial abnormalities. A language delay or disorder is common. Abnormal voice and resonance features may also be present. (Shipley and McAfee 1992: 53–54)

Ingram (1976b: 125–26) analyzes the nature of what he refers to as the deviant phonology of children with Down's syndrome and its implications for linguistic research:

Children with Down's syndrome are generally considered to have harsh voice qualities (sometimes called "husky voice"), abnormal intonation and a pre-dominance of grunts in their speech. Speech production is complicated by the existence of an unusually large tongue. This results in a frequently high level of unintelligibility and a poor prognosis for ever attaining effective speech (*cf.* Strazulla 1953).

Recently a detailed linguistic analysis of the speech of two mongoloid boys has appeared by Bodine (1974). Despite the claim that the speech of mongoloid children is by and large gibberish, she found a great deal of systematicity in the speech of the two children, even in their use of grunts.

Grunwell (1987: 245–46) discusses the role of what she refers to as phonological processes and the theoretical and methodological implications of their application to the analysis of the speech of Down's syndrome children as well:

As was indicated earlier, phonological process analysis has achieved a pre-eminent position as the most common analytical procedure employed in the investigation of children's developmental phonological disorders. Given this position it is rather surprising to find that there are relatively few studies employing phonological processes in the analysis of other types of speech disorders. The most prolific area is the study of the pronunciation patterns of mentally retarded children and Down's syndrome children (Prater 1982; Stoel-Gammon 1980; Mackay & Hodson 1982; Smith & Stoel-Gammon 1983; Bleile 1982; Bleile & Schwartz 1984). All of these studies consistently point to the normality of the phonological processes observed. Indeed unlike the studies of developmental phonological disorders no salient qualitatively different characteristics appear to emerge from these studies.

Down's syndrome children have delayed development in all areas including language and speech, in which their development is believed to be particularly low (Fraser 1978; Gunn 1985). Wetherby, Yonclas, and Bryan (1989) carried out a comparative communication profile of handicapped and normal kindergarten children and found that Down's syndrome children showed a normal distribution in the communicative parameters on the pragmatic level of language.

In a broad survey of aspects of learning and language, Buckley (1985) discovered that, when learning to read, Down's syndrome children do not use the normal strategy of combining a series of perceptual orthographic visual symbols in a word to get its expressed meaning but rather go directly from the holistic visual form—the written word—to its meaning. Down's syndrome children learning to read make semantic rather than phonological errors, which are usually attested to in the early reading acquisition of normal children. Down's syndrome children learn to read logographically, as with a picture language, rather than connecting writing to sound.

Buckley cites researchers who claim that Down's syndrome children have a right hemisphere dominance in language. She proposes that their left hemisphere does not function properly and that they have to rely on the language possibilities offered by the right hemisphere. Therefore, their speech and language development is deviant. In the right hemisphere, there is a specific lexicon of spoken and written words, but the ability to decode a grapheme-to-phoneme correspondence is lacking. There is a brief and limited retention of verbal material; there are also problems with understanding long and complex sentences that go beyond basic syntactic structures. There is a problem in raising the phonemic image of a word. One of the most problematic aspects found when testing Down's syndrome children is their low level of speech and articulation (Le Prevost 1983).

Characteristics of Down's Syndrome Children's Speech Patterns

According to Penrose and Smith (1975), Down's syndrome affects speech and language skills because of disturbances in the development of the oral mechanism (disability in the function of the articulatory mechanism, breathing, and phonation) and, secondarily, as a result of the mental retardation characteristic of the syndrome. There are oral anomalies that are part of the physical and functional disabilities related to the shape, size, position, and development of the lips, tongue, teeth, palate, jaw, etc. As a result of early hypotonia and a smaller than normal cerebellum, Down's syndrome children have slow motor development, awkward and impaired coordination, low reflexes, and a long and slow reaction time.

Functional Processes of Down's Syndrome Children

Research has shown that Down's syndrome children are capable of developing phonological strategies. Grunwell (1981) claims that functional articulatory problems may be used as a diagnostic classification and that the errors of Down's syndrome children are organic in origin (i.e., a secondary symptom of an identified organic problem).

Dodd (1975) claims that the differences between Down's syndrome and normal children's speech are qualitative; the Down's child has a similar system as the normal child but adds his or her own rules, produces errors that cannot be formulated systematically, uses normal rules inconsistently.

The majority of researchers claim that the gap between Down's syndrome and normal children is primarily quantitative: the Down's child follows the same phonological development as normal children but exhibits a longer continuation of the phonological rules (Bodine 1974; Smith and Stoel-Gammon 1983).

The most common errors made by Down's syndrome children are fronting, devoicing, stopping, gliding, deletion of unstressed syllables, deletion of word-final consonants, and consonant cluster reduction (similar to normal functional errors/processes), but these are also accompanied by idiosyncratic processes, the inconsistent use of normal processes, and a wide variety of substitutions of the same phoneme in the same utterance.

According to Moran (1986) the nasal, hoarse, and rough characteristics of Down's syndrome children's voices, characteristics that may be organically connected to the structure of the sinus cavities, are related to the hypotonic tongue, the jaw, etc., which affect the resonance of speech as well as articulatory precision.

Case Study (Adapted from Hagoel 1993)

Sarit (female, 6:4), a Down's syndrome child whose speech was scrutinized 2 years, began treatment at 3 years of age, after a year of advising and training her parents. S. tests 3 months behind her chronological age in language comprehension and a year behind in speech production. S. has a large and developed active and passive lexicon. Her major problem is in continuity in various developmental areas: auditory, verbal, instructions, visual motor. S. still suffers from light hypotonia. S.'s problems in continuity and hypotonia result in unclear speech, which is in sharp contrast to her high language level and fluency. Her extremely low level of speech intelligibility disturbs her functioning in kindergarten and at home. She attends a regular kindergarten with children a year younger than herself. She is well integrated socially, accepted by her peers, and actively participates in all activities. She also receives treatment in occupational therapy. S. has three older brothers and lives in a warm, supportive, and accepting family.

S. was recorded in two thirty-minute speech therapy sessions consisting of spontaneous interpretations of pictures, spontaneous conversation among S., her therapist, and her father, who was invited to create a free and natural situation, and language games. The recording took place in the therapy room in which S. has been treated for three years. The recordings were transcribed, and a selection of thirty words with one or two errors per word was culled for the sample.

Analysis of S.'s Speech and Explanations Based on Phonology as Human Behavior

Almost all the errors were made in phonemes of constriction (consonants), which require greater motor control and play a greater communicative role. There was only one error in a phoneme of aperture (vowel): e → a (in a dorsal environment), *lexem* → [laʃem] (bread). The more syllables per word, the more errors: six bi-/polysyllabic words had two errors, and twenty-four mono-/bisyllabic words had one error only. There were fourteen substitutions (40 percent) (which require greater effort) and twenty-one deletions (60 percent) (which require less effort) in the thirty-five (100 percent) errors found in the thirty-word sample.

All substitutions were made either in word-initial position or in stressed syllables (the communication factor). Of the fourteen substitutions, eight retained the same degree of stricture, airflow, and turbulence (the communication factor), and six simplified the manner of articulation or number of sets of articulators (the human factor): stopping (from stable to mobile), which requires less motor control: ʃ → t, *ʃote* → [tote] (he drinks); deaffrication, which requires less motor control: t͜s → s, *tsalaxot* → [salaxot] (plates), and *kofetset* → [kofeset] (she jumps); gliding, which requires less motor control: *halax* → [hayax] (he walked); and devoicing (control over one set of articulators only): *dubi* → [tubi] (teddy bear).

The substitutions clearly indicate a simplification of the choice of active articulators as well (the human factor): fronting (dorsal consonants are replaced by apical consonants): ʃ → θ, *yoʃen* → [yoθen] (he sleeps); ʃ → t, *ʃote* → [tote] (he drinks); and x → ʃ, *lexem* → [laʃem] (bread). There is a tendency for simplification even for apical sounds; the anterodorsum sibilant phoneme (ʃ) is most frequently reduced to the voiceless apical-interdental fricative (θ) (not a Hebrew phoneme), which is easier to control than apical-alveolar or apical-dental sounds /s, z/ (which are Hebrew phonemes): ʃ → θ, *yoʃen* → [yoθen] (he sleeps); and *teʃev* → [teθev] (you will sit). Some of the substitutions result in a sequence of the same phoneme (the very same articulatory gestures), which requires less motor control, planning, and organization than it would take to exploit different active articulators: *yeled* → [yeyed] (boy); and ʃ → t, *ʃote* → [tote] (he drinks).

The majority of phonemic deletions are made in word-final position (low communication load): *ʃaloʃ* → [talo] (three), *sefeɤ/sfaɤim* → [sefe/sfaɤi] (book/books), *menagen* → [menage] (he plays [musical instrument]), *va-doɤ* → [va-do] (and generation), and *maɤak yeɤakot* → (maɤa yeɤako] (vegetable soup). Unstressed syllables of polysyllabic words are also deleted (low communication load): *mexonit* → xonit (car), and *metapelet* → tapelet (nanny).

S. has particular difficulty with the stable apical lateral consonant /l/, which requires a high degree of articulatory control, and she opts for different strategies in different phonetic environments, all of which can be explained by the interaction of the human and communication factors as opposed to being considered inconsistent: /l/ is replaced by the semivowel /y/, which requires less articulatory control in a phonetic environment containing neutral or back vowels and dorsal consonants (gliding): *halax* → [hayax] (he walked). /l/ is replaced by an excrescent glottal stop intervocalically: *agala* → [agaʔa] (wagon), and *ve-lo* → [veʔo] (and-no). /l/ is deleted in word-medial (i.e., syllable-final [to avoid a potential consonant cluster]) and word-final positions: *axalti/axalnu* → [axati/axanu] (I/we ate), *yalda* → [yada] (girl), *igul* → [igu] (circle), and *gadol* → [gado] (big). /l/ is retained either in word/syllable-initial position or, usually, in the stressed syllable of bi- or trisyllabic words where there is another error in the word: *lexem* → [laʃem] (bread), *ʃaloʃ* → [thalo] (three), *yeɤuʃalaim* → [yeɤuʃalai] (Jerusalem), and *tsalaxot* → [salaxot] (plates).

S. has particular difficulty with the /r/ phoneme, a voiced postdorsal fricative /ɤ/ that requires high articulatory control, and she opts for different strategies in different phonetic environments, all of which can be explained by the interaction of the human and communication factors as opposed to being considered inconsistent: /ɤ/ is deleted in unstressed word-final position in words/expressions: *sefeɤ* → [sefe] (book), and *va-doɤ* → [va-do] (and generation). /ɣ/ is retained in stressed word-final position in words where deletions are made in unstressed word-initial position: *maheɣ* → aheɣ (fast). /ɣ/ is replaced by a glottal stop before back vowels or intervocalically: *efɣonot* → [efʔonot] (pencils), and *maɣak* → [ʔaʔak] (soup). /ɣ/ is retained in polysyllabic words/expressions in which deletions are made in word-final position: *sfaɣim* → [sfaɣi] (books), *yeɣuʃalaim* → [yeɣuʃalai] (Jerusalem), and *maɣak yeɣakot* → [maɣa yeɣako] (vegetable soup).

The fewest errors are made in word-initial position (eight of thirty-five, or 22 percent), most of which (five of eight, or 60 percent) are substitutions, which require more effort and control (the communication factor). The most errors (fourteen of thirty-five, or 40 percent) are made in word-final position (the communication factor), most of which (twelve of fourteen, or 85 percent) are deletions, which require less effort and control (the human factor). The number of errors in word-medial position is also very large (thirteen of thirty-five, or 38 percent) and is almost equally divided into seven substitutions and six deletions. However, this should not be viewed as a random distribution: the substitutions requiring more effort and control appeared in stressed syllables (with a higher communication load), and the deletions requiring less effort and control appeared either in unstressed syllables (with lower communication load) or in sequences of two consecutive consonants requiring greater effort and control (the human factor).

Down's syndrome presents an even more extreme version of the minimax struggle for maximum communication with minimal effort found in normal functional errors in language acquisition.

The data taken from Bodine's (1974) study of two Down's syndrome children, which were summarized and adapted to functional processes in Ingram (1976b: 126–27), revealed the following for the first child (male, 5:9): There was a large amount of consonant and consonant cluster deletion in initial position. Nasals and vowels were considered to be more stable aspects of the child's phonology, with a larger degree of instability in vowels. Glottalization was also widespread. Final consonant deletion was prevalent. Final consonants that did occur were devoiced. And fricatives and affricates were reduced to /θ/. The following functional processes were found in the speech of the second child (male, 6:2): deaffrication and voicing; fronting/apicalization; devoicing in word-final position; vocalization; assimilation of obstruent in cluster; gliding; and liquid deletion.

Once again, we see a large number and concentration of decontextualized and unexplained functional processes, including individual or idiosyncratic ones. It is also interesting to note that the first child had a set of ten different communicatively distinct glottalized grunts, which, together with all the other data collected, indicate an extreme case of the search for maximum communication with minimal and organically limited effort.

Mental Retardation

In one of the earlier books that I have consulted, Carrell (1968: 46–47) says the following regarding deficiencies and defects of intelligence, language, and speech, some of which may still be relevant today:

> Speech is generally said to be a form of learned behavior. To be entirely accurate, it is not wholly learned since some components of the total speech responses are unlearned behavior acquired through maturation. Nevertheless, learning problems associated with defects and deficiencies in intelligence are a major cause of impaired communication. We will have to broaden our discussion to include language learning since the acquisition of verbal symbols and learning to articulate them are not wholly separable processes.
>
> Articulation disorders are much more frequent among mentally retarded than among normal children. Furthermore, the severity of the articulation defects increases with the degree of retardation. For instance, Burt [1937] found that the incidence of defective articulation was 14 per cent in a group of school children with IQ's from 70 to 85 and nearly 25 per cent in those with IQ's from 50 to 70. He also found "severe" disorders in 5 and 13 per cent of the two groups respectively. Other studies have reported similar findings, and in some cases the reported frequency of speech defects in the mentally retarded population was even higher.

Carrell also discusses the problems of defining intelligence:

> What exactly is meant by intelligence? Psychologists find it difficult to agree on a definition of the term, but for our purposes a person behaves "intelligently" in the broadest sense, if he is able to solve problems through perceptual, cognitive, and verbal processes, and if he can perform certain tasks involving learning.
>
> But as Hebb [1966] has pointed out, the term *intelligence* can be understood in two different senses, and at any given time one must understand which meaning he has in mind. What Hebb calls *Intelligence A* is the individual's innate potential: the level of performance of which he would be capable under the most favorable circumstances. *Intelligence B,* on the other hand, is his average level of performance at a given time. The latter is measured by intelligence tests or estimated from some other

observation of his behavior. Intelligence A can be inferred from Intelligence B, but one must give careful consideration to those variables that can cause discrepancies between the two. It cannot be assumed that the two are always the same.

It follows, then, that the terms *mental retardation* and *mental deficiency* should be defined with care. The professional literature is confusing because it often fails to do so. *Mental retardation* is frequently used as a general term for any intellectual disability without recognizing the value of a separate meaning for the term *mental deficiency.* A child should be thought as *mentally deficient* if his innate potential is limited either by heredity (*endogenous* or *familial* mental deficiency), or by some *exogenous* cause (pre- or postnatal brain damage, for instance). Mental deficiency, is, then, a limitation of Intelligence A.

By *mentally retarded* one means that a child's measured intelligence is below the expected level for his age; this is Intelligence B. The degree of retardation depends on how far below the average he falls. If performance is less than potential, we say the child is *functionally retarded* to that extent and the condition is, at least in theory, reversible. Functional retardation can be the result of emotional disturbance, deprivation, sensory or perceptual deficit, insufficient motivation, and the like. Moreover, defective speech and language can be a prime cause of functional retardation.

The American Association on Mental Deficiency (AAMD) defines retardation as a general intellectual functioning below the average, accompanied by impairments in adaptive behavior discovered during a child's developmental period. Mental deficiency is defined by *Webster's* as a failure in intellectual development that results in social incompetence and is held to be caused by a defect in the central nervous system and to be incurable. Intellectual performance is usually related to the results of standardized intelligence tests. The standard measurement is usually made in terms of mental age or intelligence quotient (IQ), which presents the proportional relation between mental age (MA) and chronological age (CA): IQ = MA/CA. It has been maintained that 3 percent of the population are mentally retarded (Grossman 1983). Schlanger (1973) explains that the cause of the impairment is generally unknown in 56 percent of cases of mental retardation. Hutt and Gribby (1973) emphasize that the levels of retardation are determined in accordance with IQ, from which the educability of the retarded child is also determined: An IQ of 25–49 is considered trainable mental retardation (TMR), or severe retardation; the individual is capable of learning essential daily tasks. An IQ of 50–69 is considered educable mental retardation (EMR), or light retardation; the individual is capable of learning an occupation in addition to essential daily skills.

The Connection between Mental Retardation and Language

There are two general theoretical approaches that can be used to explain the language of mentally retarded children: as being either delayed or different from that of normal children. The former approach considers the acquisition process of the retarded child to be delayed or slightly slower than that of normal children: Some scholars found a delayed babbling stage starting at 20–25 months and the use of words beginning at 2:3–4:5 years (Karlin and Strazulla 1952). Others found similar developmental stages as with normal children, but the stages were considered to be delayed from the point of view of the sensorimotor functions in the language of retarded children (Lachner 1968). The latter approach considers the process of language acquisition to be different for retarded children than for normal children: Scholars who support this hypothesis relate this difference to different cognitive or neurological disorders. Bliss, Allen, and Walker (1978) found that the language of EMR children was delayed and the language of TMR children different because of the difficulty the latter had producing syntactic constructions. Further difficulties were found in the abilities of abstraction and symbolization and in short-term memory. There is also a clear focus on the here and now, resulting in an impaired and concrete language for the retarded (Bowles, in Spreen 1965).

Characteristics of Mentally Retarded Children's Speech Patterns

The mentally retarded child has many problems communicating. Spreen (1965) classifies the frequency of speech, voice, and language problems in various populations according to IQ: 5–7 percent of the normal population has language problems; 45 percent of the lightly retarded (EMR) population with IQs of 50–70 has language problems; and 90 percent of the severely retarded (TMR) population with IQs of 25–49 has language problems. The degree and range of language problems also rise in accordance with the level of IQ: the lightly retarded (EMR) population with IQs of 50–70 has problems with articulation, prosody, and voice quality, limited vocabularies, and low levels of abstraction; the severely retarded (TMR) population with IQs of 25–49 has more serious problems with all the above, displays a more limited and stereotypical use of syntactic constructions, and shows language characterized by perseveration (i.e., the retention and repetition of the same articulatory gestures in a word or utterance) (Schlanger 1973).

Wilson (1966) examined the speech of 777 retarded children, of whom 53.4 percent were found to have articulation problems of substitutions and deletions. There was, once again, an inverse ratio between the amount of misarticulations and IQ: the lower the IQ, the higher the amount and degree of deviations in speech. It was also found that the functional development of normal children until the age of 3 persevered much later in mentally retarded children. Similar percentages (56.7 percent of seventy-seven children) and findings were also reported in Schlanger (1973). Higher percentages (57–72 percent) of language disorders were reported in Spradlin (1963), who took into account differences in the type of populations studied and the variation in the criteria used in judging language disorders in the speech of institutionalized mentally retarded children.

All the research reviewed above has shown that the language of the mentally retarded child is impaired in all the traditional and neotraditional categorizations of language: phonology, morphology, syntax, semantics, and pragmatics. Despite the dichotomous approaches to the language of the mentally retarded as either delayed or different from that of normal children, it is generally assumed that each category of language disorders is different. However, it is also generally held that, the greater the linguistic or communicative demand, the more difficult it will be for the retarded child to meet the task. Milgram (1973) raises the hypothesis that there is a developmental gap between the verbal medium and the cognitive abilities of the retarded child. It is possible that the child has the mental but not the linguistic abilities to solve the problem. Therefore, the more abstract the linguistic task, the more difficult it will be for the retarded child to handle.

Functional Processes of Mentally Retarded Children

Ingram (1976b: 122) states the following concerning the prevalence and types of what he refers to as phonological processes found in the speech of mentally retarded children in comparison with normal and deviant children: "Studies on the articulation of mentally retarded children include those of Irwin 1942, Bangs 1942, Karlin and Strazulla 1952 and Schlanger 1953a and b. In general, each indicates that retarded children show similar substitution patterns to those of normal children, i.e. that they have similar phonological processes. Also, they show the persistent use of the common processes of deviant children. . . . Mentally retarded children, then, appear very like the deviant children with phonological disorders already discussed." This supports the findings of the other cases discussed here.

The most common functional processes that Ingram found (1976b: 115) when classifying seventeen deviant children culled from different studies were cluster reduction, stopping, depalatalization, fronting, gliding, deletion of final consonants, voicing processes, assimilation in clusters, and velar assimilation. The phonological patterns that Ingram (1976b: 118) found in eighteen deviant children studied by Weber (1970) include fronting of velars, fronting of palatals, loss of affrication, stopping, gliding, affrication, devoicing, and final consonant deletion.

Ingram (1976b: 122–23) summarized Bangs's (1942) comprehensive study in terms of natural functional processes and compared and contrasted these processes with normal and deviant language development in the following way:

> Bangs 1942 is in many ways the most comprehensive of these studies [of mentally retarded children]. He studied 53 subjects who were residents of a custodial school. He chose only subjects "whose speech defects could not be attributed to factors which are known to be of etiological significance in articulatory disorders" (343). They were tested by a naming task, using 65 cards with pictures of common objects. Transcriptions were made at the time of testing.
>
> Bangs analysed the most common substitutions by position and gives figures for the most frequent of them. These data are restated in terms of the processes described in this book. . . . They are very similar to the processes used by deviant children. . . . This leads Bangs to conclude, "the sounds most frequently substituted for each sound by the ament also are very similar to those used by the normal child" (356). In section 5.3 it was pointed out that some of the patterns of deviant children were not typically normal, Bangs also notes in his data. "Many of the minor substitutions made by aments are not in accordance with the usual ones made by children with normal intelligence" (356).

The most common substitution processes shown by the fifty-three mentally retarded children and the position in which these processes occurred are as follows:

1. gliding (favored in initial, then medial, then final position);
2. labialization (favored in initial, then medial, then final position);
3. fronting of velars (favored in initial, then final position);
4. stopping (found in all positions, but most prevalent in medial position);

5. fronting of palatals (not found in initial position; favored in medial, then final position);

6. devoicing, from fricative to sibilant (found in all positions; favored in medial position);

7. vocalization (found in final position); and

8. final consonant deletion (adapted from Ingram 1976b: 123).

Once again, we see the recurrence of many of the functional processes of various degrees of commonness and uniqueness in a fairly dense concentration in the output of mentally retarded children. Concerning the interaction between the human and the communication factors, it should also be noted that consonant deletions and vocalizations appear exclusively or predominantly in final position, which has the lowest communicative force. Substitutions, on the other hand, appear in all positions and are favored in initial and medial positions, which have the highest or a higher communicative force. Labialization was also slightly favored in initial position, as we have previously seen in the slight preference of visual phonemes in and across languages. Prosodic, syllabic, and other factors were not included in the data presented, which also may have been significant regarding the favorings or disfavorings in the various word positions.

Ingram (1976b: 123) also notes that a large number of the functional processes found in Bangs represent deletions (omissions): "There is one aspect of the data that Bangs feels is especially noteworthy. A large number of the errors are those of omission rather than substitution. Twenty-one per cent of all errors are by omission, and thirty-five per cent of the final errors are also omissions. 'This fact indicates that omissions are one of the most significant characteristics of the articulating errors found in the feeble-minded' (356). Since data on omissions is not given in the earlier studies, it is not possible to see if this is greater than that done by deviant children. A glance at the rule system, however, does not show an excessive number of deletion rules. It may be that omissions will prove to be a characteristic of retarded speech. Omission is also found to be a common error pattern in Karlin and Strazzula (1952)." I have already established that deletions and omissions indicate a clear favoring of the human factor over the communication factor, and it is not surprising that they should characterize the speech of the mentally retarded.

Case Study (Adapted from Segal 1992)

A. (female, 7:5), the youngest child of a lower-middle-class family, had two siblings aged 11 and 12; all attend regular schools. A. had a very late motor development, including a very late language development as well: first isolated words appeared at the age of 4:5; sentences appeared a little later (no record in the file). She was referred for therapy by the school psychologist, who reported general developmental problems (delayed development in all areas) and delayed language development in particular. She was found to have severe verbal communication problems and was capable of using short words and very short sentences only. She had severe learning problems, did not make any social contact with her peers, and remained on the periphery of social situations. She was also diagnosed as having emotional problems.

The intake in the speech clinic revealed a low level of language and many language errors as well as memory difficulties for words and numbers. A. recognized and used only a very limited number of lexically simple verbs. In the interpretation of pictures, she used only 2- and three-word sentences, and even those were on the most basic lexical level, without function words such as conjunctions. She had many misarticulations (particularly deletions in word-initial and word-final positions), a seemingly random set of substitutions, and careless speech with a very low level of intelligibility. The /r/ phoneme /ɣ/ was consistently omitted. She almost never used inflectional morphemes.

A. began speech therapy twice a week. During the therapy, it was apparent that she was learning. A. internalized what she was learning both in language in general and in articulation in particular. She was, however, not capable of generalizing what she had learned and could not apply the principles learned in one situation to another, except for specific things that were practiced in the clinic. Progress was shown in all areas, albeit very slow and limited, and her general level of language remained very low.

Two exemplars of A.'s speech containing characteristic misarticulations were selected for analysis and compared: the standard articulation test administered to A. during the intake and an example of her speech during one of her most recent therapy sessions (after approximately a year and a half of therapy). These exemplars will be used to explain two kinds of processes: an analysis of the processes containing A.'s characteristic misarticulations found in both exemplars and an attempt to explain them according to the

Table 8.1 Deaffrication in a Mentally Retarded Child

	Exemplar 1	Exemplar 2
Initial position	(*a*) *tsipoɤ* → [sipo] (bird) *tsav* → [sav] (turtle)	*tsipoɤim* → [sipoim] (birds)
Final position	(*b*) *rats* → [as] (he runs)	
Maintaining the affricate	(*c*)	*tsɤixim* → [tsiim] (they have to)

theory of phonology as human behavior; an analysis of changes (should there be any) that occurred in A.'s speech during her therapy and an attempt to explain them according to the theory of phonology as human behavior. The data will be presented according to the accepted functional processes that are used in the clinic and then will be analyzed according to the principles of phonology as human behavior.

Analysis of A.'s Speech and Explanations Based on Phonology as Human Behavior

Deaffrication The examples in table 8.1 indicate the following general tendencies of deaffrication (*a, b*) versus the maintaining of the affricate (*c*), which can be explained by the interaction of the human and communication factors: The use of the same active articulators in the same immediate environment is disfavored unless their juxtaposition is, by virtue of some other factor, mutually beneficial, which—because of the communication factor—explains why the homorganic affricate /ts/ is a phoneme in Hebrew in the first place. Transitions from one distinct constriction to another within a single phoneme are disfavored, which explains why there is only one affricate in the phonemic inventory of Hebrew. The use of additional articulators is disfavored, which is why the single affricate in Hebrew is voiceless. The single affricate in Hebrew is made by the apex, the most flexible, adroit, sensitive, and precise articulator and the easiest active articulator to control. The apical affricate /ts/ was deaffricated to [s] in all cases when it appeared alone in all word-order positions (*a–b*). The rather unusual deletion of the easier to control mobile phoneme rather than the more difficult stable pho-

Table 8.2 Consonant Cluster Reduction in a Mentally Retarded Child

		Exemplar 1	Exemplar 2
Initial position	(*a*)		*(t)stakli* → [sakli] (look)
			stam → [sam] (ordinary)
	(*b*)	*glida* → [lida] (ice cream)	*ktana* → [tana] (little)
		kviʃ → [vi] (road)	*bgadim* → [badim] (clothes)
	(*c*)		*tmuna* → [tuna] (picture)
Medial position	(*d*)	*miʃkafayim* → [mikafayim] (glasses)	*yalda* → [yada] (girl)
		bakbuk → [babuk] (bottle)	*simla* → [sila] (dress)

neme may be compensated for (the communication factor) by the fact that the stable phoneme (a voiceless silibant) provides clearer acoustic information by virtue of its high frequency (Hz). In this case, the communication factor may have motivated the fact that A. maintained the more difficult stable phoneme of constriction, which provides more acoustic information, particularly in word-initial position. The affricate /t͜s/ was maintained only when it formed part of a consonant cluster (*c*) in order to give maximum information and maintain the phonetic structure of the word in the communicatively crucial initial position.

Consonant Cluster Reduction The examples in table 8.2 indicate the following general tendencies of A.'s reduction of consonant clusters, which can be explained by the interaction of the human and communication factors: The articulation of two consecutive phonemes of constriction (both within and without syllable boundaries) either as single juxtaposed phonemes or in a cluster (CC) requires greater muscular control than a CVC combination; that is, consonant cluster reduction minimizes human effort at the expense of the communication factor. In initial consonant clusters containing mobile and stable consonants (*a*), the mobile rather than the stable consonant was deleted just as in the deaffrication (discussed above). In the initial clusters containing a posterodorsal consonant and a labial, labial-dental, or apical consonant (*b*)—[gl], [kv], [kt], [bg]—the posterodorsal consonant was deleted in favor of the easier to control labial, labial-dental, or apical, which in all these cases gave additional visual input in initial

Table 8.3 Deletion of Velar Fricatives in a Mentally Retarded Child

	Exemplar 1	Exemplar 2
Word-initial position	(*a*) *ɣakevet* → [akevet] (train)	
	ɣats → [as] (he runs)	
		ɣakdu → [adu] (they danced)
		xadaʃim → [adaim] (new)
/ɣ/ as part of an initial CC	(*b*) *pɣaxim* → [paim] (flowers)	*tsɣixim* → [tsiim] (they have to)
Word-medial position	(*c*) *pɣaxim* → [paim] (flowers)	*tsɣixim* → [tsiim] (they have to)
	midɣaxa → [midaa] (sidewalk)	*gaɣbayim* → [gabayim] (socks)
	aɣye → [aye] (lion)	*haɣbe* → [abe] (a lot)
	aɣnevet → [anevet] (rabbit)	*taɣnegolet* → [anegolet] (a hen)
		uɣva → [uva] (stable)
		tsipoɣim → [sipoim] (birds)
Word-final position	(*d*) *tsipoɣ* → [sipo] (bird)	
	kaduɣ → [kadu] (ball)	
	mafteax → [matea] (key)	

position (/v/, /b/, and even /l/). In the initial [tm] cluster (*c*), the nasal requiring the simultaneous excitation of three sets of articulators is deleted in favor of the apical mobile consonant, requiring the excitation of one set of articulators only. The deletion of the nasal may also be viewed as the human factor being stronger than the communication factor since the nasal provides important transitional acoustic information (has formants like vowels). The retention of the apical and more visual /l/ in the initial [gl] cluster indicates two elements of the human factor being stronger than the communication factor since the "sonorant, liquid" /l/—like the sonorant nasal—provides important acoustic information by virtue of having formants (albeit weaker formants than vowels). In the noninitial, medial consonant deletion (or consonant-cluster-across-syllable-boundaries deletion), the consonant in syllable-final position with a lower communicative load was consistently deleted, and the consonant in syllable-initial position with a higher communicative load was consistently maintained.

Deletion of Velar Fricatives (x, ɣ) in All Phonetic Environments The examples in table 8.3 indicate the following general tendencies of the deletion of what is traditionally called voiced and voiceless velar fricatives, which can be explained by the interaction of the human and communication factors: As was pointed out in the intake, the voiced velar fricative /ɣ/ (the Israeli /r/ phoneme) was not part of A.'s phonemic repertoire. This particular phoneme is clearly a problematic one for many children acquiring Hebrew both with and without organic difficulties. The data in table 8.3 also indicate that the same probably holds true for /x/, the voiceless counterpart of /ɣ/ (but this might be harder to verify since there might have been a slight turbulence of air that was not investigated spectrographically for both the anterodorsal voiceless sibilant /ʃ/ and /x/). It is not surprising that the posterodorsal, stable phonemes of constriction, which are harder to make than their more flexible labial-dental and apical counterparts, are those that A. cannot articulate. It is also not surprising that the voiced /ɣ/ requiring the simultaneous excitation of two sets of articulators should be the one that is most clearly missing in A.'s (as well as others') phonemic repertoire. I would like to point out that, in exemplar 2, there was evidence that both the posterodorsal stable phonemes /x/ (which may have been articulated previously with very slight turbulence) and /ɣ/ were beginning to be acquired: /ɣ/ was replaced by the glottal stop /ʔ/ preceded by the low central vowel /a/, which replaced /e:/ in pe:ɣot → [paʔot] (fruits); /ɣ/ was articulated in the name *kaɣin* (Karin).

Deletion of Unstressed Initial Syllables in Polysyllabic Words The examples in table 8.4 indicate the following general tendencies of the deletion of unstressed syllables, which change the phonetic structure of the word and can be explained by the interaction of the human and communication factors: It is obvious that, in general, the more syllables per word, the more control is needed to produce it, and the more communicative information there is in the word itself. Therefore, it is not surprising that, in these polysyllabic words of four and five syllables, the human factor should prevail in the deletion of one or two syllables in order to maintain minimal effort. It is equally not surprising that the syllables that are deleted will be those with the least communicative load, that is, the unstressed syllables.

Table 8.4 Deletion of Unstressed Initial Syllables in a Mentally Retarded Child

Exemplar 1	Exemplar 2
televizia → [vizia] (television)	*taɤnegolet* → [degolet] (hen)
mixnasaim → [masaim] (pants)	*mixnasaim* → [nasaim] (pants)

Inconsistent Articulations of the Same Word in Different Contexts It should also be noted that, in the examples considered immediately above, the deletion of unstressed initial syllables in polysyllabic words, there are two cases of alternative pronunciations of the same word or, in other words, inconsistent articulations: The first is *mixnasaim* → [nasaim]/*mixnasaim* → [masaim] (pants). In the first instance, the initial unstressed syllable [mi(x)] is deleted, and the articulation of the rest of the word remains unchanged. In the second instance, the /n/ is replaced by the visual bilabial nasal /m/ after the initial unstressed syllable [mi(x)] is deleted. Another possible explanation could be that only the "consonant cluster" in [i(x)n] is deleted and that the initial /m/ is retained. In all three instances involving unstressed syllable or consonant cluster reduction with or without the /n/ → /m/ substitution, there is a compromise between the human and the communication factors in the production of this difficult polysyllabic word.

The second is *taɤnegolet* → [degolet]/*taɤnegolet* → [anegolet] (chicken, hen) (cf. the *c* examples in table 8.3 above). In the first instance, the initial unstressed syllable [taɤ] is deleted, and the apical nasal /n/ requiring the excitation of three sets of articulators is replaced by its homorganic voiced stop /d/, requiring the excitation of two sets of articulators only. In the second instance, both the /t/ and the consistently unarticulated /ɤ/ are deleted, but the phonetic structure of the polysyllabic word is maintained by the vowel or the nucleus of the initially unstressed syllable, which in this case is not deleted. Once again, these so-called inconsistent articulations represent alternative strategies of reaching an efficient compromise between the human and the communication factors in the production of this difficult polysyllabic word.

It should also be noted that these different articulations were uttered in different speech situations (an intake test and a conversation) and in different phonetic contexts (a list of individual words and part of a phrase in natural or spontaneous speech).

As was previously discussed in the sections on apraxia, dyspraxia, and Down's syndrome, inconsistent articulations of the same word have been viewed as a kind of marker for delayed, deviant, and organic speech disorders; this approach could also apply to general functional processes as well. And, as was previously explained, very often a closer look at the larger contexts in which the same word was uttered in different ways reveals that this "inconsistency" merely illustrates the same speaker applying different strategies to solve the problem of achieving or maintaining maximum communication with minimal effort in different phonetic environments or in different speech situations.

Perhaps one of the problems of clinical phonology based on natural or formal generative and postgenerative phonological theories is that the "rules" of these theories do not always take context into account. The theory of phonology as human behavior might be criticized for applying different or even contradictory strategies to explain the same or similar phenomena in what might appear to be an ad hoc way from a formal point of view. Another way of viewing this, however, is to see that formal rules have their inevitable exceptions and cannot always be applied across the board precisely because intelligent human beings may solve similar problems in different contexts and situations in diverse ways.

Other Processes Found in A.'s Speech A.'s speech also revealed devoicing, glottalization, the "inconsistent" deletion of certain consonants in initial and medial positions (in accordance to context), and assimilations, reduplications, or perseverations where more difficult phonemes were replaced by easier phonemes or by phonemes readily available in the immediate context: *naalayim* → [lalaim] (shoes) and *degel* → [dedel] (flag).

A.'s speech as well as other examples of the speech of mentally retarded children analyzed by functional processes can be explained by the theory of phonology as human behavior as a most extreme example of the struggle between the human and the communication factors. In these cases, the various principles of the theory outlined in the beginning of this chapter, as well as the additional principles postulated by Katz (1993, 1995) in the clinic, can be employed to explain the nonrandom distribution of all the consistent and seemingly inconsistent phonetic phenomena found in the speech of patients considered to have organic disorders.[5]

Summary and Conclusions

Let me conclude this chapter with a brief summary of the major theoretical principles underlying the theory of phonology as human behavior for phonological analysis (in the clinic):

1. One begins with the phonetic observations, articulatory and acoustic, within which there are no observable phonemic units (clinical intake).

2. By means of the communication orientation, one can establish the *number* of distinctive units of a language (or for a client via discrimination tests).

3. Consideration of the acoustic and physiological characteristics of the units (and the client) suggests a variety of characterizations.

4. In choosing among these characterizations, it is apparent that the characteristics of the units must be of such a kind that the human user can learn them (in usual and unusual circumstances of first language acquisition).

5. One does not know in advance, deductively, in exactly what way the human factor will interact with the communication and other factors.

6. Phonotactic skewings in language (and in the clinic), both diachronic and synchronic, reflect the learning process of the speakers (and clients).

7. This skewing, viewed consistently with the human factor against the background of the other factors of communication, acoustics, and physiology, informs one of the characteristics with which one is confronted.

8. Phonology is not random but motivated; the frequencies of the phonological units and the ways they combine are determined both by their phonetic makeup and by the speaker's (or client's) exploitation of—or coping with—that makeup in the act of communication.

9. Gestures enhancing communicative distinctiveness are favored, and articulatorily more difficult gestures are disfavored.

10. There is a conflict between the communication and the human factors in the search for maximum communication with minimal effort in the diachronic development of a language and its current synchronic state.

11. This conflict is even more keenly felt in language acquisition, where functional processes and errors may be observed, and even more so in the clinic, where functional and organically motivated processes and errors show an even more extreme conflict between the communication and the human factors.

12. The theory of phonology as human behavior can explain the connections and

interactions of the phylogeny, ontogeny, and pathology of the development of sound systems in human language in a principled way.

In the following chapters, I will continue to apply the theory of phonology as human behavior to the clinic, namely, the speech of the hearing impaired (including analyses of the results of audiological discrimination tests as well as their articulatory processes and errors), the speech of a patient who has had a cochlear implant, and the speech of aphasics.

V

Phonology as Human Behavior

Audiology and Aphasia

The dissolution of the linguistic sound system in aphasics provides an exact mirror-image of the phonological development in child language. Thus *e.g.*, the distinction of the liquids *r* and *l* is a very late acquisition of child language, and, as Froeschels observes, it is one of the earliest and most common in aphasic disturbances.
—Roman Jakobson (1941/1968: 60)

The order in which speech sounds are restored in the aphasic during the process of recovery corresponds directly to the development of child language.
—Roman Jakobson (1941/1968: 62)

The linguistic progress of the child and the regression of the aphasic are, in essence, direct and particularly concrete consequences of this principle. The stratified structure of language is in this way revealed. The more data linguistics makes available, from different peoples, on the speech of children and aphasics, the more significant and thoroughly can it handle the structural laws of particular languages and language in general.
—Roman Jakobson (1941/1968: 93–94)

9 Audiology, Hearing Impairment, and Cochlear Implants

Distinctive feature theory quickly became implicit in the minds of most of us. For the doubters, it was at least a provocative oversimplification to question or to argue against. The theory also has affected clinical practices in speech/language therapy (Winitz 1975). It has not yet significantly affected the audiology clinic. Another application has been in the diagnostic testing of voice transmission systems (Voiers 1977). Perhaps theory has not completely revolutionized phonetics, especially not the important questions in the brain-motor organization of speech, but it has greatly and beneficially affected the study of speech communication. —J. M. Pickett (1988: 6)

Theories are ways to try to comprehend highly complex large-scale interactions. Comprehension is motivated by the scientist's desire for understanding, by the scientist's need to teach others (both practitioners and scientists) and to provide rationales for use in improving practices. Speech communication involves such large-scale interacting phenomena that a wide variety of explanatory theories can be effective for comprehension, even of a given subdomain, such as the perception of speech. Thus some constraints on what we wish to understand, and thereby be able to control in practice, are necessary to limit the number of current theories. Put another way: our particular domains of investigation determine the related theories used to guide our investigation. —J. M. Pickett (1988: 5)

Audiology and Hearing Impairment

Hearing is the principle sensory channel through which children acquire language and speech. A deficit in hearing inhibits the reception of auditory feedback of the vocal or verbal behavior of the individual and his or her surroundings. The entire linguistic development of a hearing-impaired child differs significantly from that of a hearing child from the earliest stages of intentional babbling up to and including all aspects of adult speech production. In general, the greater the hearing loss, the more difficult and problematic the acquisition and production of language.

In this chapter, I will apply the theory of phonology as human behavior to the field of audiology and hearing impairment. Audiology is the science that deals with the receptive or perceptual aspects of the speech chain (Denes and Pinson 1963); it is clearly related to and plays an underlying background role in the work of the speech clinic. Grunwell (1987: 9) describes this symbiotic relationship as follows: "The clinician must also make a comprehensive assessment of a person's speech production abilities, including not just an examination of the speech production mechanism and its phonetic functioning, but also an assessment of the aural reception mechanism and its auditory functioning. This latter should include an auditory phonemic discrimination test, i.e. an investigation of the person's ability to perceive the phonological contrasts used in the normal pronunciation of his language. These procedures are, however, well-established clinical practice."

More often than not, however, the work of the audiologist in the speech and hearing clinic is viewed separately from that of the speech pathologist. Shipley and McAfee (1992: 342) reflect this aspect of the state of the art:

> The assessment of hearing is within the professional province of the audiologist, not the speech-language pathologist. However, the speech-language clinician is interested in clients' hearing abilities since hearing loss directly affects the development or maintenance of optimal communicative skills. Specifically, we are interested in the effects of hearing-impairment:
>
> —On the assessment of communicative development and disabilities,
> —On the development or maintenance of communication disorders,
> —On treatment recommendations and the selection of appropriate treatment procedures and target behaviors, and
> —On communicative and academic development.
>
> Speech-language pathologists are limited to screening their clients' hearing, but it is also vitally important for the speech-language pathologist to understand hearing loss, audiological assessment procedures, interpretations of findings, and implications of hearing loss on speech and language development.

Yet, even when the specific functions of speech pathologists and audiologists are clearly distinguished, their symbiotic and synergetic cooperation is still recognized as part of a holistic kind of therapy advocated by Shipley and McAfee (1992: 364): "Hearing is an extremely important factor in the development and maintenance of communicative abilities. A hearing loss can contribute to or even be the single cause of many communicative disorders. The audiologist is responsible for evaluating and diagnosing hearing loss. The speech-language pathologist is responsible for understanding the audiological assessment results and their impact on a client's speech and language. A client's best interests are clearly served when audiologists and speech-language pathologists pool their knowledge, abilities and clinical skills on the client's behalf."

In this chapter, I will first discuss and analyze the speech of hearing-impaired children in terms of the theory of phonology as human behavior. I will then show how the theory can be applied to the work of the audiologist or hearing clinician in discrimination tests. Finally, I will apply the theory to the speech of a deaf woman who had a cochlear implant.

Cochlear implants have been defined by Martin (1990: 386) in the following way: "Cochlear implants consist of one electrode or an array of electrodes that are placed surgically into the cochlea of the inner ear. The electrodes are attached to an internal receiver that is implanted in the bone behind the external ear. The acoustic signal is received by an externally worn microphone, which feeds a speech processor, which, in turn, amplifies and filters the sound and sends the electric impulses to a transmitter that converts the signal to magnetic impulses. The connection between the external and internal components of the cochlear implant is made either by an induction system or by a direct plug-in arrangement through the skin. When the cochlea is severely damaged, the cochlear implant can provide electric stimulation to the auditory nerve for transmission to the brain." In short, the purpose of this chapter is to apply the theory of phonology as human behavior to the various aspects of the auditory side of clinical phonology.

The Speech of the Hearing Impaired from a Traditional Point of View

People with hearing losses are considered to have sensory and perceptual deficits. Hearing sensitivity can be evaluated by an audiogram, which is a graphic illustration of hearing sensitivity. An audiogram depicts hearing levels (in dB, or decibels, a measurement of intensity or loudness) at different frequencies of sound (Shipley and McAfee 1992: 388). The human ear can hear frequencies in the range of approximately 20–20,000 Hz (or hertz, the measurement of frequency). Human speech lies in the range of 125–8,000 Hz, with the most essential communicative information being contained between 300 and 3,000 Hz. Children suffering from hearing loss do not receive the same auditory feedback as normal hearing children; this affects both the way they acquire and the way they monitor their own speech. Carrell (1968: 22) states the following regarding the connections between hearing loss and misarticulations:

> The nature of misarticulations secondary to sensory hearing loss is governed by a number of variables. They depend first on the frequencies at which the individual's threshold is impaired. A *flat audiogram,* in which the loss is approximately the same from 125 Hz to 8,000 Hz [i.e., the frequencies of human speech], may reduce the child's ability to hear, and therefore learn, any of the sounds of speech. A *high frequency* loss confined to, or greater in, the frequencies lying above 2,000 Hz will have a relatively greater effect on the reception and learning of the fricative, plosive, and affricate sounds, than on vowels and diphthongs. The severity of the loss is, of course, of great importance. In addition there are subtle factors, many of them poorly understood, that cannot be deduced from inspection of a routine audiogram, but which nevertheless are critical to the functional efficiency of hearing. Age, intelligence, extent of previous speech learning, and what might be called *phonetic aptitude* are influential variables.
>
> For these and other reasons one must not be too hasty in reaching conclusions about the relationship between auditory acuity and articulation status. . . . However, we can say generally that a hearing loss present at birth or acquired early in life must be considered one of the significant reasons for misarticulation, and that the patterns of speech are somewhat distinctive for different degrees and kinds of loss.

Hearing loss and its effect on speech have been classified according to the various hierarchical degrees determined for different levels of hearing loss. Carrell (1968: 22–23) defines mild hearing loss and discusses the phonemic errors characteristic of it from a traditional point of view: "By a mild hearing loss we mean one in which the threshold, while not normal, is still not raised to the point where the child has any significant difficulty in acquiring the ability to talk. The errors in mild hearing loss are primarily on the nonsyllabic fricative, plosive and affricate sounds. Vowels and other syllabic sounds are little affected because they contain sufficient acoustic energy to bring them above the threshold. Consonants are more difficult to hear and discriminate. Fricative sounds are more vulnerable in this respect than plosives and affricates, again because of their differences in acoustic energy." Carrell also mentions the similarity between the misarticulations associated with mild hearing loss and early (or what he refers to as "infantile") language acquisition: "Actually, the errors in mild hearing loss are much the same as those of infantile speech, which is what one would expect if he accepts the premise that lack of good auditory discrimination is among the major reasons for phonetic delay. Specifically, a child with a mild hearing loss is likely to exhibit [θ]/[s], [ð]/[z], [θ]/[ʃ], [ð]/[ʒ], [s]/[ʃ], [z]/[ʒ], [f]/[θ], [v]/[ð], and similar confusions. Some distortions or inaccurate approximations of the sibilants may be heard, and there may even be a kind of generalized imprecision in articulation. Omission of sounds is not particularly typical."

At the opposite extreme of severity of hearing loss are those diagnosed as being profoundly deaf. Profound deafness and the phonemic errors associated with it are identified and discussed in Carrell (1968: 23):

Since deafness is defined educationally as a degree of hearing loss so great that the individual has too little hearing to acquire speech (at least without special training), it follows that the associated articulation problems will be severe. Indeed, a failure to develop standard speech sounds is one of the typical signs of deafness in a young child. Among untrained children whose deafness dates from birth (*congenital deafness*) or is acquired shortly thereafter, any attempts at vocalized communication usually consist almost entirely of undifferentiated vowel-like sounds, or of syllables in which the initiating or terminating "consonant" movements are generalized lip and front-tongue [apex] adjustments. The signals so produced only remotely resemble familiar speech sounds. Frequently the vowel or vowel-like resonances are conspicuously nasal.

Those deaf children who do acquire some degrees of oral speech (and most of them can be taught a great deal) will nevertheless continue to have articulation defects of a kind consistent with the fact that they get few or no auditory cues. The quality of their vowel resonance is almost never accurate enough to make the vowels indistinguishable from those of a normal speaker, although front vowels are often better than back vowels. Consonant articulation is almost certain to be inaccurate, except possibly for the visual sounds, such as [f], [v], [m], [w], [p], [b], and perhaps [θ] and [ð]. Speech sounds ordinarily made with contact between the front of the tongue and the anterior portion of the upper dental arch (*linguapalatal* and *lingua-alveolar* sounds) such as [t], [d], [l], and [n] will usually be better pronounced than *linguavelars* such as [k], [g], and [ŋ], which the deaf child is likely to produce with a fronted position of the tongue. Indeed, all of his *lingual* nonsyllabics are usually made with *lingua-alveolar, linguapalatal,* or *linguadental* positioning.

The specific case studies that I will be presenting in this chapter, however, belong to the intermediate ranges between the above extremes, that is, what is referred to in the literature as moderate to severe hearing loss, which is defined and whose phonemic errors are discussed by Carrell (1968: 24–25) in the following traditional way:

> *Moderate to severe hearing loss* covers the range of auditory disability between mild hearing loss and deafness. Since the range is great, the kind and amount of speech handicap varies [*sic*] considerably. In general, a moderate to severe loss is sufficiently great to interfere appreciably with language learning and social functioning, and it usually calls for special education and management. The phonemic errors of children with this degree of loss (if congenital, or acquired early) will fit into the patterns described for mild hearing-impairments, but will be aggravated in degree. As the severity of the loss approaches deafness, the speech characteristics will naturally become more like those of the deaf.
>
> Retardation in the rate at which phonetic skills are developed is thus more marked than among children with mild hearing loss, but less, of course, than among the deaf. In contrast to mild hearing loss, a moderate to severe loss is likely to cause some misarticulation of the vowels, particularly when the loss of acuity approaches the upper limits of the range. Confusions and misarticulations involving such relatively high energy sounds as [l], [r], [j], [w], [m], [n], and [ŋ] will begin to appear at progressively higher levels of loss; errors on the nonsyllabic sounds will become more nearly like those heard in deaf speakers. Errors in the production of the sibilants and on [f], [v], and [θ], and [ð] become more marked, and most of the phonemic confusions characteristic of infantile speech will appear to an aggravated degree. The prosodic elements of speech will also be affected to an extent consistent with the severity of the loss.

Carrell's traditional descriptions and explanations have been adapted to the theory of natural processes by Ingram (1976b) and others.

The Speech of the Hearing Impaired and Functional Processes

Ingram (1976b: 123) discusses the speech of the hard of hearing as part of a larger chapter on the nature of deviant phonology. He compares and contrasts the speech of the hearing impaired with that of normal and deviant children and comes to the conclusion that the speech of the hearing impaired is unique:

> Just as the deletion of consonants seems to characterize the speech of the mentally retarded, there appear to be certain characteristics that set the hard-of-hearing apart from both normal and deviant children. Studies of the speech of hard-of-hearing children have been numerous (Hudgins 1934, Hudgins and Numbers 1942, Carr 1953, Calvert 1962, Fry 1966, John and Howarth 1965, Markides 1970, Levitt and Smith 1972, West and Weber 1973, Oller and Kelly 1974, Oller and Eilers 1975). In these studies several factors recur indicating that hard-of-hearing speech has a nature of its own.
>
> By far the most extensive of these studies is that of Hudgins and Numbers (1942). In an early study, Hudgins (1934) had noted five particular aspects of deaf speech: (1) extremely slow, laboured and excessively breathy speech; (2) prolonged production of vowels, resulting in either distortion or the creation of a new syllable; (3) a tendency to devoice stops in all positions; (4) excessive use of nasality with vowels and consonants; and (5) abnormal rhythm across an utterance. The study of Hudgins and Numbers was undertaken to examine more closely the validity of these observations.
>
> Hudgins and Numbers made phonograph records of the speech of 192 deaf pupils between 8 and 20 years of age. This resulted in a total of approximately 1200 sentences of 6 to 12 words each. These were examined for the most common errors in both consonants and vowels. They analyzed the consonant errors into seven types and the vowel errors into five types.

The functional processes and the percentage of their use in the speech of deaf children is shown in table 9.1.

Ingram (1976b: 124) then compares and contrasts the speech of the mentally retarded (a discussion based on Bangs [1942], which is discussed in the previous chapter) and normal children with that of the hearing-impaired children according to the theory of phonological processes:

> The first striking finding is the large number of errors in the production of vowels. Bangs (1942), for example, finds few vocalic errors in his study, and normal children acquire vowels quite early. Secondly, the devoicing of stops is not like the normal processes of assimilation. Normally stops tend to be voiced before vowels. A third unusual process is the deletion of initial consonants. Normal children usually overcome this quite early. A widespread characteristic of several of the processes

9.1 Functional Processes in the Speech of Deaf Children

Consonants		Vowels	
Process	%	Process	%
Devoicing of stops	20	Mixed substitutions	55
Mixed substitutions	7	Simplifications of diphthongs (creation of two syllables, reduction to one vowel)	9
Cluster reduction (vowel insertion, liquid deletion, /s/ deletion)	18	Creation of two syllables	10
Denasalization	12	Vowel neutralizations	19
Vowel insertion (between consonants, across a syllable)	6	Vowel nasalization	7
Final consonant deletion	13		
Initial consonant deletion	23		

Source: Ingram (1976b: 124), which is based on Hudgins and Numbers (1942).

is the creation of CV syllables. When two consonants come together, either in a cluster [process iv] or across a syllable boundary [process v], there is a tendency to insert the [ə] vowel and create a new syllable. This also occurs with vowels where two syllables would be created from one (e.g. *boy* [bawi]). These can be explained as resulting from the earlier noted tendency towards slow, drawn out speech. This is generally described as inability to produce correct timing in the production of speech (*cf.* John and Howarth 1965).

It is clear that the theory of natural phonological processes provides a rich set of criteria that allow us to describe, compare, and contrast the speech patterns of individuals and of groups in a very detailed, systematic, and comprehensive manner.

The Speech of the Hearing Impaired and Phonology as Human Behavior

The descriptive data presented above concerning what Ingram refers to as "unusual processes" can be explained by the interaction between the human factor and the communication factor, where, in this case of hearing impairment, the human factor is greatly minimized at the expense of the communication factor:

1. Distorted phonemes of aperture that serve as the nuclei of syllables, provide fundamental acoustic information, and maintain the phonetic structure of the word most naturally lead to a high degree of unintelligibility and severely hinder communication.

2. Normal assimilation processes—particularly the voicing of obstruents, the only phonemes of constriction where the voiced-voiceless dichotomy provides a phonemic distinction—may be viewed as a safety valve for, or a compromise between, the human and the communication factors.

3. Wholesale or across-the-board devoicing of stops—tipping the balance in favor of the human factor at the expense of the communication factor—will halve the number of communicative distinctions provided by stops by restricting the sets of articulators that are being exploited by the speaker.

4. The deletion of consonants—the human factor—always reduces maximum communication and does so even more in word-initial position, which has the highest communicative load.

5. The creation of additional or epenthetic syllables, which eases difficult transitions (the human factor), also distorts the phonetic structure of the word, thus reducing communication.

Therefore, in the light of the above, the speech of hearing-impaired children can be seen as an even greater distortion than many of the organic clinical processes that were discussed in the previous chapter. Yet it must be remembered that both hearing-impaired children and children with deviant and normal language development all share similar natural functional processes. Ingram (1976b: 124) brings this familiar point to our attention again: "While pointing out how hard-of-hearing children differ from other deviant types, it is also important to mention that many of the processes are similar to those of both normal and deviant children. This was emphasized in Oller and Kelly (1974). Also, there is one characteristic that hard-of-hearing children share with deviant children. Oller and Eilers [1975] found that the speech of two young [hearing-impaired] girls was much more unstable than that of two matched normals. This compares favorably with Edwards and Bernhardt's (1973a) findings on deviant children." These and other studies of the segmental characteristics of the speech of the hearing impaired have indicated the following errors, tendencies, or processes that can be explained by the theory of phonology as human behavior as well.[1] Let us first consider phonemes of constriction.

Deletions. The most characteristic and frequent functional processes in the speech of the deaf are consonant deletion in all word and syllable positions and consonant cluster reduction, that is, a clear favoring of the human factor over the communication factor. Markides (1970) points out that the deaf generally delete consonants while the hard of hearing have a stronger tendency for substitutions; that is, the degree of sensory deficit of the human factor has a direct and causal consequence for the kinds of errors made: the more severe the deficit, the stronger the effect on intelligibility and communication. There is general agreement that consonant deletion in word-final position is greater than in word-initial position; that is, the communication factor is at work to regulate the deficiencies of the human factor in the most efficient and synergetic way possible.

Substitutions. Substitutions in turbulence and airflow have been shown to be the most frequent (Smith 1975): that is, the extremes in aperture and constriction are favored in their respective phonetic environments (e.g., stopping, deaffrication, gliding, etc.): the human factor striving for minimal (easy to control) gestures at the expense of maximum communication. Substitutions of active articulators are also found with the strongest tendency to exploit the most visual active articulators and passive receptors: the lips, the lips and teeth, and the apex and teeth for certain gestures; the importance of visual rather than auditory perception of language for the hearing impaired is obviously crucial and influences both encoders and decoders synergetically.

Glottalization. Glottalization is another functional process associated with the speech of the deaf that severely affects the intelligibility and the communication of the speaker, giving very few clues to the addressee as to what the target phoneme is likely to be.

Voicing. There appears to be no agreement concerning voicing: certain scholars claim that the tendency is to add voicing to voiceless phonemes (Smith 1975), while others claim that the opposite tendency is prevalent (Markides 1979). Taking into account the individual variation among speakers and the role of context in phonetic environments and their possible influence on voicing and assimilatory processes in general, it is not surprising that both tendencies can be attested to and defended.

As was stated in the previous chapter, one should not assume that these functional processes (as well as formal generative and postgenerative phonological rules) can and should work across the board for all speakers in all situations. Language is a tool of human communication, and different speakers may exploit different communicative strategies in different linguistic and situational contexts. In all cases, however, it may prove fruitful to explain the seemingly contradictory phenomena by searching for the particular strategies being employed by the individual speaker in specific linguistic and situational contexts as part of an attempt to achieve maximum communication with minimal effort.

Moving to phonemes of aperture, the errors in vowels are generally less frequent than in consonants, which can be explained in the following ways:

1. *acoustically,* vowels have greater energy, which makes them easier to perceive than consonants;
2. from the point of view of *articulation,* vowels generally require fewer and less precise gestures than consonants and are therefore easier to produce;
3. from the point of view of *communication,* vowels are the nuclei of syllables and preserve the phonetic structure of words;
4. the speech of the deaf has been characterized as being extremely slow and labored and excessively breathy, all of which may affect the production of phonemes of aperture.

Therefore, it is not surprising that the hearing impaired make more errors in vowels than the non–hearing impaired but still make more errors in consonants than in vowels.

Centralization. The most frequent vowel process is *centralization:* central vowels require the least precision and the least control over the tongue, but they also provide the least distinct communicative oppositions. A more extreme case of centralization is the neutralization of vowels to schwa [ə];

Tense-lax substitutions. Tense-lax substitutions for vowels have also been reported.

Reduction of diphthongs. More complex diphthongs are monophthongized.

Nasalization. A general nasalization has been attested to in the speech of the deaf, including the nasalization of vowels. It has already been established that nasals require the simultaneous excitation of three sets of articulators, on the one hand, but are considered to be natural sounds and may provide important acoustic cues, on the other, thus making nasalization a reasonable process to be found in the speech of the hearing impaired from the synergetic point of view of achieving maximum communication with minimal effort.

We have already seen in the previous chapter that the difference between functional and organic clinical cases is based on the number, frequency, concentration, type, and degree of errors, on a range from common to unusual, found in the individual speaker. This recurrent leitmotiv of showing the similarity of processes might merely illustrate how different individuals—just as different language communities—employ diverse strategies to achieve maximum communication with minimal effort, the underlying motto of the theory of phonology as human behavior.

Case Study

Eyal (male, 4:0) is an extremely charming hearing-impaired twin.[2] E.'s hearing impairment is hereditary and has no other accompanying problems. He has been diagnosed as being moderately hearing impaired (pure tone average = 55 dB, frequency mean average of 500, 1,000, 2,000 Hz) and has been using hearing aids since the age of 2. The family is of a low socioeconomic background, and the parents' consciousness of matters dealing with language and speech is low.

E. studies in a special kindergarten for the hearing disabled four days a week, in which he meets with a speech pathologist twice weekly. He is also integrated in a regular kindergarten for two days a week. He communicates with a combination of sign language and speech. He is not easily understood by those who are untrained or who do not know him. The factors contributing to the low level of intelligibility in E.'s speech and language are a large number and wide variety of misarticulations and such language problems as a limited and general vocabulary, the use of simple and general verbs, and syntactic difficulties. In addition, E. speaks very softly and has a hoarse, raspy voice.

The data to be analyzed from E.'s speech consist of a corpus of mainly isolated words because most of his speech is composed of one-word utterances only. The intelligibility of his spontaneous speech is low for a listener who has no specific reference or clear contextual clues. Therefore, the corpus was elicited through the use of pictures and questions and answers such as, "What do we see here?" in order to provide the necessary background reference and context.

It could be argued that this elicitation method reduces the communication element of E.'s speech. He may be aware that both he and the clinician have the pictures before them, and he therefore has no urgent need to get his message across. The clinician, Tsuf-Mosisko (1993), points this out because E.'s mother informed her of the following incident of homonymic clash that clearly illustrates the synergetic connection between the human and the communication factors in E.'s speech: E. uses the same word [ʔina] both for *gvina* (cheese) and *margarina* (margarine); however, in a specific situation where E. had a pressing need to demand cheese he said *geʔina!* which he had never used before and has not used since in any other context.

E. appears to have acquired and produced all the phonemes of Israeli Hebrew save for the posterodorsal voiced stable /r/ phoneme /ɣ/, which is either deleted, glottalized, or devoiced in the corpus.

Analysis of E.'s Speech and Explanations Based on Phonology as Human Behavior

The corpus and the distribution of processes and percentages. Thirty-three words were analyzed in the corpus, among which forty-four errors were made. Of those errors, twenty-five were substitutions (56 percent), and nineteen were deletions (44 percent). From this we see that E.'s speech is fraught with errors: one or more error per word. Most of the errors are substitutions rather than deletions, reflecting E.'s attempt to achieve a balance between the human and the communication factors: that is, in more cases than not, he will put in the effort to replace certain difficult sounds with other easier ones in order to maintain the phonetic structure of the word and preserve as much as possible the minimal number of communicative distinctions in his speech.

The number and percentage of deletions according to word/syllable position. E.'s speech showed thirteen deletions in final position (70 percent), five in medial position (roughly 26 percent), and one in initial position (roughly 4 percent). From this we see that E.'s speech shows a direct connection between the communicative load of the position in the word or syllable and the number of deletions representing minimal effort: the lower the communicative load, the greater the number of deletions.

The number and percentage of substitutions according to word/syllable position. E.'s speech showed thirteen substitutions in initial position (55 percent), six in medial position (25 percent), and five in final position (20 percent). From this we see that E.'s speech shows a direct connection between the communicative load of the position in the word or syllable and the number of substitutions requiring more effort: the higher the communicative load, the greater the number of substitutions.

The number and percentage of distinctive features that were substituted. One distinctive feature was substituted in seventeen words (71 percent), two in seven words (29 percent), and there were no examples of the substitution of three distinctive features. From this we see that E. attempted to substitute more difficult sounds with less difficult sounds (the human factor) while maintaining as many distinctive features as possible in the substitution (the communication factor).

Substitutions of stricture and airflow. There were twenty substitutions of stricture and airflow in all: fifteen involved stopping (f/s → p; s/ʃ → t; z → d; x → k), three deaffrication (t͜s → t), one consonant cluster reduction (dv → b), and one affrication (x → k͜x). From this we see that E. almost exclusively favors mobile phonemes of constriction (over homorganic stable phonemes), which have been shown to require less effort to produce and maintain. E. also prefers singleton mobile phonemes rather than more complex units such as affricates and consonant clusters of the mobile-stable type, which are disfavored because they contain transitions of different types of airflow in the same phoneme or in the same immediate phonetic environment. In the single case of affrication (x → k͜x), it is the more difficult posterodorsal (rather than labial or apical) stable phoneme that is substituted for by a homorganic affricate, which provides an easier transition in initial position, where mobile phonemes are preferred. In the single case of a nonhomorganic substitution (s → p), we have a case of both substitution and reduplication in the same word: *sefe*ɤ → [pepe] (book), where the visual bilabial mobile sound is reduplicated and placed in initial position. It should also be noted that all the substitutions in stricture and airflow always preserve the same number of sets of articulators, which further enhances communication.

Substitutions of active articulators. There were eleven substitutions of active articulators in all: five anterodorsum → apex (fronting/apicalization), three apex → labial (labialization), one posterodorsum → apex (fronting/apicalization), one posterodorsum → glottis (glottalization), and one apex → anterodorsum (backing). From this we see that E. has different degrees of control over the musculature of all the active articulators. His speech shows a stronger tendency for fronting—including apicalization and labialization for obstruents (ʃ → t; g → d; d, v → b) and one instance for nasals (n → m). He generally substitutes the active articulator of a target phoneme with a proximate but more visual active articulator. The one exception is his general avoidance of the anterodorsum, except for one case of backing from the apex to the anterodorsum for the approximants = semivowels (l → y), where the lateral /l/ requires more effort and musculature control than /y/, resulting in reduplication in the word *yeled* → [yeyed] (boy). This familiar example represents a case where the repeated use of the same active articulator in an easier gesture is mutually beneficial. The single instance of glottalization (/ɤ/ → /ʔ/) involves the particularly difficult posterodorsal, voiced stable /r/ phoneme [ɤ] in the word *puɤim* (Purim) after a back vowel. The case of the n → m substitution appears in the word *balon* → [balom] (balloon), which indicates the avoidance of the use of the same active articulator in a proximate phonetic environment. Once again, we see general tendencies and strategies that are exploited in various ways in different contexts, all of which consistently indicate an attempt to reach maximum communication with minimal effort whereby there is a synergetic interaction and compromise between the human and the communication factors.

Devoicing. E. showed one instance of devoicing (/ɤ/ → /x/). From this we see that E. consistently maintains the number of sets of articulators being exploited. There is only one phoneme that E. does not produce, /ɤ/, which he substitutes for with its voiceless counterpart, /x/, once in the corpus.

Deletion of unstressed syllables. There was only one instance of the deletion of an unstressed syllable. From this we see that E. consistently maintains the expected number of syllables per word for both bisyllabic and polysyllabic words. In the corpus, the vast majority of the words (twenty-eight of thirty-three) were bisyllabic, three of thirty-three were polysyllabic (three to four syllables), and one of thirty-three was monosyllabic. Only in the four-syllable word *taɤnegolet* (hen, chicken), which was discussed in the previous chapter, do we have an instance of the deletion of initial unstressed syllables: *taɤnegolet* → [golet].

Once again, it is evident that E.'s speech has a relatively high concentration of various general and unusual processes that contribute to the low intelligibility of his speech. One can uncover a systematic distribution of these functional processes by applying the basic principles underlying the theory of phonology as human behavior.

Other studies that have applied the theory to moderately to severely hearing-impaired children have produced similar results. Perhaps owing to the relative simplicity of the Israeli Hebrew vowel system, there were very few, if any, vocalic misarticulations. Some of the functional processes or errors for phonemes of constriction discussed in these studies include: the deletion of sibilants (high acoustic frequency), a high degree glottalization (particularly of all posterodorsal as well as of other consonants), nasalization (particularly of the lateral /l/), gliding, lack of posterodorsal fricatives (/ɣ/ and /x/), reduplication to preserve an available and relatively easy articulation, fronting (particularly apicalization), deaffrication, consonant cluster reduction, and devoicing (adapted from Diamant 1994; Heres 1993; Kaplan 1990; Rothschild 1992; Segal 1990; Z. Sharoni 1992; and Walgren 1989).

Once again, in all cases, similar strategies were employed to achieve maximum communication with minimal effort. One also could find that what appeared to be random anomalies of idiosyncratic speech could be reevaluated and seen as context-specific strategies used to maintain the synergetic relation between the human and the communication factors. When comparing and contrasting some of these seemingly irregular or random phenomena among different children, the supposed exceptions in one child's output turned out to be repeated in the same contexts for several children, indicating a systematic distribution of the phenomena after all.

Audiology and Phonology as Human Behavior

The importance of hearing and hearing assessment and the integral connection between audiology and speech pathology has been established in the beginning of this chapter. This relation can be likened to the need to study both articulatory and acoustic phonetics together in a phonetics course in order to get a full understanding of both the production and the perception of speech, as was discussed in chapter 6 (on teaching phonetics as human behavior). In the previous sections on audiology and hearing impairment, the different classifications of hearing loss and their effects on communicative development were discussed. Shipley and McAfee (1992: 344) summarize this connection between type of hearing loss and communicative development as follows:

> Hearing losses vary in severity from individual to individual. . . . The classifications [for describing severity levels of hearing loss] are related to average hearing levels

obtained during pure tone audiometry. As hearing losses vary immensely, their influence on speech and language development also varies. Logically, the greater severity of the hearing loss, the greater its potential negative impact on speech and language. . . . Hearing loss affects individuals differently, regardless of severity, and specific intervention is dependent on:

—The type of loss;
—The dB levels and frequencies affected;
—Age of onset;
—The client's age when the loss was diagnosed;
—Previous intervention (e.g., therapy or educational placement, type of intervention, communication mode);
—Medical intervention (e.g., ongoing or sporadic, etc.);
—The client's intelligence;
—The client's motivation;
—The client's general health;
—Care and stimulation provided by caregivers. For example, caregivers may provide speech and language stimulation in the home, learn sign language, learn how to "trouble shoot" hearing aid problems, include the client in family activities, etc.

One of the ways that clinicians evaluate the hearing of clients is by screening, which is defined as follows and illustrates the integral connection between speech pathology and audiology that was mentioned in the beginning of this chapter: "Speech-language pathologists often provide a hearing screen as part of the complete diagnostic evaluation to identify a potential peripheral hearing loss that may affect a client's communicative development or abilities. When a client fails a screen, he or she should be referred to an audiologist for further evaluation. Screens are typically administered at 20 or 25 dB for the frequencies of 1000, 2000, and 4000 Hz. For some clients, particularly children, . . . more conservative criteria [are used]—15dB at 500, 1000, 2000, 4000, and 8000 Hz—to reduce the risk of missing someone with a mild hearing loss" (Shipley and McAfee 1992: 346).

Another way that a client's aural reception mechanism and its auditory functioning are assessed in the speech and hearing clinic is an auditory phoneme discrimination test. The latter has been defined as an investigation of the person's ability to perceive the phonological contrasts used in the normal pronunciation of his or her language. One of the ways that a client's ability to hear and understand speech is assessed is by means of speech audiometry, which is defined by Shipley and McAfee (1992: 358) as follows: "Speech audiometry evaluates a client's ability to hear and understand speech. It can also be used for assessing the effects of amplification. Two important speech audiometric findings are *Speech Reception Threshold* (SRT) and *Speech Recognition* scores. An SRT indicates the lowest decibel level at which a client can correctly identify a standard list of two syllable words (called *spondees*) 50% of the time. *Cupcake, baseball,* and *hotdog* are examples of spondee words. A normal SRT is within plus-or-minus 6 dB from the pure tone average (average of pure tone thresholds at 500 Hz, 1000 Hz, and 2000 Hz). The speech recognition score reveals the client's ability to recognize words. The test is administered at a comfortable decibel level above the SRT. The client is asked to select the correct word from similar-sounding pairs (*cat-bat, beach-peach,* etc.), or repeat back single words (*day, cap,* etc.). A normal score is 90–100% correct."

In this chapter, I will analyze the results of such recognition and discrimination tests according to the principles of phonology as human behavior. The discrimination tests used (e.g., the Pal PB-50 Word Lists, which have been translated and adapted for Hebrew) meet the following criteria: they contain familiar and frequent lexical items; they have a phonetically dissimilar structure (e.g., no repeated phonemes in a word or reduplications); they represent a normal sampling of speech sounds; and they are homogeneously audible. It should be mentioned that the specific tests used in most Israeli speech and hearing clinics for Hebrew consist of four lists of fifty phonetically balanced monosyllabic rather than bisyllabic spondaic words.[3]

Case Study

Rovel (1990) examined the errors made by subjects identifying words that they did not hear under optimal conditions. The subjects in her study (all adults) were divided into two groups, five hearing impaired and five with normal hearing. Both ears were tested separately; that is, ten hearing-impaired and ten normal hearing ears were tested.

Two lists of twenty-five monosyllabic (mostly CVC) words were presented to each subject (one list in each ear) to be identified, and the errors were recorded and transcribed. The lists were presented to the hearing-impaired group at thirty-five dB above the threshold and to the normal hearing group at fifteen dB above the threshold. (The reason for this difference in intensity or loudness is that, if normal hearers were presented with the list at thirty-five dB above the threshold, there would probably be no errors in their performance.) The errors were analyzed for the following criteria: word position and error type (substitution, deletion, addition). Errors of substitution were further analyzed for the following criteria: active articulators; stricture and airflow; voicing; and nasality.

Analysis of Auditory Discrimination Tests Based on Phonology as Human Behavior

Number of words with errors according to word position. Eighty-one words with errors were found for the hearing-impaired group, sixty-one (roughly 75 percent) in word-initial position and twenty (roughly 25 percent) in word-final position; these data include eight words with errors in both initial and final positions. Fifty-six words with errors were found for the normal hearing group, thirty-nine (roughly 70 percent) in word-initial position and seventeen (roughly 30 percent) in word-final position; these include seven words with errors in both initial and final positions. These results indicate that, for both the hearing impaired and those with normal hearing, hearing difficulties created by adverse acoustic conditions create a serious problem in communication. The majority of errors for both groups appear in word-initial position, which carries the greatest functional communicative load. Words with errors in both initial and final position, indicating an even greater potential breakdown in communication, were also found in both groups. However, the number and percentage of errors made by the hearing impaired were greater in general and in word-initial position than those made by those with normal hearing, indicating an even more extreme case of the synergetic principle of maximum communication with minimal effort.

Errors according to phoneme type. The hearing impaired made errors both for phonemes of aperture and for phonemes of constriction; those with normal hearing made errors for phonemes of constriction only. From this we see that the errors made by the hearing impaired opened the way for even greater potential breakdowns in communication because they appeared in all word positions—initial and final for phonemes of constriction and medial for phonemes of aperture. Vowels constitute the nucleus of the syllable and provide important acoustic information regarding the identification of adjacent phonemes of constriction. Once again, there is evidence of an extreme version of the synergetic principle of maximum communication with minimal effort.

Errors in phonemes of aperture. The hearing impaired made seven vocalic errors, six instances of o → a and one instance of i → ε. From this we see that the majority of errors favored the substitution of a mid-back tense vowel with the low central vowel /a/. The single instance of a front vowel substitution favored a mid-front lax vowel over a high front tense vowel. In all cases, vowels requiring less effort were favored over vowels requiring greater effort, at the expense of the communication factor.

Results for Those with Normal Hearing under Nonoptimal Conditions

Simple (one feature only) word-initial substitutions. Taking substitutions of active articulators only first, there were five instances of backing (considered to be an idiosyncratic process) (three of t → k [backing-velarization] and one each of s → ʃ [apex-anterodorsum] and m → n [backing-apicalization]), one instance of backing in a consonant cluster (tl → kl [backing-velarization]), and no instances of fronting only. Turning to substitutions of stricture and airflow only, there was one instance of stopping (x → k [stable → mobile]) and one instance of deaffrication (t͜s → t). From this we see that there was a limited number of simple substitutions either in active articulators or degree of stricture and type of airflow only. The majority of substitution errors involved complex substitutions of more than one distinctive feature per sound, clearly an even greater potential breakdown in communication.

Complex (two to three features) word-initial substitutions. Under consideration here are substitutions of active articulators + stricture and airflow. There were five instances of fronting + a substitution of degree of stricture and type of airflow: one each of s → p (labialization + stopping [stable to mobile]), ʃ → t (apicalization + stopping [stable to mobile]), and g → n (apicalization + nasalization) and two of ʃ → t͜s (apicalization + affrication). There were three instances of backing + a substitution of degree of stricture and type of airflow for simple phonemes: ʃ → k (backing + stopping [stable to mobile]), p → x (backing + mobile to stable [unusual]), and t → h (glottalization + mobile to stable [unusual]). There were two instances of backing + a substitution of degree of stricture and type of airflow for affricates: t͜s → ʃ (backing + deaffrication) and t͜s → x (backing + deaffrication). There was one instance of backing + devoicing: b → k (backing + fewer sets of articulators). And there was one instance of fronting + stopping + voicing:

x → d (apicalization + stopping + voicing [unusual]). From this we see that there are a large number and wide variety of simple and complex substitutions of one to three distinctive features involving active articulators, different degrees of stricture and airflow, and the number of sets of active articulators some of which even change the phonetic structure of the word—and all this in word-initial position—indicating a most extreme example of the mini-max struggle between the human and the communication factors.

Additions in word-initial position. There were two instances of creating a C-VC syllable (in a historical ?VC—today oVC) word: o → p (preceding a front vowel), o → t (preceding a front vowel), and o → k (preceding a back vowel). There was one instance of homorganic consonant cluster formation of different degrees of stricture + airflow: l → dl. There were two instances of nonhomorganic consonant cluster formation of different degrees of stricture + airflow: p → pt and l → kl. There was one instance of stopping + the addition of a syllable: *sam* (he put) → *ta'am* (taste). There was one instance of consonant cluster reduction + the addition of a syllable + a consonant substitution: *ptil* (cord, fuse) → *patiʃ* (hammer). From this we see that there are also several additions involving two or three distinctive features that also change the phonetic structure of the word in crucial word-initial position, further indicating a most extreme example of the mini-max struggle between the human and the communication factors.

Deletions in word-initial position. There was one instance of initial consonant deletion: *gir* (chalk) → *ir* (city). There was one instance of consonant cluster reduction: *ptil* (cord, fuse) → *pil* (elephant). The fact that there were far many more substitutions in initial position shows the importance of the role of the communication factor. Deletions in initial word-order position indicate the strength of the human factor. The errors of those with normal hearing in word-initial position clearly illustrate the importance of the underlying principle of the theory to characterize and explain the extreme case of minimal perceptual acoustic and audiological information causing poor speech performance for those with normal hearing. Not unsurprisingly, we will find fewer and less complex errors in word-final position.

Simple and complex word-final substitutions. For active articulators only, we find t → p (fronting-labialization) and n → m (fronting-labialization). For stricture and airflow only, we find d → l (gliding of stops [unusual]), p → f (mobile to stable [in final position]), and d → z/ʒ (mobile to stable [in final position]) ([ʒ] is not a phoneme in Hebrew). For voicing only, we find f → v (increase of number of set of articulators). For active articulator + stricture and airflow, we find f → t (backing-apicalization + stopping) and two instances of f → k (backing + stopping). And for active articulator + stricture and airflow + voicing, we find ʃ → d (fronting-apicalization, stopping + voicing). Not unsurprisingly, we find fewer and less complex (but still rather unusual) errors in word-final position, which has a lower communicative force.

Additions in word-final position. Here we find only *po* (here) → *xor* (hole) (CV → CVC), or misperceptions in active articulators, stricture, and airflow plus a possible search for a typical CVC syllable.

Deletions in word-final position. Here we find *mit͡s* (juice) → *mi* (who/from). The deletion of a complex affricate in final position indicates the role that word position has in the interrelation between the human and the communicative factors.

Results for the Hearing Impaired

Simple (one feature only) word-initial substitutions. Taking substitutions of active articulators only first, there were four instances of backing (considered to be an idiosyncratic process) (one of p → t [backing-apicalization], two of t → k [backing-velarization], and one of b → d [backing-apicalization]), two instances of fronting (k → p [fronting-labialization] and x → s [fronting-apicalization]), and one instance of fronting in a consonant cluster (tl → pl [fronting-labialization]). Turning to substitutions of stricture and airflow only, there was one instance of stopping: s → t (stable → mobile). There were multiple errors in the same word as well: s/f → ʃ (backing-lips/apex to anterodorsum) and *sof* (end) → *ʃoʃ* (a nickname for ʃoʃana, "Rose"). And there were two instances of voicing: t → d and k → g (activating two sets of articulators rather than only one [unusual]). From this we see that there was an even more limited number of simple substitutions either in active articulators or in degree of stricture and in type of airflow only for the hearing impaired. In addition, there were simple voiceless-voiced errors as well. Furthermore, there was an example of two errors of backing in the same word. The vast majority of substitution errors involved the complex substitutions of more than one distinctive feature per sound, clearly an even greater potential breakdown in communication for the hearing impaired. It may be that some of these unusual substitutions (particularly the backing) may have provided tactile cues necessary for the hearing impaired.

Complex (two to three features) word-initial substitutions. As far as substitutions of active articulators + stricture and airflow were concerned, there was one instance of fronting + affrication (x → t͜s [apicalization + affrication (unusual)]), there were no instances of backing + a substitution of degree of stricture and type of airflow for simple phonemes, there were nine instances of backing + a substitution of degree of stricture and type of airflow for affricates (t͜s → ʃ [backing + deaffrication]), there was one instance of backing + devoicing (z → x [backing + fewer sets of articulators]), and there was one instance of fronting + stopping + voicing (x → d [apicalization + stopping + voicing (unusual)]). From this we see that there are a larger number and wider variety of simple and complex substitutions of one to three distinctive features involving active articulators, different degrees of stricture and airflow, and the number of sets of active articulators, some of which even change the phonetic structure of the word for the hearing impaired. There are more complex errors in word-initial position, indicating a most extreme example of the mini-max struggle between the human and the communication factors for the hearing impaired. It may be that some of these unusual substitutions (particularly the backing) may have provided tactile cues necessary for the hearing impaired.

Additions in word-initial position. There were six instances of homorganic consonant cluster formation of different degrees of stricture + airflow (l → dl) and one instance of backing + change in stricture and airflow + devoicing + vowel substitution + addition of a syllable (*zer* → [bouquet] → *xaver* [friend]). From this we see that there were more frequent additions involving even more distinctive features that also change the phonetic structure of the word, indicating a most extreme example of the mini-max struggle between the human and the communication factors for the hearing impaired.

Deletions in word-initial position. There was one instance of consonant cluster reduction: *ptil* (cord, fuse) → *til* (rocket). The fact that there were far many more substitutions in initial position for the hearing impaired shows the greater importance of the role of the communication factor. Deletions in word-initial position indicate the strength of the human factor. The more complex errors of the hearing impaired in word-initial position clearly illustrate the importance of the underlying principle of the theory to characterize and explain the extreme case of minimal perceptual acoustic and audiological information causing an even poorer speech performance for the hearing impaired. Not unsurprisingly, we will find fewer and less complex errors in word-final position than in word-initial position, but to a greater degree than for those with normal hearing.

Simple and complex word-final substitutions. For active articulators only, we find f → ʃ (backing-lips to anterodorsum [unusual]), f → x (backing-velarization), two instances of d → g (backing-velarization [unusual]), and n → m (fronting-labialization). For active articulators only for affricates, we find t͜s → t͜ʃ (backing-apex to anterodorsum [unusual especially since t͜ʃ is not a phoneme in Hebrew]). For active articulators only for deaffrication, we find t͜s → t. For active articulators only for voicing only, we find k → g (increase of number of set of articulators) and t → d (unusual in word-final position). And for active articulator + stricture and airflow, we find g → n (fronting-apicalization + nasalization), f → t (backing-apicalization + stopping), and two instances of f → k (backing + stopping). Not unsurprisingly, we find fewer and less complex (but still rather unusual) errors in word-final position, which has a lower communicative force in general and slightly more so for the hearing impaired. It may be that some of these unusual substitutions (particularly the backing) may have provided tactile cues.

Additions in word-final position. Here we find *po* (here) → *tor* (turn) (CV → CVC), a result of misperceptions in active articulators, stricture, and airflow plus a possible search for a typical CVC syllable similar to those with normal hearing. The hearing impaired made an easier substitution than those with normal hearing (*tor* vs. *xor*).

Metathesis and change of stricture and airflow. Here we find *po* (here) → *of* (fowl). Metathesis, which might be considered unusual, was not found for those with normal hearing. It should also be noted that the change in stricture and airflow preserves the principle that explosive-mobile phonemes are favored in word-initial position and that stable phonemes are favored in word-final position.

In addition to all the errors listed above for phonemes of constriction, it must be remembered that errors of substitution for phonemes of aperture were also found in the data of the hearing-impaired subjects. These errors usually appeared in the medial position of words containing other errors for phonemes of constriction in word-initial and/or word-final positions as well, indicating that the number of errors per word was much greater for the hearing impaired than for those with normal hearing.

It must always be remembered that semantic and pragmatic factors such as frequency, ease of retrieval, and familiarity of the lexical items found in the discrimination lists present additional linguistic and extralinguistic factors that may also have affected the different errors and processes that were made by both subjects with normal hearing and the hearing-impaired subjects as well. Furthermore, in many, if not most, audiological clinical situations, speech samples are elicited from identification, repetition, or other fixed tasks, which may reduce the communication factor, as was previously mentioned. The speech situation in general, and the differences between spontaneous and nonspontaneous speech in particular, should be researched as well. It should also be remembered that the hearing impaired often rely on tactile rather than auditory cues, which is an additional factor that should be studied. However, in most of the cases examined, it has been shown that the underlying principles of the theory of phonology as human behavior can be applied as a means of describing and explaining the speech of both those with normal hearing and the hearing impaired.[4]

Cochlear Implants and Phonology as Human Behavior

In the beginning of this chapter, cochlear implants were defined. I shall now briefly review their current status in the medical and audiological fields on the basis of the discussion in Shipley and McAfee (1992: 363): "Cochlear implants are still being developed and refined. At the time of this publication, some of the best results have been for clients with profound sensorineural hearing loss, who have acquired the loss after the development of speech and language. There is also increasing implant work with young non-hearing children (see Owens & Kessler, 1989). These implants do not create or restore normal hearing but, minimally, provide awareness of sound to the once-silent world of the deafened client (Bess & Humes, 1990). A cochlear implant is presently an alternative for only a small percentage of the hearing-impaired population—while research and refinement of the procedure continues. Candidates are very carefully selected, and extensive pre- and postoperative counseling and habilitation/rehabilitation for clients and their families is necessary (Bess & Humes, 1990; Martin 1990, 1991)." [5]

Case Study

Teitelbaum (1990) applied the theory of phonology as human behavior to the speech of Simha (female, 40), a graphic artist in an advertising agency, after a cochlear implant. S. suffers from a hearing loss that began at the age of two as a result of taking large amounts of antibiotics, that is, a possible toxic etiology. Since then, she has had a gradual loss of hearing that has left her totally deaf in her right ear and with a severe hearing loss in her left ear. Over the years, S. has worn a hearing aid on her left ear, which had helped her to the point that she could understand words at forty-five dB through the auditory channel only. Approximately two years before her implant, S. suffered from a sudden hearing loss in her left ear, which left her totally deaf in both ears. She began to wear a hearing aid on her right ear as well, but it did not help her understand speech through the auditory channel only. She could perceive very loud sounds principally through feelings of vibrations rather than by hearing. S. was tested to see whether she was a suitable candidate for a cochlear implant and was found to be so.

Potential candidates for cochlear implants must pass a battery of audiological tests that require the perception of minimal auditory cues such as the identification of environmental sounds, the identification of men's and women's voices, the identification of spondaic words in opened and closed sets, the identification of vowels, the identification of consonants in all word positions, and the identification of familiar sentences via the auditory channel only and the auditory and visual channels. In general, the preoperative results of these tests are very poor, and there is a significant improvement in the postoperative results.

In July 1989, S. underwent a successful cochlear implant, which has left her with the ability to understand conversations even on the telephone. Approximately four months after the implant, she was given audiological tests requiring the perception of minimal auditory cues, and the results were satisfactory in relation to the basic situation prior to the implant. Teitelbaum examined the errors that S. made on the tests for consonants in word-initial and word-final positions. These tests consisted of thirty-five monosyllabic words of the CVC type where either the initial or the final consonants were changed per word and the subject was required to identify the word in a closed test. The words were formed with all the five basic vowels and all the consonants of Hebrew. The errors were analyzed for the following criteria: the type of error, active articulators, mobile versus stable, voicing, and nasality.

Analysis of Auditory Discrimination Tests after a Cochlear Implant Based on Phonology as Human Behavior

Number of words with errors according to word position. Fourteen (roughly 40 percent) errors were made in word-initial position and thirteen (roughly 37 percent) in word-final position; there was only one error per word. Both the number and the percentage of errors in general show that S. successfully identified most of the words presented to her. Indeed, her performance was significantly better for the errors made in word-initial position and just a little worse for the errors made in word-final position than both the hearing-impaired subjects and those with normal hearing discussed in Rovel's (1990) study. It is also significant that she had only one error per word, which was not the case for the subjects in Rovel's study, where both groups made more than one error per word in seven to eight words. It should also be noted that, like the subjects with normal hearing, S. made errors only in phonemes of constriction while the hearing-impaired subjects in Rovel's study made errors in phonemes of aperture as well. The number of errors that S. made in both word-initial and word-final positions are almost equal, with a slight favoring for initial position (which is more crucial for maximum communication) indicating a slightly stronger influence for the human factor—a tendency that I have consistently found to be true in the clinic.[6]

Error type. S. had only errors of substitutions and no errors of deletions or additions; she had both simple (one feature only) and complex (two to three features) errors. Errors of substitutions indicate a stronger investment in the human factor, which is motivated by the desire for maximum communication. In contrast with Rovel's subjects, who had errors of substitutions, deletions, additions, and metathesis, S. seems to be more motivated by the communication factor. The fact that there were both simple and complex substitutions shows the interaction between the human and the communication factors. There were only two complex errors with more than two distinctive features (while there were several for Rovel's subjects), which may further indicate a slightly stronger influence of the communication factor.

Simple (one feature only) word-initial substitutions. Taking substitutions of active articulators or number of sets of articulators only first, there was one instance of backing (considered to be an idiosyncratic process) (b → g [in the environment of a back vowel]), and there were no instances of fronting only. Turning to substitutions of stricture and airflow only, there was one instance of deaffrication (t͜s → t). Finally, for voicing only, we find one instance of x → ɤ (increase in number of articulators). There was a limited number of simple substitutions in either active articulators or degree of stricture and type of airflow or voicing only. The majority of substitution errors involved the substitutions of more than one distinctive feature per sound, indicating an even greater potential breakdown in communication. This is the case both for S. and the subjects of Rovel's study. The single instance of backing may have provided tactile cues.

Complex word-initial substitutions. For substitutions of active articulators + number of sets of articulators, there was one instance of fronting + devoicing (g → t [apicalization + fewer sets of articulators]), there were two instances of fronting + voicing (unusual) (t → b [labialization + additional articulators]), there was one instance of backing + voicing [unusual] (p → d [apicalization + additional articulators]), there was one instance of stopping + voicing (s → d [mobile to stable + voicing (unusual)]), and there were two instances of backing + mobile to stable + devoicing (unusual) (d → ʃ [apex to anterodorsum + fewer articulators] and b → x [apex to posterodorsum + fewer articulators]).

Denasalization for all nasals. There were two instances of denasalization + backing + changes in stricture and airflow (from nasal to fricative)[7] (m → z [apicalization + fewer sets of articulators] and m → ɤ [backing + fewer sets of articulators]), and there were two instances of denasalization + backing + devoicing + a stronger decrease in airflow (from nasal to stop) (m → t [apicalization + fewer articulators (unusual)]). There are a large number and wide variety of simple and complex substitutions of distinctive features involving active articulators, different degrees of stricture and airflow, and the number of sets of active articulators, none of which change the phonetic structure of the word, as in the case of Rovel's subjects—and all this in word-initial position, indicating a most extreme example of the mini-max struggle between the human and the communication factors. It may be that some of these unusual substitutions (particularly the backing) may have provided tactile cues.

Simple and complex word-final substitutions. For voicing only (unusual in word-final position), we find f → v. For active articulator + stricture and airflow, we find ɤ → l (fronting-apicalization + gliding) and v → l (backing-apicalization + gliding). For active articulator + number of sets of articulators, we find g → t (fronting-apicalization + devoicing). For deaffrication + active articulator, we find t͡s → f (fronting-labialization + visibility factor). For deaffrication + active articulator + number of sets of articulators, we find t͡s → g (backing + voicing [unusual]). And for active articulator or passive receptor + stricture and airflow + number of sets of articulators, we find two instances of f → d (apicalization + stopping + voicing), p → v (bilabial to labio-dental + mobile to stable + voicing [unusual]), and k → v (fronting-labialization + mobile to stable + voicing [unusual]).

Denasalization for all nasals. For denasalization + change in passive receptor + changes in stricture and airflow (from nasal to fricative) + devoicing, we find two instances of m → f (unusual). Not unsurprisingly, we find fewer and perhaps less complex (but still rather unusual) errors in word-final position, which has a lower communicative force, and even fewer errors for the person with the cochlear implant.

The fact that S. had fewer errors than the other hearing-impaired subjects that have been studied indicates the relative success of the cochlear implant especially when we consider the fact that S. was diagnosed as being deaf in both ears prior to the implant.

Summary and Conclusions

In this chapter, I have applied the basic principles of the theory of phonology as human behavior to the hearing impaired, audiology, and cochlear implants. I have discussed and analyzed data derived from the speech of a hearing-impaired child and from language discrimination tests administered to subjects with normal hearing under adverse acoustic conditions and to the hearing impaired. I have also compared and contrasted these errors derived from discrimination tests with those of a subject who successfully underwent a cochlear implant. In all cases, we have seen that the basic principles of the theory of phonology as human behavior are fundamentally supported by the clinical data and may even serve as a means to explain the data. It should be noted that, the more severe the organic damage, the more external variables may play a part in the distribution of the data. Bearing this in mind, I shall analyze data derived from aphasics in the last chapter and thus continue the original Jakobsonian tradition of applying phonological theory to aphasia and the Diverian tradition of viewing phonology as human behavior.

10 Aphasia

As the developments of the last decades prove, aphasia is an extremely productive field for linguistic study; furthermore, the cooperation of linguists, psychologists, psychiatrists, neurologists and other experts is of ever increasing value here. —Roman Jakobson (1971: 37)

Linguistic research on aphasia may follow different paradigms. This volume represents examples of two approaches. In one approach, concepts of linguistic theory are the starting point and are then related to aphasic language. Language data from aphasics thus provide one type of substantial data for linguistic theory.

In the second approach, the emphasis is on the aphasic's language-processing abilities. Within this framework of research, linguistics is viewed as a necessary tool for describing the aphasic's intact processing abilities and processing deficits. —Wolfgang Dressler and Jacqueline A. Stark (1988a: xi)

Any classification must have a purpose and must be based on an underlying theory. The classification presented here has a . . . purpose: . . . To show how a phonological approach may contribute to a better understanding of aphasic disturbances of sound structure, that is, to convince the reader that there is much more to phonology than is often thought. Phonology seems to be gravely underrated not only by neurologists, neuropsychologists, and speech therapists, but also by neurolinguists. Phonological concepts or criteria currently used are few and rather superficial; otherwise phonology is reduced to, and replaced by phonetics. —Wolfgang Dressler (1988: 1)

Aphasia: Definition and Classification

In this chapter, I will briefly define aphasia and discuss the specific kinds of aphasia that have been studied according to the theory of phonology as human behavior. Shipley and McAfee (1992: 387) define aphasia in general simply as the "loss of language abilities and function as a result of brain damage. It may affect comprehension and/or expression of verbal language, as well as reading, writing, and mathematics." There are various classifications of aphasia, which are linked to linguistic functions; these have been briefly summarized by Shipley and McAfee (1992: 300) as follows:

> Aphasia is defined as a loss of language function secondary to an injury of the brain. Two of the most common causes are strokes (cerebral vascular accident, or CVA) and accident (Boone, 1987). Aphasia can have multiple ramifications:
>
> —Impaired understanding and/or expression of complex language.
> —Impaired ordering of the sequenced elements of language including words, phrases, and sentences.
> —Difficulties remembering words, producing the correct words, or saying words in syntactically correct orders.
> —Difficulty with expression in grammatically correct manners.
> —Difficulty reading and writing in conjunction with verbal language.
> —Impaired ability using or understanding gestures (adapted from Hedge, 1991).
>
> MacNeil (1988) notes that more than two dozen classifications of aphasia have been developed over the years. Currently, one of the most commonly used classification systems is the Boston Classification (Goodglass & Kaplan 1983[b]), in which aphasia is broken down into two broad categories—fluent and nonfluent. Each of these categories has three subtypes.

The following are the three general subtypes according to the Boston classification of fluent and nonfluent aphasia: nonfluent aphasia: Broca's aphasia, transcortical motor aphasia, and global aphasia; and fluent aphasia: agrammatism, conduction aphasia, and anomic aphasia.

In this chapter, the speech of two aphasic patients, each representing one of these categories, will be analyzed. The first case study (from Ani 1990) will be of Broca's aphasia, a nonfluent aphasia. The second case study (from Gvion 1989) will be of conduction aphasia, a fluent aphasia according to the standard categorization.

Linguistics, Phonology, and Aphasia

As the epigraphs that opened this chapter indicate, aphasia and the relation between linguistics and aphasia in general and phonology and aphasia in particular are among the most provocative, productive, and exciting domains in interdisciplinary research. The role of linguistics, however, in aphasic research should always be kept in the proper perspective, as is prudently pointed out by Crystal (1987 [1981]: 7): "This book, then, is not about the application of clinical language data to linguistic ends: it is about the application of linguistics to clinical ends. But there is an important consequence of this change of direction: the decision to apply these ideas in the first place, the way in which the ideas came to be applied, and the final evaluation of their efficiency all lie in the hands of the clinician. There is one main reason for this, namely that linguistics is only one of a whole range of disciplines which contribute to the understanding and management of linguistic disability. It may be felt to be the central contributing discipline, as Jakobson (1955) argued with reference to aphasia, but as Lesser points out, 'Although aphasia may be a linguistic problem, the aphasic patient is a medical problem' (1978: 20)."

Aphasia, like—and perhaps even more than—the other topics discussed in this book, is vast and complex. It is the object of much interest, debate, and interdisciplinary research. As was stated in chapter 8, apraxia and aphasia have traditionally been linked in the speech clinic. From the clinical point of view, Collins (1989: 87) states: "Apraxia of speech, Broca's aphasia, and conduction aphasia theoretically represent independent clusters of identifiable and classifiable speech and language behaviors. Unfortunately, these clusters are, and have been perceived differently with resulting semantic polarization. The terms 'apraxia of speech', 'conduction aphasia', 'Broca's aphasia', and 'literal paraphasia' frequently elicit a cacophony of alternatives, including 'phonetic disintegration', 'motor aphasia', and 'sensory aphasia'. In this chapter, we try to avoid the terminological morass, but do not suggest that the semantic differences are trivial."

As we have seen from the above, another term frequently used in discussions of apraxic and aphasic speech is *paraphasia.* Collins (1989: 90) presents and explains paraphasias as follows:

> Goodglass and Kaplan (1983[a]) define paraphasia as ". . . the production of unintended syllables, words, or phrases during the effort to speak" (p. 8). In their view, paraphasia is characteristic of speakers whose speech sounds are uttered fluently. They do not include the distorted pronunciation of patients with "poor pronunciation". This exclusion may signal a crucial distinction.

Goodglass and Kaplan list four specific varieties of paraphasias. *Literal (or phonemic) paraphasia* refers to a paraphasia in which, in spite of "easy" articulation of individual sounds, the patient produces syllables in the wrong word order or embellishes his words with unintended sounds. For example "pipe" may become "hike . . . no pike . . . pipe". Some phonemic features of the intended word are usually preserved. *Neologistic distortions* are words which are gross, literal paraphasias, or "extreme" literal paraphasias. *Verbal paraphasias* are real words used inadvertently in place of another. *Paragrammatism,* or extended paraphasia, refers to running speech which is logically incoherent either because the phrases do not make sense together or because of intrusions of misused words, neologisms, or all of these features.

In the confines of this chapter, I will concentrate on only a very small and limited amount of all of the issues outlined above, those that are relevant to the theory of phonology as human behavior as it may be applied to the language of apraxia, aphasia, and paraphasia.[1]

Phonetics versus Phonology and Aphasia

Phonology has played a fundamental role in aphasic research and is directly related to the recurrent questions concerning phonetics versus phonology in general and the distinction between phonetic versus phonological errors and functional processes in both developmental and clinical phonology—especially in aphasic language—in particular.

In the discussion of dyspraxia and dysphasia in chapter 8, Grunwell's (1987: 276) view of these issues, in which she also includes her own and others' views of phonetic versus phonological aphasic errors and their prime importance in clinical treatment, was cited:

> It must be appreciated that many of the errors in acquired dyspraxia are in fact similar to the phonological errors in dysphasia. Indeed the majority of patients with dyspraxia also have some degree of dysphasic impairment. This leads MacKenzie (1982) to use the term aphasic articulatory defect and aphasic phonological defect. Along the lines indicated above she also identifies two distinct impairment patterns—one articulatory and one linguistic. However, she highlights the necessity to include the term *aphasic* with reference to both patterns: "a sparing of the phonological level in the patient with aphasic articulatory impairments is unlikely. Those

with language defects [aphasic phonological defects] do not necessarily have articulatory impairments, but if aphasia exists, phonological level disruption is likely to be present" (MacKenzie op cit.: 44). It is essential therefore that the characteristically different phonetic errors are recognised, since they are the basis of this differential diagnosis and are crucial for devising treatment strategies (see further MacKenzie op cit.). A detailed impressionistic phonetic transcription and analysis are obviously required; a phonetic representation that records the data in terms of the phonemic categories of normal speech will be completely inadequate and will fail to identify the characteristics of the phonetic/aphasic articulatory disorder.

Dressler (1988: 1) presents a history of what he refers to as *phonological paraphasia,* which he defines according to the following conditions, conditions that are directly related to the question of phonology versus phonetics: "(i) There is an aphasic disturbance of the phonemic setup of a (morphologically) simple or complex word. (ii) The target word or morpheme is identifiable. (iii) The produced erroneous sequence can be derived from the target sequence via one or more phonemic replacements (including sequential replacements [movements] and replacement with zero or of zero [omissions and additions, respectively]). (iv) The describer can classify and justify the assumed error path from target to produced sequence." Dressler also presents a brief history of the research in phonological paraphasia from its very beginning up to and including generative and natural phonological approaches. Dressler points out, for example, that Jakobson was not really the first to link linguistics and phonology to aphasia; rather, "the great forefather of phonology, Baudoin de Courtenay [1886–1972], was the first linguist to publish on phonological paraphasias, [although] his contributions were entirely forgotten in later decades" (p. 2).

Naturally, Dressler also pays tribute to Jakobson's (1941/1968, 1971) pioneering work on developmental phonology and aphasia; he argues, however, that Jakobson's primary error was to view aphasic disturbances as being phonemic rather than phonetic: "In 1941 Jakobson emphasized the disturbance of phonemic systems (inventories) as a main feature of aphasia. This is quite incorrect, as shown by Lebrun (1970; Lebrun, Lenaerts, Goiris, & Demol, 1969; cf. also Kotten, 1984, p. 86), for only in the limited recordings of severe aphasics may phonemes be entirely missing, for example, the rather rare affricate /p͡f/ in German" (1988: 2). Dressler, of course, credits Jakobson for introducing the concepts of distinctive phonological features and the notion of markedness to phonology in general and to aphasiological studies in particular in what he refers to as the framework of structural phonematics. Dressler then summarizes and evaluates the role that these specific theoretical and methodological concepts have played in aphasiological studies: "The later development of aphasiological studies in terms of structural phonematics may be characterized by the systematic account of phonological substitutions in terms of phonematic oppositions (with or without the use of distinctive features) and markedness theory (cf., e.g., Blumstein 1973, 1981; Lecours & Lhermitte 1969; Mierzejewska, 1977; Nuyts, 1982, p. 47; Pilch & Hemmer, 1970)" (1988: 3).

Concerning the concepts of distinctive features and the theoretical and methodological status of the phoneme in general and their primary place in aphasiological studies in particular, Dressler claims the following on the basis of what may be termed the classic work of Blumstein (1973): "As far as distinctive phonological features are concerned, Blumstein (1973) concluded that aphasic substitutions point to the necessity for changes in the specification and hierarchy of Jakobson's features. . . . The only rather undisputed heritage of structural phonematics in current neurolinguistic research is the notion of phoneme and the segmentation of sound sequences into phonemes, but even this has been criticized by Lebrun et al. (1969) and relativized by phonetic work on transitions such as voice onset time (VOT) (Blumstein et al., 1980)" (Dressler 1988: 3–4).

Dressler is a strong advocate of natural phonology and, at the end of his article, returns once again to the fundamental question of phonetics versus phonology and aphasic research from this theoretical and methodological point of view as well:

> Phonology must not be reduced to phonemic representations with the result that all phonological rules/processes have to be assigned to phonetics (as Kohn et al., 1984, seem to believe necessary). Evidently phonological paraphasias do not comprise phonetic disturbances such as VOT (Blumstein et al., 1980) or of other fine articulatory detail (e.g. Blumstein & Shinn, 1984; Harmes et al., 1984).
>
> Although most neurological authors explicitly distinguish phonetics and phonology, . . . there are authors who propose phonetic explications for these phonological substitutions that I have accounted for in terms of natural phonology (cf. Blumstein, 1981, p. 138) particularly for those of Broca's aphasics. . . . And whereas Blumstein et al. (1980) and Shinn and Blumstein (1983) meticulously distinguish

between phonemic and phonetic errors in their VOT studies, Gandour and Dardarananda (1984) tried to subsume them into phonetic etiology. This strategy threatens to reduce phonology completely to phonetics. (1988: 19)

The major issue is, of course, at what level the errors and functional processes are derived and motivated. Do we have misarticulations or distortions of allophones or rather deficits in the phonemic inventory? Are the disorders merely on the motor level, or can they be traced to higher levels? As we have already seen, there is no clear-cut and simple answer to these questions. Should the determination of phonetic versus phonological processes and errors be based on the "competence" and "performance" of the encoding patient, and, if so, how is this information to be obtained accurately and objectively? Or, on the other hand, should the more subjective judgments of decoders be the determining factor of establishing the phonetic, or phonemic, or phonological status of the sound units of patients? Once again, I believe that phonetics and phonology are interrelated, feed into each other, and cannot be easily separated. Indeed, the integral connection linking them is especially crucial to the work done in the speech, language, and hearing clinics and may, in turn, shed light on these problematic issues in the field of linguistics.

The Language of Apraxia and Aphasia and Phonology as Human Behavior

As we have previously mentioned, there is much theoretical as well as clinical debate concerning the mechanisms responsible for the problems associated with the apraxia of speech, aphasia in general, and Broca's and conduction aphasias in particular. One of the major issues in this debate is, of course, whether the problems of apraxic and aphasic speech are phonological or phonetic in nature and how these questions affect the diagnosis, assessment, evaluation, and treatment of aphasics in the clinic.

Many differences have been found in the speech of patients suffering from different kinds of aphasia as well as in that of individuals diagnosed as having the same kind of aphasia. This large interpersonal and intrapersonal variation has led researchers and clinicians to assume that the errors in aphasic speech both within individuals and across the different classifications of aphasia are basically random and inconsistent. As we have previously seen in the chapters on functional and organic clinical applications of the theory, including analyses of the hearing impaired, these claims of randomness and inconsistency are often based on the same word being produced differently by the same speaker or speakers in different contexts or speech situations.

Certain generalizations have been made about the speech of aphasics in general and those suffering from Broca's aphasia and conduction aphasia in particular. Not unsurprisingly, many of these generalizations can be described and explained from the point of view of phonology as human behavior. The speech of Broca's aphasics, for example, is considered to be awkward and poorly controlled: vowels are considered to be the easiest to produce, followed by consonants and consonant clusters. Mobile phonemes of constriction are considered to be easier than stable phonemes of constriction.

According to Blumstein (1973, 1978) and others, the four basic functional processes found in the disordered speech of Broca's aphasics (as well as in the functional, organic, and hearing-impaired clients that we have examined) are substitutions, deletions, additions, and assimilatory processes. The following general principles have also been found in studies of aphasia across languages (e.g., Blumstein 1973, 1981; Keller 1978; and others); they support the approach to phonology as human behavior as it has been developed and applied in this volume:

1. More errors are made in consonants than in vowels (the human factor).

2. There are usually more errors of substitutions (the communication factor), although we have found that there may also be a marked prevalence for deletions (the human factor), particularly in word/syllable-final position (the communication factor).

3. Aphasics appear to have more difficulty producing consonants in word-initial position than in word-final position (the human and communication factors).

4. Consonant clusters are simplified by reduction (the human factor).

5. More errors are made in marked structures (requiring greater control over the musculature of different sets of articulators simultaneously) than in unmarked structures (the human factor).

6. There is a tendency to replace phonemes with other phonemes that differ in one distinctive feature only rather than in more than one (the communication factor).

7. The more frequently a phoneme is used in the language, the lower the relative frequency of errors for that phoneme (the human and communication factors).[2]

Similar conclusions and generalizations concerning apraxia of speech support the underlying tenets of the theory of phonology as human behavior as well. Darley (1982) summarizes some of them:

1. Articulatory errors increase as the complexity of motor adjustments required of the articulators increases (the human factor).

2. Consonants in the initial position may be misarticulated more often than consonant phonemes in other positions (the communication factor).

3. There is some evidence that phonemes with a higher frequency of occurrence may be more accurately articulated than phonemes that appear less frequently (the human and communication factors; cf. n. 2, this chapter).

4. Errors are variably related to the target sounds, with the percentage of the errors differing by one or two distinctive features (the human and communication factors).

5. The most common types of sequencing errors observed are anticipatory, reiterative, and metathetic (the human factor).

6. Performance on automatic and reactive speech production is relatively better than performance on volitional purposive speech production. Imitative responses frequently contain more articulatory errors than spontaneous production (the communication factor).

7. As words increase in length, so do articulation errors (the human factor).

8. Articulatory errors in oral reading are not random (and not just in oral reading!)—they are more frequent on words that carry linguistic or psychological "weight" and that are more essential for communication (the human and the communication factors).

Aphasia and Phonology as Human Behavior

Broca's Aphasia

Collins (1989: 87–88) defines Broca's aphasia as follows:

Goodglass and Kaplan (1983[a]) tell us that Broca's aphasia most commonly results from a lesion or lesions involving the third frontal convolution of the left hemisphere, the subcortical white matter, and extends posteriorly to the inferior portion of the motor strip, or precentral gyrus. Its essential characteristics are awkward articulation, restricted vocabulary, restriction of grammar to its simplest, most overlearned forms, and relative preservation of auditory comprehension. Writing is usually impaired at least as severely as speech, and reading is only mildly affected. This profile is typical, but not invariant. Mohr *et al.* (1978), for example, suggest that there may be both a "big" and "little" Broca's aphasia, which depend upon an interaction of size and location of lesion. They have suggested that lesions restricted to the inferior frontal cortical areas of the left hemisphere yield fairly rapidly to a picture of mild impairment of language with "speech apraxia" as the principal distinguishing characteristic. [They suggest] that a true Broca's aphasia results when lesions extend far beyond Broca's area into the operculum, insula, and adjacent cerebral regions. The typical picture resulting from this extensive lesion is one of global aphasia initially, which evolves over time to a Broca's aphasia.

Broca's aphasia mainly affects the expressive aspects of language, that is, spontaneous speech and writing. Other names given to Broca's aphasia include *expressive aphasia, motor aphasia, anterior aphasia* (because the injury is in the front of the brain), and *verbal aphasia*. Broca's aphasia is defined as having the following characteristics (according to Hegde 1991: 334): agrammatism, effortful speech, short phrases, a lack of the usual patterns of intonation, nonfluency, presence of apraxia, good comprehension, and mostly motor problems.

I will concentrate here on the clinical aspects of the speech of patients with Broca's aphasia. The spontaneous speech of Broca's aphasics is nonfluent, hesitant, fragmented, and monotonous. The disturbance in the verbal output is expressed by difficulty starting words and passing from one phonetically different syllable to another. The result of the disturbance is the mispronunciation of the "target word" by omissions, substitutions, additions, lengthenings, reduplications, and assimilatory processes, including anticipations, perseverations, metathesis, or blends on the phonological and syllabic levels rather than morphological. There are many instances of literal paraphasias usually on the syllable rather than the word level and perseverations (repetitions of a phoneme, word, or sentence).

Case Study

The patient (male, 41) whose spontaneous speech is to be analyzed was born in Romania and has lived in Israel since 1961. He had native fluency in Hebrew for all four of the basic language skills—speaking, comprehension, reading, and writing—and no known language difficulties prior to his brain injury. He was diagnosed with Broca's (expressive) aphasia with receptive elements of listening and reading comprehension as well.

During the period of his confinement in the hospital, there was an improvement in his language skills: his receptive language problems disappeared, and his speech became more fluent and functional. During the period of this improvement (after he was diagnosed with Broca's aphasia), his speech was analyzed.

A corpus of forty spontaneous utterances was taken from a recorded conversation between the clinician and the patient in which the patient was describing a set of pictures. The utterances were transcribed on the same day that they were recorded. Twenty-four errors were found, of which twenty-two have been analyzed. For two of the utterances it was impossible to determine with certainty what the target word was supposed to be. The analysis was based on the entire utterance in context, not on individual and isolated words. The patient spoke Hebrew with a native (Sabra) accent, and the analysis was based on the phonological system of Israeli Hebrew.

Analysis of the Speech Errors of Broca's Aphasia and Explanations Based on Phonology as Human Behavior

Number and type of errors. There were three types of errors: deletions (eleven); substitutions (ten); and additions (one). There was only one error per word. All the errors were in phonemes of constriction.

Number and type of errors according to word position. In initial position, there was one error of substitution. In medial position, there were eight errors of deletion, eight of substitution, and one of addition. In final position, there were three errors of deletion and one of substitution.

Number and type of errors according to the structure of the phonetic environment within which the errors were made in the utterance. In CV environment, there were two errors of deletion and eight of substitution. In CC environment, there were seven errors of deletion, two of substitution, and one of addition. In CCC environment, there were two errors of deletion.

Number and type of errors according to the number of syllables per word. In monosyllabic words, there was one error of deletion and one of substitution. In bisyllabic words, there was one error of deletion and two of substitution. In trisyllabic words, there were six errors of deletion, five of substitution, and one of addition. In four syllable words, there were three errors of deletion and two of substitution.

Position of the word with an error in the utterance. In initial position, there were two errors of deletion and one of substitution. In medial position, there were six errors of deletion, four of substitution, and one of addition. In final position, there were three errors of deletion and five of substitution.

Most of the errors were either deletions or substitutions of phonemes of constriction in almost equal amounts indicating the patient's attempt to reach a compromise between the forces of the human and those of the communication factor. Most of the errors and all error types were in word-medial position (in a corpus of many polysyllabic words containing errors), with an equal distribution of deletions and substitutions. Fewer errors (four) were found in word-final position, with a favoring of deletions. There was only one error of substitution in word-initial position. This shows that the force of the communication factor had a strong influence on the human factor. Almost half (ten) the errors were made in CV syllable structures, eight of which were substitutions. There is the same number of errors in the more difficult CC structure (consonant clusters either within or across syllables and affricates), where all error types were found, but eight of ten were deletions. In the even more difficult CCC structure (within and across syllable boundaries), there were only two errors, both deletions. The majority of the errors were made in polysyllabic words in utterance-medial and utterance-final positions. All these data indicate that the structure of the phonetic environment, the size of the word, and word and utterance position affect the number and type of error in a way in which maximum communication is obtained through minimal effort.

Simple (one feature only) substitutions. Taking substitutions of active articulators only, we find s → ʃ (backing [apex to anterodorsum]) and ʃ → s (fronting [anterodorsum to apex]). These apparently inconsistent substitutions appear to be more consistent when viewed in context. Each phoneme was replaced by the other in an utterance where the replaced phoneme appeared twice or thrice in the same context, that is, the exploitation of the same set of articulators in an adjacent phonetic environment when it is beneficial, or perseveration (keep on doing the same thing once you're in control). Taking substitutions based on number of sets of articulators, we find b → p, ɣ → x, and m → b (devoicing and denasalization [control of fewer sets of articulators]) and s → z (voicing [control of additional set of articulators]). The voicing (greater relative effort) occurred in the medial position of a word that was part of a five-syllable utterance that was totally voiced, that is, the exploitation of the same set of articulators in an adjacent phonetic environment when it is beneficial, or perseveration (keep on doing the same thing once you're in control).

Complex (two- to three-feature) substitutions. Taking active articulator, stricture, and airflow, we find ɣ → b (fronting + stopping [unusual]) and y → g (backing + stopping [unusual]). In both cases, the replaced phoneme was in close proximity to the phoneme that replaced it, that is, the exploitation of the same set of articulators in an adjacent phonetic environment when it is beneficial, or perseveration (keep on doing the same thing once you're in control). Taking fronting-apicalization + nasalization (unusual), we find ʔ (intervocalically) → n and y → n. In both cases, the nasal replaced a nonnasal sound in an utterance containing three other proximate nasals, that is, another assimilatory process indicating the exploitation of the same set of articulators in an adjacent phonetic environment when it is beneficial, or perseveration (keep on doing the same thing once you're in control).

Deletions, omissions, and reductions. Taking deaffrication and consonant cluster reduction, we find t͜s → s (deaffrication). In all three cases, the affricate /t͜s/ was reduced to /s/ (rather than the more usual and easier /t/). In one case, the affricate appeared in word-final and utterance-final position, which naturally favors stable phonemes of constriction. In the other two cases, it appeared as part of a CCC across a syllable boundary of the [t͜s-t] type, making the deletion of the [t] element of the affricate the more efficient one to drop in order to maintain the phonetic structure of the word. Taking consonant cluster reduction in CCC environment, we find [t͜s-t] → [t͜s + o]. In the single case where the affricate remained and the [t] was deleted (in the phrase *le-hit͜staer al ze,* "to be sorry for this"), had the patient been "consistent" in his deaffrication, he would have said *le-histaer al ze,* "to attack this," giving a totally different and antonymous message: the communication factor at work! Taking consonant cluster reduction in CC environment, we find [ɣt] → [ɣ], [mk] → [m], and [lt] → [l]. In these cases, a syllable-final stable or nasal phoneme of constriction employing two to three sets of articulators was deleted in favor of a mobile phoneme of constriction employing only one set of articulators in preferred syllable-initial position. Taking utterance-final consonant deletion, we find that two of the same final stable or nasal phonemes of constriction employing two to three sets of articulators (/ɣ/ /m/) were deleted in utterance-final position, the position with the lowest communicative load. Finally, taking "normal" deletions, we find that two other deletions that are prevalent in colloquial Israeli Hebrew also appeared in the patient's speech in familiar expressions: *yeʃ(l)anu* → [yeʃ anu] (we have) and *ma ha-ʃa'a* → [ma (a)–ʃa'a] (what time is it?). It would be difficult to determine that these deletions are a result of Broca's aphasia rather than an instance of normal, colloquial Israeli Hebrew, which reduces consonant clusters across syllable boundaries, drops /h/, or deletes unstressed function words in specific idioms.

Additions. Here we find [xn] → [xsn], from CC → CCC (unusual). The patient added [s] to the cluster [xn] in the word *ha-toxnit* → [(h)a-toxsnit] (the program). However, what appears to be an increased difficulty (CC → CCC) should rather be viewed as the creation of an excrescent homorganic [s], which facilitates the transition from [x], a posterodorsal fricative, to [n], an apical nasal, via the apical fricative [s], whose voicing value might be unclear. It is also significant that the phoneme /s/ substituted for /z/ appears almost immediately after this addition in the same utterance.

In all the instances given above, it is clear that the data indicate diverse strategies that are being employed in various ways in order to achieve maximum communication with minimal effort. The addition of context aids in the explanation of what might appear to be unusual, idiosyncratic, inconsistent, or random errors. The context provides additional information that supports an analysis based on the underlying principles of the theory of phonology as human behavior.

Conduction Aphasia

Collins (1989: 87–88) defines conduction aphasia as follows: "Geschwind (1965) attributes conduction aphasia to a lesion in the arcuate fasciculus, the fiber pathways believed to carry information from Wernicke's area to Broca's area. Goodglass and Kaplan (1983[a]) apply this term to the syndrome in which repetition is disproportionately and severely impaired in relation to the level of fluency in spontaneous speech and to the near normal level of auditory comprehension. It is considered a "fluent" aphasia because the patients usually produce well-articulated sequences of English phonemes with normal intonation, and initiate a variety of syntactic patterns. This is contrasted with the awkward articulation and paucity of grammatical form and restricted vocabulary seen in Broca's aphasia. And yet, according to Goodglass and Kaplan, spoken output may range from fluent to nonfluent. Thus, there may be a fine line between the nonfluent speech of the Broca's aphasic and the nonconfluent conduction aphasic."

Conduction aphasia is diagnosed according to the criterion of good (sometimes almost normal) receptive abilities but difficulty repeating words and phrases. Conduction aphasia is considered to have the following characteristics (according to Hegde 1991): relatively fluent speech, only minor comprehension problems, and difficulty repeating words and phrases. Hegde (1991: 334) goes on:

> The speech of conduction aphasics, particularly in repetitions, is known to be rife with literal paraphasias, neologistic distortions and what Albert *et al.* (1981) refer to as jargon. Friedrich *et al.* (1984) have discussed some of the various theoretical approaches that have been used in attempts to define these phenomena. In conductive aphasia all the functions involving speech production (spontaneous and automatic speech, repetition and naming) primarily will be characterized by literal (phonemic) paraphasias and less so by verbal paraphasias and searching for words (Albert *et al.* 1981, Benson 1979).
>
> The large number of phonemic paraphasias exists despite the fact that the speech of conduction aphasics is well articulated and "clean," without any dysarthric distortions (in which the errors themselves are not always clear); displays no weakness in the muscles exciting the articulatory organs; and has normal prosody. The conduction aphasic is usually aware of his errors and will try to make several attempts to repair them which will either take him further away from or closer to the target word (Albert *et al.* 1981, Kohn 1984). Conduction aphasics generally are known to be able to produce the same phonemes easily and correctly that have been misarticulated previously in other linguistic and situational contexts which is not typical of the kinds of articulation disorders derived from motor disturbances (Benson 1979).
>
> Conduction aphasics also are characterized by dysgraphia which is expressed by replacing a target word with another (verbal paragraphia similar to verbal paraphasia), particularly by literal paragraphias (similar to literal paraphasias), namely: deletions, substitutions, additions and metatheses of letters. It is generally believed that their dysgraphic errors reflect the articulation errors of their spontaneous speech (Albert *et al.* 1981, Gandour *et al.* 1982).
>
> As has been previously stated, conductive aphasia is considered to be a fluent aphasia. Other aphasias such as Broca's aphasia are also characterized by phonemic paraphasias but, unlike the conduction aphasic, the speech of Broca's aphasics is usually considered to be nonfluent, aprosodic and awkward, showing signs of effort

in articulation, sometimes accompanied by motor disturbances such as dysarthria and apraxia. However, Collins (1989) has suggested that these aphasias may be part of a cline or continuum of fluency which seems to be the case for the patients that have been analyzed here.

Case Study

Gvion (1989) chose to apply the theory of phonology as human behavior to a patient diagnosed with conduction aphasia. Her rationale was that conduction aphasia is considered to be more of a phonological than a phonetic disorder. In other words, unlike Broca's aphasia, conduction aphasia is believed to be, not the result of motor disorders in articulation, but rather a disorder in the phonological programming of the language influencing the selection and placement of phonemes in continuous sequences (Monoi et al. 1983; Kohn 1984). The question is whether the difficulties at this "higher" level can be seen to be systematic and nonrandom on the basis of explanations derived from the interaction of the human and the communication factors despite the impression that they may not be "consistent" (partially based on the clinical and research work done by Blumstein [1981] and others).

The patient (male, 50), a native Israeli, whose spontaneous speech is to be analyzed, had full control of all four of the basic language skills and no known language difficulties prior to his brain injury. The data for the analysis were culled from a recording of approximately fifty utterances that was transcribed immediately after the event. Twenty-six "phonological" errors and processes were found in the corpus. Of those twenty-six errors, five were discarded. In these instances, it was not possible to determine the target word on the basis of the possibility of verbal paraphasia. Words that the patient attempted to correct, and sometimes succeeded in correcting, were also included in the analysis. The analysis was based on the entire utterance in context, not on individual and isolated words. The patient spoke Hebrew with a native (Sabra) accent, and the analysis was based on the phonological system of Israeli Hebrew.

Analysis of the Speech Errors of Conduction Aphasia and Explanations Based on Phonology as Human Behavior

Number and type of errors. There were four types of errors: fourteen substitutions, five deletions, one addition, and one metathesis. In the vast majority of words, there was only one error per word, save for one word with multiple errors. All the errors were in phonemes of constriction.

Number of errors according to word position. There were four errors in initial position, fourteen in medial position, and four in final position. From this we see that there is a clear favoring of substitutions for phonemes of constriction in word-medial position, indicating an awareness of the communication factor, possibly at the expense of the human factor.

Simple (one feature only) substitutions. Taking substitutions of active articulators only, we find one instance of s → ʃ (backing [apex to anterodorsum]), three instances of ʃ → s (fronting [anterodorsum to apex]), and one instance of t → k (backing [unusual]). These apparently inconsistent substitutions appear to be more consistent when viewed in context. For the unusual s → ʃ, t → k (backing) substitution and one of the three ʃ → s (fronting) substitutions, each phoneme was replaced by the other in an utterance where the replaced phoneme appeared twice or thrice in the same utterance, that is, the exploitation of the same set of articulators in an adjacent phonetic environment when it is beneficial, or perseveration (keep on doing the same thing once you're in control). The remaining two instances of fronting appeared in a syllable boundary consonant cluster [xʃ], where the patient chose to activate the more flexible, easier to control, and more precise apex, which is further away than the anterodorsal /ʃ/ immediately following a posterodorsal articulation and preceding a labial-dental articulation: *maxʃev* → [maxsev] (computer). It is also interesting to note that this particular pronunciation is well known among children and even some adults (particularly among the kibbutz born and bred). Taking substitutions of stricture and airflow only, we find l → d (stopping). This is a familiar and prevalent functional process favoring an easier gesture and maximum closure over a more difficult gesture and incomplete closure. Taking substitutions based on number of sets of articulators, we find d → t (devoicing [control of fewer sets of articulators]). This, too, is a familiar and prevalent functional process favoring the excitation of fewer sets of articulators at the expense of the communication factor. We also find l → n (nasalization [control of additional sets of articulators]). This rather unusual process appeared in an utterance where another /n/ appeared in successive proximity, that is, perseveration or assimilation for mutual benefit.

Complex (two- to three-feature) substitutions. Taking active articulator, stricture, and airflow, we find ɣ → y (fronting + gliding [unusual]) and y → g (backing + stopping [unusual]). In both cases, the replaced phoneme was in close proximity to the same phoneme that replaced it or to a phoneme sharing the same active articulator, that is, the exploitation of the same set of articulators in an adjacent phonetic environment when it is beneficial, or perseveration or assimilation (keep on doing the same thing once you're in control). Taking fronting-apicalization + denasalization, we find /ŋ/ → d. In this case, the posterodorsal nasal was replaced by an apical stop in word-final position: fewer sets of articulators and a preference for apicals in word-final position. Taking stricture and airflow + number of sets of articulators, we find t → z, *mitbax* → [mizbax] (kitchen) (mobile to stable + additional articulators). This unusual process appeared in a word with almost total voicing and might be considered a case of voicing assimilation. However, the mobile to stable substitution is unusual particularly since it appears in a syllable boundary containing a mobile-mobile consonant cluster. However, it must be noted that the word ends with another stable phoneme, /x/. Therefore, a possible explanation is the preference of a stable fricative in both syllable and word-final positions and the continuation of voicing at the expense of a similar articulatory gesture.

Deletions, omissions, and reductions. Taking deaffrication and consonant cluster reduction, we find t͜s → s (deaffrication). There was one instance where the affricate /t͜s/ was reduced to /s/ (rather than the more usual and easier /t/). In this case, it appeared as part of a CCC word-inital mobile-mobile-stable cluster—*kt͜sat* → [ksat] (a little)—making the [t] element of the affricate the more efficient one to drop in order to maintain the phonetic structure of the word. Taking consonant cluster reduction in CCC environment, we find [t͜s-l] → [t͜s-o]. In this case, the affricate remained intact, and the /l/ was deleted in the word *le-hat͜sliax* → [le-hatsiax] (to succeed), which maintained the phonetic structure of the word and reduced a difficult CCC combination. Taking consonant cluster reduction in CC environment, we find [xk] → [k]. In this case, the stable-mobile cluster was reduced in a word boundary, preserving the stable phoneme of constriction in preferred final position. It is also worthy to note that the utterance contained two sets of repeated phonemes in adjacent environments—/k/ + /k/ and /l/ + /l/—and that the patient chose to drop the third /k/ in an unstressed postero-dorsal environment and maintain the easier apical repetition instead in a stressed syllable: *lo kol-kax kulam* → [lo kol-kax ulam] (not so much all of them). Taking "normal" deletions, one other deletion prevalent in colloquial Israeli Hebrew that also appeared in the first aphasic patient's speech was the familiar expression: *yeʃ (l)anu* → [yeʃ anu] (we have). It would be difficult to determine whether this deletion is a result of Broca's aphasia and/or conductive aphasia rather than an instance of normal, colloquial Israeli Hebrew.

Additions. Here we find [xn] → [xsn], from CC → CCC (unusual). This conduction aphasia patient made the exact same addition to almost the identical word as the Broca's aphasia patient. He added [s] to the cluster [xn] in the word *toxna* → [toxsna] (computer program). However, once again, what appears to be an increased difficulty (CC → CCC) should rather be viewed as the creation of an excrescent homorganic [s], which facilitates the transition from [x], a posterodorsal fricative, to [n], an apical nasal, via the apical fricative [s], whose voicing value was unclear. It is also interesting to note that the added phoneme, /s/, was preceded by two others and then followed by /s/ in the same utterance (perseveration?).

Multiple errors. The patient had one four-syllable word with three errors in it: *hitɣaxat͡sti* → [isgaxasti] (I washed myself). The processes include t → s (from mobile to stable [unusual]) and ɣ → g (stopping [from stable to mobile]). The strategies employed by the patient allowed him to place a stable rather than a mobile phoneme in preferred syllable-final position and a mobile rather than a stable phoneme in preferred syllable-initial position in the phonetic context of a consonant cluster at a word boundary. Although he preserved the voicing values, communication suffered owing to the human factor. The next process was deaffrication: t͡s → s. This can be explained by the similar example of deaffrication previously discussed: the affricate /t͡s/ was reduced to /s/ (rather than the more usual and easier /t/) when it appeared as part of a CCC mobile-mobile-stable cluster, in this case toward the end of the word and the utterance. The deletion of the initial /h/ in this word is probably characteristic of native Israeli speech and may not be a result of conductive aphasia. It also is not by chance that such a highly complex word marked morphologically, syntactically, and semantically should also be polysyllabic in form and have so many misarticulations in it: we have here a supreme case of isomorphism and iconicity.

Metathesis. Here we find *akabel tosefet maskoret* → [akabel sotefet maskoret] (I'll receive additional pay). It may not be by chance that the metathesis appears in the pragmatically and semantically crucial concept of *more* or *additional* pay. It may also not be coincidental that the metathesized word occurs in the middle of the sentence rather than in the more crucial beginning of the sentence or in the less communicatively crucial end of the sentence. At any rate, metathesis is listed as one of the characteristic processes of aphasic speech, although it also appears rather frequently in normal phonological development as well as in the clinic for both functional and organic cases. Our experience has shown metathesis to be prevalent among the learning disabled as well.

It is most interesting to note that the same strategies for the same errors in similar contexts were found for both the patient diagnosed with Broca's aphasia and the patient diagnosed with conduction aphasia. Assuming that these disorders are related and are part of a nonfluent to fluent continuum and that these patients were correctly diagnosed, these data further appear to support the underlying premise that the interaction of the human factor and the communication factor is working in aphasia. It is also obvious that taking the linguistic and situational contexts into account aids in the analysis of what appear to be inconsistent articulations made by the same as well as by different speakers.

Summary and Conclusions

This chapter—indeed, this entire volume—has been dedicated to presenting a specific theoretical approach to phonology that is part and parcel of a larger linguistic theory. Throughout this book, the theory of phonology as human behavior has been placed in its historical, theoretical, and methodological framework; introduced and applied to solve the problems of the nonrandom distribution of phonemes in a specific class of consonant clusters in English, Italian, Hebrew, Yiddish, and other languages; presented as a theoretical and methodological framework to explain the nonrandom phonotactic distribution of phonemes in a wide variety of languages based on different linguistic units such as words, stems, and roots; used to explain a particularly problematic synchronic and diachronic problem in Hebrew phonology by providing principles that can be applied in a panchronic way; suggested as a source for the teaching of phonetics as human behavior and for analyzing texts in general and a unique poetic text in particular; applied to the areas of developmental and functional clinical phonology and compared and contrasted with other phonological theories in general and natural phonology in particular; and further applied to organic clinical problems as well as the speech of the hearing impaired, audiological discrimination tests, cochlear implants, and, finally, aphasia.

Although I have done my best to advocate this larger view of language in general and phonology in particular, I have never claimed that this is the only correct or the best theory there is. All of human behavior and scientific inquiry are open to a myriad of diverse theoretical and methodological approaches. This book presents just one approach in an attempt to see how far one might go in its application with the hope that it may inspire further and even better research in the future.

One of the advantages of the theory of phonology as human behavior—at least as I see it—is that it provides a single set of principles with synchronic, diachronic, panchronic, developmental, and clinical applications. This may be an exemplification of what Jakobson (1941/1968: 64) has said: "The development of child language, the dissolution of aphasic language, and the synchrony and diachrony of the languages of the world exhibit a sequence of common laws of solidarity."

One of the goals of twentieth-century linguistics has been to provide a theory that makes sense out of the chaos of human linguistic behavior. The theory of phonology as human behavior seems to look for precisely those kinds of principles that were originally proposed by Jakobson (1941/1968: 58) for phonology to explain invariance and variation: "Only in the light of inherently linguistic and comprehensive procedure does the sequence of stages of phonemic systems turn out to be meaningful and rigorously consistent. This sequence obeys the principle of maximal contrast and proceeds from the simple and undifferentiated to the stratified and differentiated."

One of the ways that this search for isomorphic principles has been done is by focusing on the human factor in an attempt to humanize a science that has become—in my opinion at least—overly formal and sterile. Such an approach has recently been advocated by other linguists such as Hagège (1993: x): "It is my conviction that the human presence in language building deserves much more attention than it has received so far on the part of linguists. Indeed, the time has come to re-humanize linguistics, and to show that this can be done in full accordance with scientific standards."

Indeed, I view linguistics as a behavioral, cognitive, empirical human science that uses actual performance data rather than a Cartesian-Chomskyan philosophical theory nurtured and controlled solely by intuition, in the sense of the words of Sir Harold Himsworth (1986): "It is only to the extent that the intellect is disciplined by factual experience at every step in its operations that man can have confidence in the validity of the concepts it produces. In short, concepts reached by abstract thought, however logical, have no title to validity save insofar as they are endorsed by factual observations. . . . Accordingly, it is only by rigorously investigating his factual experiences, and following his findings wherever they may lead, that man can provide himself with the requisite information on which to develop his understanding. Therein lies the difference between the scientific and the philosophical approaches to the advancement of knowledge." It is precisely for this reason that, in conclusion, I pass on to the reader and to my own students the following advice:

> Do not believe in anything merely on the authority of your teachers and elders.
> —Kalama Sutta

Appendix 1

Phonology as Human Behavior: Take-Home Assignment

I. Preliminaries: Getting Started

1. Summarize *in your own words* the basic theoretical and methodological principles of the theory of phonology as human behavior from the articles in the reader and the class lectures and discussions.
2. Choose a spoken or written text composed of 100 distinct words (add an additional word for each word that is repeated) to be known as your "corpus." The text must be approved by me. Each student must work on a different text.
3. Write the "identity card" of every phoneme that appears in your text. If a phoneme is repeated, you only have to write it once, but apply it each time in its immediate phonetic environment every time it appears. The identity card includes all the primary distinctive features of phonemes of constriction and phonemes of aperture (including diphthongs) that we have learned according to the theory of phonology as human behavior:

a) Phonemes of constriction: the number of sets of articulators, direction of airflow, kind of obstruction of air (degree of stricture and airflow), active articulators/passive receptors, mobile versus stable, etc.;

b) Phonemes of aperture: active articulator of tongue, tongue height, tongue position, lip rounding/spreading (degree of aperture); and

c) Diphthongs: falling, rising, central.

II. The Analysis

1. Divide your corpus into words of one syllable (monosyllabic words), two syllables (bisyllabic words), and three or more syllables (polysyllabic words). Do you find a random or nonrandom distribution of the number of syllables per word in your corpus? Relate this distribution to the human and communication factors and the principles of the theory of phonology as human behavior.
2. Divide your corpus into words that are stressed initially, medially, and finally. Is the stress per word position random or nonrandom? Relate this distribution to the human and communication factors and the principles of the theory of phonology as human behavior.

3. Examine your corpus for the following principles; present your results, and explain them according to these or other principles of the theory:

a) The disfavoring of additional articulators (0, +1, +2) (remembering that there are more voiced consonants and vowels in the system than voiceless consonants, which appear distinctively only in the class of obstruents);

b) Is there a tendency for similar sets of articulators (0, +1, +2) to be collocated in adjacent environments, and, if so, why?

c) The disfavoring of the coarticulation of the same articulators (or near articulators) in adjacent environments;

d) The disfavoring of the same phoneme in adjacent environments;

e) Is there a difference in the random or nonrandom distribution of phonemes in word-initial and word-final positions, and, if there is, why?

i) Is there a favoring of visible phonemes and/or apical (or other) phonemes in word-initial position, and, if so, why?

ii) Is there a favoring of explosive phonemes of constriction (mobile stops or other mobile sounds) in word/syllable-initial position, and, if so, why?

iii) Is there a random or nonrandom distribution of the number of sets of additional articulators (0, +1, +2) in word-initial position, and, if so, why?

iv) Is there a favoring of apical articulators in word-final position, and, if so, why?

v) Is there a favoring of stabile phonemes of constriction in word/syllable-final position, and, if so, why?

vi) Is there a random or nonrandom distribution of the number of sets of additional articulators (0, +1, +2) in word-final position, and, if so, why?

4. If your corpus contains consonant clusters of the type discussed in Diver (1979) or Davis (1984/1987), do they uphold the principle of the preferred coarticulations of like stability and mobility? (*Extra credit:* Are the preferences of the coarticulation of like stable and mobile phonemes of constriction found in your corpus in other environments as well?)

III. Summary and Conclusions

On the basis of the data that you have collected from your corpus, would you say that your analysis has supported or contradicted the theory that we have learned?

Appendix 2

Le Jaseroque[1]

Il brilgue: les tôves lubricilleux
Se gyrent en vrillant dans le gauve,
Enmimés sont les gougebosqueux,
Et le mômerade horsgrave.

Garde-toi du Jaseroque, mon fils!
La gueule qui mord; la griffe qui prend!
Garde-toi de l'oiseau Jube, évite
Le frumieux Bands-à-prend.

Son glaive vorpal en main il va-
T-à la recherche du fauve manscant;
Puis arrivé à l'arbre Té-té,
Il y rest, réfléchissant.

Pendant qu'il pense, tout uffusé
Le Jaseroque, à l'oeil flambant,
Vient siblant par le bois tullegeais,
Et burbule en venant.

Un deux, un deux, par le milieu,
Le glaive vorpal fait pat-a-pan!
La bête défaite, avec sa tête,
Il rentré gallomphant.

As-tu tué Le Jaseroque?
Viens à mon coeur, fils rayonnais!
O jour frabbejeais! Calleau! Callai!
Il cortule dans sa joie.

Il brilgue: les tôves lubricilleux
Se gyrent en vrillant dans le gauve,
Enmimés sont les gougebosqueux,
Et le mômerade horsgrave.

Der Jammerwoch[2]

Es brillig war. Die schlichte Toven
Wirrten und wimmelten in Waben;
Und aller-mümsige Burggoven
Die mohmen Räth' ausgraben.

Bewahre doch vor Jammerwoch!
Die Zähne knirschen, Krallen kratzen!
Bewahr' vor Jubjub—Vogel, vor
Frumiösen Banderschnätzchen!

Er griff sein vorpals Schwertchen, zu
Er suchte lang das manchsam' Ding;
Dann, stehend untern Tumtum Baum,
Er an-zu-denken-fing.

Als stand in Tief in Andacht auf,
Das Jammerwochen's Augen-feuer
Durch tulgen Wald mit wiffek kam
Ein burbelnd ungeheuer!

Eins, Zwei! Eins, Zwei! Und durch und durch
Sein vorpals Schwert zerschnifer—schnück,
Da blieb es todt! Er, Kopf in Hand,
Geläumfig zog zuruck.

Und schlugst Du ja den Jammerwoch?
Umarme mich, mien Böhm' sches Kind!
O Freuden-Tag! O Hallooo-Schlag!
Er chortelt froh-gesinnt.

Es brillig war. Die schlichte Toven
Wirrten und wimmelten in Waben;
Und aller-mümsige Burggoven
Die mohmen Räth' ausgraben.

Notes

1 Phonetics versus Phonology
The Prague School and Beyond

1. The term *European structuralist framework* is being used here as an umbrella term that comprises the specific phonological theories dealt with in this chapter as opposed to such other schools of phonology as American descriptivism and generative and postgenerative phonological theories. The latter may have different definitions of language than the theories discussed in this chapter and therefore different theoretical and methodological goals. For example, the holistic concept of isomorphism or the postulation of the same set of theoretical principles for all levels of language typifies this semiotic approach (Andrews and Tobin, in press; Aphek and Tobin 1988, 1989; Tobin 1985, 1988b, 1989, 1990c, 1993a, 1994). The European structuralist framework has been defined and discussed in Bierwisch (1971), Lepschy (1970), Le Roy (1967), Pomorska et al. (1987) (reviewed in Tobin 1988c), and Sampson (1980) (reviewed in Tobin 1986).

2. The concept of *langue* vs. *parole* is not identical to Chomsky's notion of *competence* vs. *performance.* These represent two different views and definitions of language. The Saussurian notions are *sign oriented,* while the Chomskyan notions are *sentence oriented.* The Saussurian notions separate the abstract code level shared by the community from the concrete and individual execution of the code. The Chomskyan notions are related to an individual speaker's rules of grammatical competence (an abstract individual notion). Competence does not necessarily reflect a speaker's concrete performance but is solely determined by the equally abstract notion of a native speaker's intuitions.

3. This has been particularly evident on the so-called morphosyntactic levels of language as illustrated in the development of sentence- vs. sign-oriented linguistic theories. Sentence-oriented theories have defined language as "a set of sentences" that reflects the rules of an individual speaker's competence and that contains within it an autonomous level of syntax. Sign-oriented or semiotic theories have defined language as "a system of systems composed of linguistic signs" that combine signals and meanings together rather than separate them into independent and autonomous levels. These issues are discussed in Tobin (1990c, 1993a, 1994).

4. The general arguments for or against an isomorphic holistic or nonholistic view

of phonetics and phonology in a larger structuralist framework are discussed in Baltaxe (1978), Bloomfield (1933: chap. 8), Délas (1973), Diver (1979: 161–63), Halle (1977: 123–27), Ivić (1965), Jakobson (1962a: 231–33, 280–310, 410–15, 464–504, and passim), Jakobson and Halle (1968), Le Roy (1967: 64–66), Martinet (1949: 1–26), Martinet (1960: 53–92), Muljačič (1970), Saussure (1966 [1916]: 30–64), Trubetzkoy ([1939] 1969: 1–14 and passim), and Zwirner and Zwirner (1970).

5. The implications of these basic theoretical and methodological tenets concerning the interaction of the communication and human factors as an ecological force in language are discussed in Diver (1974, 1975, 1979), Davis (1984/1987), and Tobin (1990a, 1990b) of the Columbia school and Jakobson (1971) and Jakobson and Waugh (1987 [1979]) of the Jakobsonian school.

6. The creation of a theoretical, explanatory structuralist model is discussed in Lepschy (1970: 25–35) and may be viewed as being originally based on the concept of the phoneme. The concept of the phoneme and its role in linguistic explanation is and has been the subject of much debate throughout the years. Generative and other formal phonologists have been officially "killing" the phoneme for years (e.g., Chomsky and Halle 1968: 11 [based on Halle 1959]; Chomsky 1964, 1966; Chomsky and Halle 1965; Postal 1962, 1968). During this early period of rejecting the phoneme, certain generative phonologists came out in its defense. Wang (1968: 707, n. 19), e.g., claims: "The speaker must have some general idea of the network of contrasts in his language as it is reflected at the phonemic level of phonological representations. In addition he must also have an implicit awareness of the morphophonemic alternations—both the kind in which a morpheme changes its own shape and the kind in which it causes an alternation in its neighbors. The morphemes which participate in alternations require morphophonemic representations, which are sometimes very abstract, as well as an associated set of morphophonemic rules. The morphemes which neither undergo nor cause alternations simply have phonemic representations and are exempt from the morphophonemic rules. Thus there are exactly two levels of phonological representation which are more abstract than the phonetic: the phonemic and the morphophonemic." A summary of the role of the morphophonemic and related levels in the early period of generative grammar is found in Tobin (1983). Szende (1976) defines distributional phenomena within and across languages, and Szende (1980) defines the phoneme according to its phenomenological aspects.

Most recently, Kaye (1989: 149–54) has declared the phoneme dead once again in light of modern generative nonlinear phonology. His arguments are based on the premise that phonology should be as abstract and as far removed as possible from phonetics, a position that I do not share. In an earlier defense of the phoneme as a viable theoretical and methodological unit of analysis, Schane (1971: 520) said: "The phoneme was the offspring of structuralism, the pride and joy of post-Bloomfieldian linguistics. Since then the child has been abandoned. Yet some of us may have felt guilty about disinheriting the child. As generativists, if we acknowledge him, then it was as an illegitimate child. Perhaps we can now recognize the little bastard for what he really is." I still consider this position to be valid today.

I support the notion of the phoneme as being crucial to phonological explanation on the basis of the role that communication plays in determining the very structure of language. This position has been explicitly stated by Jakobson and Waugh (1987 [1979]: 3): "We object to the abandonment of the notion of phoneme: even though the distinctive features are primordial, the phoneme has its place in language structure." The notion of the phoneme as a signal composed of a bundle of distinctive features signifying "mere otherness" in opposition to other phonemes and the mediating relation that phonemes have to meaning as opposed to the immediate relation of morphemes and words to meaning have been discussed in Jakobson and Waugh (1987 [1979]) in general and in Linda Waugh's app. 2 of the 2d ed. (1987) in particular. These issues, particularly the concepts of mediacy and immediacy, have been further discussed and debated in van Schooneveld (in press). The issue of phonology vs. phonetics is discussed at greater length in the following chapter under the rubric of the identification of unobservable units.

7. As pointed out by Sampson (1980: 246, n. 4): "Saussure did not invent the term 'phoneme'—it was first used by the French phonetician Dufriche-Desgenettes in 1873; but it seems to have been Saussure's *Mémoire* of 1878 that brought the term into common use to indicate an element of the sound-system of a language as opposed to a speech-sound considered apart from its role in the phonology of a particular language." A new psychologically based view of the phoneme as a less abstract prototypical segment that produces contrasts on the phonological rather than the lexical level is offered in Berg (1993). I reject that position because I believe that all the levels of language interact isomorphically on both the abstract and the concrete levels. Berg's article also mentions further arguments for and against the phoneme, such as Studdert-Kennedy (1987), Elman and McClelland (1986), Schane (1971), Levitt (1984), Johns (1969), and Sapir (1933) pro and Chomsky (1964), Griffen (1984), Bailey (1980), Lindblom (1986), Kaye (1989), and Manaster-Ramer (1988) contra. Yehene (1994, 1995) discusses two different kinds of memory processes connected to phonemes and allophones from an evolutionary point of view in light of the theory of phonology as human behavior underlying this book. A similar approach to developmental phonology is found in Kent (1992).

8. The Prague school in general may be viewed as the natural successor to Saussure or as his immediate heir. What is often referred to as the Geneva school is really a group of scholars (e.g., Godel, Bally, Sechehaye, Frei, and others) who have edited or elaborated on Saussure's original writings and are affiliated with Saussure's institution, the University of Geneva.

9. The fact that speakers are unaware of the *phonetics* (the allophones) of what they actually say (*parole*) but are conscious of the *phonological system* (the phonemic oppositions on the lexical level of *langue*) is further examined by Catford (1988) with regard to the Praguian notion of functional load and diachronic sound change. His quantitative data support the view that the potential lexical level of *langue* is of greater psychological importance than the realized textual frequency of *parole*. My own experience in the teaching of phonetics intuitively favors this claim. I have

always found that native speakers are clearly aware of the *phonemes* of their language but are both unaware of and even shocked by the plethora of *allophones* and the minutiae needed to distinguish between them. It should also be noted that the complementary distribution of allophones represents a clear-cut example of the role of the human factor: each allophone is found in the particular phonetic environment in which it is easiest or most natural to produce. These issues are discussed at greater length in the next chapter under the rubric of the identification of unobservable units.

10. Distinctive feature theory in general (including the Praguian notions of markedness, neutralization, the archiphoneme, functional load, etc., the Chomsky-Halle [1968] system, and comparing and contrasting Trubetzkoy and Jakobson and generative treatments) is the subject of Baltaxe (1978) as well as Akamatsu (1988), who was also influenced by the work of Martinet. A most interesting and innovative discussion claiming that distinctive features not only mark oppositions (in the traditional Praguian view) but also unify phonemes that behave in a similar way on both the synchronic and the diachronic levels, specifically through the processes of alternation and assimilation, is presented in Liberman (1988). Tobin and Segev (1983a, 1983c, 1984a, 1984b) have applied the Praguian concepts of functional load and distinctive feature theory to the field of forensic spectrographic voice identification. These concepts also have wide and far-reaching implications for clinical phonology that will be discussed later in this volume.

11. Diver's quantitative analysis goes beyond the work in the area of functional load done by the Prague school, Martinet, and Catford (1988); Eberhard Zwirner's approach to "phonometrics" (Zwirner 1938a, 1938b, 1963; Zwirner and Zwirner 1970), which was compared and contrasted with Diver's quantitative analysis in Tobin (1988d); as well as Gabriel Altmann's approach to quantitative phonology (Altmann and Lehfeldt 1980).

12. The concept of language synergy with regard to invariance vs. variation in general and the synergetic relation between the sign-oriented notions of signals and meanings and lexicon and grammar in particular are discussed in Tobin (1990c: chap. 3) and Tobin (1994: chap. 2).

13. It is interesting to note that most discussions of minimal pairs usually present phonemes in word-initial position only (e.g., *pin* vs. *bin*), often giving the impression that this is the only environment where minimal pairs can be tested. This, of course, is probably the ideal environment, where the force of communication is the highest and the environment that first comes to a native speaker's mind. However, it should be remembered that, even in less ideal environments such as word-medial and word-final positions, minimal pairs can be attained (e.g., *pun* vs. *pan, act* vs. *apt,* and *pin* vs. *pit*) for both consonants and vowels.

14. I have been informed by students that they are usually taught that the aspirated [p^h] appears in word-initial position, which is probably the most frequent place for stressed syllables in English. However, not all words containing aspirated voiceless stops are initially stressed: e.g., *apart, support, hypothesis,* etc. The controversial concepts of stress-timed vs. syllable-timed (where all syllables regardless of stress

have equal time) languages are discussed in Hall (1964: 80) and may be illustrated in the alternative pronunciations of the English and Italian words *laboratory* and *laboratorio,* respectively. The nonrandom, predictable relation of the synergetic distribution of allophones will be discussed at greater length for a specific diachronic problem in Hebrew in chap. 5.

2 Phonology as Human Behavior

1. For the interested reader, I will limit myself here to listing book-length works representing the theory that analyze a wide variety of languages (Swahili, Spanish, Serbo-Croatian, Dutch, and English, respectively): Contini-Morava (1989), García (1975), Gorup (1987), Kirsner (1979), and Reid (1991). The Columbia school approach, combined with other sign-oriented approaches (such as the Jakobsonian–van Schooneveldian school and the Guillaumean school of the psychomechanics of language), was employed in Tobin (1990c, 1993a, 1994), which analyze aspects of English, Hebrew, and selected Romance languages. Andrews and Tobin (in press), Contini-Morava and Sussman Goldberg (1995), and Tobin (1989) are state-of-the-art sign-oriented anthologies that include representative analyses of the three above-mentioned sign-oriented theories applied to a wide variety of languages. Givón (1979) and Klein-Andreu (1983) are anthologies that contain several articles representing the Columbia school.

2. Sign-oriented linguistic theory in general and the specific linguistic schools mentioned above have been described and discussed at greater length in Tobin (1990c: chap. 4) and Tobin (1994: chaps. 1, 2). The Columbia school in particular is more fully discussed in the works cited in n. 1 of this chapter, and in them more extensive bibliographies of that school can be found.

3. This statement is fundamentally crucial to the orientations of the theory of phonology as human behavior. The communicative distinctness of the phoneme as a signal or even a sign meaning "mere otherness" was discussed in the previous chapter and at greater length by Jakobson (summarized in Sangster 1982; and Jakobson and Waugh 1987 [1979]). The actual number of phonemes in all languages (about twenty to sixty, with most languages having between thirty and forty) is based on the mini-max struggle for maximum communication with minimal effort. Fewer than twenty phonemes would not provide an adequate or efficient number of communicative distinctions, and more than sixty would be too hard to learn and remember. Most languages have developed various compromises between the two extremes, having twenty or more consonants (which require more effort) and five or more vowels (which are easier to make) as their basic phonemic inventory. The development of larger and more complex phonemic units such as affricates in consonants and diphthongs in vowels may also be viewed as a means of resolving the mini-max struggle of language.

4. Elsewhere, Diver (1974: 20–24) applies the same underlying principles involved

in his definition of phonology to explain the nonrandom distribution of other phenomena such as Trubetzkoy's neutralization of the bilateral voiced/voiceless stop opposition (*d/t*) etc., in word-final position in German.

5. The statistical count made by Diver consists of all the monosyllabic words in his active vocabulary (roughly 2,500) arranged so that the number of phonemes can be recovered in any position, either alone or in combination with any other phoneme (Diver 1979: 171, 1995: 71). A database composed of monosyllabic words has the methodological advantage of reducing the number of variables that could influence the results of the study such as mixing different morphological levels, syllable stress, and, in English at least, vowel reduction in nonstressed syllables. Diver's corpus is large enough to allow for a reasonable statistical analysis of the data as well.

6. Not only are the apical sounds used more frequently (as pointed out by Diver in his corpus and in language in general), but there are also more of them. A quick glance at the consonant chart of the International Phonetic Alphabet immediately reveals that there are more apical consonants than any other kind. This can be explained not only by the superior adroitness of the apex but also by the fact that it has more proximate "places of articulation," or what Davis (1984/1987: 49) refers to as passive receptors to join up with: interdental, dental, alveolar, hard palate, etc. Furthermore, according to Daniloff and Adams (1985), the apex contains more sensory receptors than the other active articulators, facilitating greater articulatory precision as well. The frequency of apical consonants is followed by labials and dorsals, which represent the extremities of the oral vocal tract and present the most efficient communication distinctions—the extremes (front and back) vs. the middle. The same holds true for the well-known, probably universal, vowel triangle:

i   u
   a

which consists of the extreme high front and back vowels and the low central vowel, providing the extreme and most efficient communicative distinctions.

7. Once again, it is not only the frequency of the voiced stops that suffers. It should be remembered, but is often overlooked, that the voiced-voiceless distinction in consonants usually is relevant only for the obstruents—stops, fricatives, affricates—which require the highest degree of muscular control and are therefore at the top of the hierarchy of constriction. The other consonants or semivowels, liquids, approximants, etc.—the resonants—those consonants at the bottom of the hierarchy of constriction usually are all voiced as are vowels. One may then ask the following question: if voiced sounds are harder to make, then why are there more voiced sounds than unvoiced ones? The answer lies in the acoustic and communication orientations. Voiced sounds provide more acoustic and perceptual information—they provide resonance and have acoustic formants that provide the primary auditory and communicative information most necessary for speech perception. Indeed, most consonants usually are identified on spectrograms or by ear through their transitions with vowels. Therefore, the need for maximum communication justifies the extra

effort necessary for making voiced sounds. In other words, they are easier to hear in general and over distances in particular. It should also be remembered that, when affricates—more difficult and complex consonants—appear in the phonemic inventory of a language, the voiceless affricates precede the voiced ones, provided that the latter become part of the inventory. Problems with voicing in Hebrew in the clinic related to phonology as human behavior are discussed in Ben-Dor (1990), Jehudah (1991), and Shachar (1990).

8. Voicing and voice-onset time can also be related to the different allophones for voiced and voiceless stops in English and other languages and the human factor. The aspirated allophones of voiceless stops in English can be seen as a direct result of the human factor. In addition to requiring the control of two sets of articulators simultaneously, voicing also hinders or impairs the airflow. Therefore, there is more air to be aspirated in the case of voiceless (traditionally referred to as fortis) rather than voiced (traditionally referred to as lenis) stops. English can also be compared with languages such as Hindi, which has voiced aspirated stops requiring both simultaneous control of two sets of articulators and maximum control of the airflow. Diver has contrasted here English with the Romance languages—which do not have aspirated allophones of voiceless or voiced stops—with regard to voice-onset time. Hebrew functions in a way similar to the Romance languages concerning voice-onset time and the lack of aspirated allophones of voiceless and voiced stops, which has been discussed in Raphael and Tobin (1983), Raphael, Tobin, and Most (1983), and Raphael et al. (1995).

9. It should be pointed out to the reader that the production of nasals involves three sets of articulators: nasals are all voiced (+1), oral stops (+2), produced with the uvula (+3), which lowers to allow most of the air to enter the nasal passage but leaves enough air in the oral passage to determine which set of active oral articulators is being used: bilabial *m,* apical *n,* or dorsal *ŋ*. Despite the fact that nasals are complex sounds articulatorily, they are also natural sounds. As we know, the vocal and nasal tracts were originally designed for eating and breathing, respectively. Talking came later and was superimposed on the same musculature. Furthermore, the bilabial nasal *m* is acquired from the onset as a natural result of an infant nursing (hence the appearance of *m* in so many languages for the word *mother* or the term *am* in baby talk across languages and cultures to indicate food). Finally, nasals have a unique pattern of formants like vowels and give strong acoustic cues (sometimes even stronger than vowels) in speech production and reception (Raphael et al. 1974; Raphael et al. 1975; Dorman et al. 1974).

10. From the point of view of phonology as human behavior, consonants are phonemes of constriction, and vowels are phonemes of aperture. In other words, consonants restrict or impede the flow of air, and vowels allow free movement of air. Consonants generally require more articulatory control and are harder to learn than vowels, which can be seen in first language acquisition and in the clinic (see chap. 7). Consonants are more distinct from each other and give stronger communicative oppositions than vowels, which form part of an acoustic continuum. Therefore, it is

not surprising that there are more consonants than vowels in languages. It is also not surprising that the ideal syllable is CVC, with the vowel serving as a nucleus (with a free movement of air) and separating two consonants (which constrict the airflow). Syllables of the CCVC are clearly much harder to make and sustain and are therefore much less frequent in languages. Halpern (1991) presents a cross-linguistic study dealing with the interplay between consonants and vowels in English and Hebrew related to the point of view of phonology as human behavior.

11. Diver (1979: 178) also points out the avoidance of the same item occurring both in root-initial and root-final position in Semitic languages: i.e., a disfavoring of the musculature at the extremes of linguistic units smaller than a word. This phenomenon as well as others (see n. 13, this chapter) were examined for the Hebrew triconsonantal (CCC) root system (Tobin 1990a, 1990b) and will be presented in chap. 4.

12. This parallel can be seen clearly in the acquisition of phonology. Jakobson (1941/1968) was the first to point out that children acquire phonemes in a hierarchical order. This order can be related to the relative difficulties of fine motor control necessary for different sounds based on their respective articulators. Developmental psychologists such as Piaget (1970) and others have established various chronological orders for the acquisition of different skills that are also based on the control of fine motor movement. It may be said that, just as toilet training and learning how to tie one's shoes are related to specific ages when certain fine motor control is acquired, the same holds true for the acquisition of different phonemes in language (Kent 1992). Developmental phonology in general and Jakobson's (1941/1968) theory of child phonology will be discussed from the point of view of phonology as human behavior in chap. 7.

13. An extreme case of the exclusive occurrence of apicals in word-final position is found in ancient Greek (Diver 1979: 179). There is also a preponderance of apicals (labeled as dental-alveolars) in the Hebrew root system in general and in root-final position of the triconsonantal (CCC) root system in particular (Morgenbrod and Serifi 1981: 14), which will be discussed in chap. 4.

14. The special communicative status of initial position can also be seen in linguistics and phonetics classes (see chap. 1, n. 13). Usually, the concept of minimal pairs is taught by presenting examples in word-initial position because they are the ones that probably are most frequent and certainly the ones that immediately come to mind. This slight preference for visible phonemes in initial position also has been found in other languages such as Italian (Davis 1984/1987) and Hebrew (Tobin 1990a, 1990b).

15. The lower status or reduced communicative role of final position and the resultant preference for apicals in this position, not unsurprisingly, has been attested to in other languages as well, such as Italian (Davis 1984/1987) and Hebrew (Tobin 1990a, 1990b). It should also be mentioned that, even when word-final position may be relatively meaningful (e.g., in English morphological inflectional suffixes—nominal plural /s/, /z/, /ɪz/; third-person, singular verb /s/, /z/ /ɪz/, genetive /s/, /z/ /ɪz/; past tense /t/, /d/, /ɪd/, etc.), over the centuries it is usually the apical phoneme of

constriction that remained while the other vocalic or nonapical inflectional endings tended to be dropped.

3 The Italian and Latin Connections

1. This is followed by a rather extensive note, comparing and contrasting the concepts of description and explanation in generative theory on the basis of Lightfoot (1982) and the Columbia school. This discussion deals with basic issues such as universals, innateness, well-formedness, rules, etc., which distinguish these two sentence- as opposed to sign-oriented approaches. Further discussion of these differences can also be found in Tobin (1990c: chap. 4) and Tobin (1994: chap. 2). Davis's note will be reproduced in full with regard to explanation and opaque rules in phonology (see chap. 5, n. 8).
2. Davis has an amusing note here, exemplifying an extreme case of avoidance found in a mathematics teacher who has difficulty pronouncing the words *twelve* and *twenty* and thus substitutes *dozen, two-zero,* and so forth for them.
3. The reader is reminded that the issue of frequency or functional load and sound change regarding the phonological system and the lexicon is dealt with by Catford (1988) (see chap. 1, n. 9 above).
4. This traditional phonemic inventory appears after a long discussion (Davis 1984/1987: 8–18) where the many problems involved in determining the phonemes of Italian as presented in Arce (1962), Camilli (1965), Castellani (1956), Hall (1948), and especially Muljăcič (1969) are considered at great length. The differences between the phonemic inventory presented in table 3.1 and the usual phonemic inventory of modern standard Italian are Davis's viewing both /s/ and /z/ as separate phonemes (1984: 11–12 and n. 6) and the elimination of /w/ as a separate phoneme, replaced by the labialized velars /k^w, g^w/ symbolized by Davis as /q, G/, respectively (p. 18). The special or problematic status of /w/ in sound patterns across languages is discussed in Ohala and Lorentz (1977). In Davis's text, the phonemic inventory of Italian is followed by a brief summary (1984/1987: 20–27) of the history of the Italian language, taken primarily from Migliorini (1966) with a note on contemporary Italian from Magister (1984).
5. I say "all human languages" despite the fact that Chinese (and possibly other tone languages) has neutralized the distinction between voiced and voiceless consonants. It should be remembered that both tone and pitch variations as well as voicing all involve control of the larynx. It may very well be that the larynx containing the vocal folds—the first articulators to produce distinctive features, usually either tone and/or voicing—may neutralize one or the other when it is not crucial to communication. The various other effects of different states of the glottis, airstream mechanisms, and phonation types (e.g., murmur, breathy voice, whisper, creaky voice, etc.) are discussed in Ladfoged (1982: chap. 6).
6. This same effect may also be seen in Hebrew. Even a cursory look at the dic-

tionary entries for *kaf* ("front *k*") and *qof* ("back *k*")—two historical phonemes in Hebrew—clearly show that the former (one oral articulator—posterodorsal), as opposed to the latter (two oral articulators—labio + posterodorsal), is much more exploited in initial position (and probably every other position) in the lexicon. Furthermore, the least exploited phoneme in word-initial position—according to the number of dictionary entries—is the letter *vav* (historically a /w/, *waw*), which is a voiced labio + posterodorsal sound involving two oral articulators as well as the larynx. Hebrew did not have a /k^w/ –/ g^w/ opposition and had only a voiceless labio + posterodorsal mobile consonant of constriction.

7. This preference for visibility also has implications in other areas of human language. In Tobin (1993a: 78), I note a far more frequent use of visual rather than auditory verbs in our corpus. I have also noted that there are many more traditional and neotraditional analyses of the lexical pair *look* and *see* than of *listen* and *hear*. One can also find a larger number of lexical entries in dictionaries in the visual than in the auditory semantic fields. This leads, of course, to the questions, Which is the most important of the five senses? or, If you had the choice, would you rather be blind or deaf? Whatever the answer is, it does appear that visual sensory verbs may be the leading ones. Once again, in all areas of human language, the same or similar isomorphic principles seem to be working in coordination.

8. The rejection of communication as a motivation for language and linguistics was one of the original pillars of generative theory and still is today. Some of the other examples given against communication as motivation for language and linguisic theory are lying and obfuscation, which represent the speaker's extralinguistic intentions rather than serving as a linguistic argument against communication. People who choose not to communicate do so by extending or violating basic communication principles that are inherent in our social use of language.

9. In a note here, Davis points out that the relevant mathematical formula for this calculation is $(19^2 - 19)/2$, or 18 + 17 + 16 + . . . + 3, + 2, + 1.

10. This is followed by a note citing Recasens (1984) as an interesting study of the acoustics of these two phonemes, /ʎ, y/, in Catalan, paying particular attention to the effects of phonetic environment and formant structure.

11. It should also be remembered that, like the nasals, the lateral approximants /l, ʎ/ provide primary auditory and perceptual communicative information in the form of acoustic formants. The postulation of a separate class of lateral vs. central is also justified by the fact that there are also lateral fricatives, /ɬ, ɮ/, thus allowing for different manners of articulation or hierarchical differentiations in stricture and airflow. The same can also be said for the various retroflexive *r* phonemes /r, ɹ, R, ʁ, ɾ/, which present different degrees of stricture and airflow as trills, glides, and even a tap that acoustically resemble fricatives, semivowels, and stops, respectively.

12. This principle for the preference for explosive phonemes in initial position is crucial in the Hebrew language as a means to explain the historical distribution of /b, g, d, k, f, t/ known as *BeGeDKeFeT,* whereby stops and fricatives were allophones of the same phoneme in biblical Hebrew. This very thorny issue in contemporary

Hebrew phonology as well as a more detailed explanation of explosive and implosive phonemes are discussed at greater length in chap. 5 below.

13. In a note here, Davis enumerates the procedures with which he selected the random number of stems and checked them according to Devoto and Oli (1967).

14. This is followed by a note explaining the statistical procedures for determining significance.

15. In a note here, Davis states that the anterodorsal 1° phoneme /ʃ/ might be compared with /tʃ/, but factor E is confounding. Also, /ʃ/ is particularly limited by its historical development from /s + t͜s/, /s + k/, and /eks + s/.

16. In a note here, Davis explains that he has raised the significance level from .05 to .1 in order to increase the statistical *power;* in other words, he does not want so much to prove that an association exists as to *detect* a possible association. Potentially, the higher significance level makes the task of explaining differences more demanding since slighter differences must be explained.

17. I have presented only a very limited account of how the theory of phonology as human behavior deals with phonemes of aperture in this already overlong chapter. I have concentrated on phonemes of constriction because of their greater number and role in human communication and the especially problematic part that they play in clinical phonology.

18. The Hebrew data have been selected because of their relevance to the material that will be presented in the clinical applications of the theory in Israel. The Yiddish data are there for comparison. The phonological system of at least one other language, Urdu, has been examined according to the Columbia school theory (Azim 1989, 1993, 1995; Jabeen 1993). Azim's (1989, 1993, 1995) analyses do not concentrate on syntagmatic phenomena such as the syllabic canon or the pattern of the consonant clusters in Urdu but rather focus on problems particularly selected for their peculiarly Indian characteristics: the opposition of apicodental to apicopalatal (retroflex), the relation of oral to nasal vowels, and especially the problems that arise in a system that is rich in aspiration and has a complex vowel system. A guideline on how to perform a Columbia school phonological analysis was presented in Davis (1989). Diver (1993) further elaborates the phonology of the extremes of word-order position by placing emphasis on the role of vowels. Diver (1995) presents a theoretical and methodological overview of the theory.

4 The Hebrew and Yiddish Connections

1. I am presenting an (oversimplified) panchronic view of Hebrew, and certain unavoidable diachronic, orthographic, and dialectal inconsistencies are therefore present. These include the biblical occlusive-spirant allophonic (today basically phonemic) alternations (p-f, b-v, k-x) (which have also been partially maintained in general Israeli Hebrew) as well as the similar (g-ɣ, d-ð, t-θ) alternations, which have been lost. Orthographically, each pair is represented by a single letter only. I

will also maintain the pharyngeal *het* /ħ/, *ayin* /ʕ/, and the glottal stop *aleph* /ʔ/, which do not necessarily appear in general Israeli Hebrew, and the (lip + posterodorsal) phonemes /w, q/, even though /w/ has been replaced by /v/ and /k/ and emphatic /q/ have merged. I list emphatic *tet* and nonemphatic *taf* as "T-t" but view them as a single sound, and ʃ representing two distinct sounds today, (ʃ + s), will be treated as a single unit. I will not deal specifically with the other emphatic or ejective consonants well known in Semitic either. It should also be noted that I have viewed the historical (and Oriental or Sephardic) Hebrew /r/ phoneme as an apical trill, although in Israeli Hebrew it is usually pronounced as a voiced posterodorsal fricative /ɣ/. (Note that Diver also considers the English /r/ as an apical mobile trill, which it was believed to be historically as well [see chap. 2 above].) I would like to add, however, that the patterns that I have uncovered for this panchronic view of Hebrew are even strengthened in general Israeli speech, where there are fewer communicative distinctions involving fewer (particularly pharyngeal and laryngeal) active articulators and no ejective or emphatic articulations.

2. As was seen in the previous chapters, Diver (1979) originally proposed two alternative distinctive features related to manner of articulation (stable + mobile) to explain all the various favorings and disfavorings of initial consonant clusters composed of "stop + r" versus "fricative + l" in English monosyllables. In Davis (1984/1987), this approach is expanded and includes these and other consonant and vowel features as part of a single continuum. In this chapter, this phonetic environment will be examined for Hebrew and Yiddish.

3. This principle may also be applied, in part, to the loss or merger of certain oral consonants. (There may be additional sociolinguistic reasons for the well-known loss of pharyngeal or laryngeal consonants in Hebrew.) Indeed, many of those consonants that have been replaced by or have merged with other consonants (e.g., /w-v/, /q-k/, /T-t/) are precisely those consonants requiring the control of more than one articulator (lips + posterodorsum, emphatic vs. nonemphatic). The reason why there are more voiced phonemes than voiceless phonemes in languages has already been discussed (see chap. 2, n. 7, and chap. 3, n. 5).

4. These data present additional problems for various diachronic, psycholinguistic, sociolinguistic, and other reasons related to the distribution of triconsonantal (CCC) roots within words. In particular, the historical occlusive-spirant allophonic alternations in opening (occlusive) and closing (spirant) syllables—referred to as *BeGeDKeFeT* because of the consonants involved—must be considered. This problem is not purely diachronic either: Schwarzwald (1981) has demonstrated that a confusion exists among many speakers of Hebrew today regarding this (and other) alternation(s). The particularly thorny problem of *BeGeDKeFeT* will be discussed at greater length in chap. 5 below. There are other methodological problems regarding the combining of historically distinct consonant phonemes (t-T, k-q) that have merged and have the same active articulators and degrees of stricture and airflow today.

5. The use of the same active articulators is disfavored for all phonemes of constric-

tion in the C-I + C-II and C-I + C-III positions, but only for sixteen of twenty-two (73 percent) phonemes of constriction in the C-II + C-III positions. Most of these "exceptional" phonemes of constriction are those that already have been determined as involving additional sets of oral articulators /T, t͡s, ʃ, q/.

6. The voiced-voiceless distinction holds for all the pairs /p-3 vs. b-1; t+T-10 vs. d-0; s-4 vs. z-2; ʃ-5 vs. j-0; k + q-3 vs. g-1/, save for the pharyngeals /ħ-0, ʕ-4/. The pharyngeal phonemes of constriction in general and determining their exact manner of articulation (stop, fricative, approximant, backed vowel?) for *ayin* /ʕ/ in different phonetic contexts are well-known problems that will not be dealt with here. The acoustic properties reflecting the variability of *ayin* in Iraqi Arabic has been discussed in Ali, Danilof, and Hoffman (1988).

7. The data for the voiced-voiceless opposition are as follows: /t+T-15 vs. d-12; s-7 vs. z-6; k+q-6 vs. g-4; ħ-6 vs. ʕ-2/, except for the labials /p-9 vs. b-14/.

8. The nasals as "temporally extended stops" may be even more visible than their oral counterparts, as may historically ejective and emphatic consonants, which were not included here. It should also be noted that the largest number of entries in the Hebrew dictionary are for /m/, followed by other labials and apicals. More detailed discussions of nasal and emphatic consonants in general and in Semitic languages in particular may be found in Fujimara (1962) and Jakobson and Halle (1962).

9. Only independent words (as opposed to construct forms of nominal compounds or bound morphemes) containing initial consonant clusters were included in the corpus. The selection of initial consonant clusters was determined by standard Israeli pronunciation. It should be noted that most of the words in the corpus have a historical *schwa* /ə/ between C_1 and C_2 that is no longer pronounced (save for the occasional use by news broadcasters on the radio, whose pronunciation is being monitored by the Hebrew Language Academy, or in formal recitations of prayers reflecting an archaic liturgical register, or, possibly, in Bible classes). The problem of the *schwa* /ə/ and the diachronic, prescriptive, descriptive, and linguistic treatments of the various kinds of *schwa* and their pronunciation—or lack thereof—has been much discussed in the literature. Muraoka (1993) refers to the *schwa* as "much ado about nothing" and a "sore point in Hebrew grammar" in an article containing a historical survey of its role in Hebrew grammar.

10. The data have been influenced by several factors previously mentioned. The pharyngeal and laryngeal phonemes of constriction (which are usually not pronounced in standard Israeli Hebrew) (see nn. 1, 6, this chapter) have not been included in the corpus, which is restricted to the oral active articulators found in the previous studies. The mergers of /T-t/ and /k-q/ (nn. 1, 3, 4, this chapter) have been maintained in this corpus as they were for the triconsonantal (CCC) root system. The number of stable phonemes in C_1 position is limited owing to the problem of *BeGeDKeFeT* (nn. 1, 4, this chapter). Just as Diver's corpus did not have /v/, /z/, /ʒ/, /ð/, in C_1 position, no examples were found for the closest voiced fricative equivalent in Hebrew (not affected by the *BeGeDKeFeT*), namely, /z/ (see table 4.1 above).

11. The reader will note that Bernholtz-Priner (1993) also collected initial conso-

nant clusters with the affricate /t͡s/ and the nasal /m/ in C_1 position, which were not included in the previous studies. The small number of examples found in the data culled for these complex sounds is not surprising and further supports the principle that additional articulators are disfavored. I have reproduced all the data that Bernholtz-Priner collected in table 4.12, but the reader should be aware of the fact that the /t͡s/ and /m/ clusters have not been included in the calculation of the totals and cross-totals or in the larger analysis.

5 Panchronic Applications in Hebrew Phonology

1. The revival of modern Hebrew at the turn of the century, and the special and controversial role played by Eliezer Ben-Yehuda, referred to as the man who was responsible for the revival, have been the subject of much research. For more thorough treatments of this issue, the interested reader should consult Bar-Adon (1975), Fellman (1973b), and Harshav (1993). Contemporary or Israeli Hebrew is defined and discussed in the first chapters of Berman (1978), Glinert (1989), and Rosén (1977) (reviewed in Tobin 1991), which present linguistically oriented analyses of this language in English.
2. The issue of language normativism and its acceptance by the Israeli educational system and the media is a—if not *the*—central question that has occupied theoretical and applied linguists for decades. Many generative-based analyses of contemporary Hebrew (e.g., Berman 1978 and Glinert 1989) have naturally had to confront the concept of native speakers' intuitions, a notion that is particularly problematic for a revived language. This problem is aggravated even further in the heavily prescription-laden atmosphere in Israel, a country that is strongly influenced by the Hebrew Language Academy. Berman (1978: 2–3) describes the problem of the pervasiveness of purism prevalent in the Israeli educational system and its detrimental effect on native speakers' intuitions, the crucial methodological control of generative theory, in the following way:

> The language this book is concerned with, then, is native Hebrew as spoken—and written—by residents of the State of Israel who were born in the country or who settled there before the age of ten or so. . . . Our analysis will devolve mainly upon the colloquial usage of Israeli high school graduates, with heavy reliance on local university students—both linguistics majors and those with no specialized knowledge of Hebrew language or linguistics—as informants. Note, however, that Modern Hebrew provides a quite unique testing-ground for processes of language change which have been accelerated and concentrated beyond what one would normally expect to find. This is due to the combined factors of Modern Hebrew's having evolved within an immigrant society, with a consequent intensification of "languages in contact" situations to which Hebrew speakers are exposed, on the one hand, and to the rapid adaptation of a recently purely literary and liturgical language to the exigencies

of contemporary spoken usage . . . , on the other. Consequently, while our study accords special attention to casual everyday usage, we will also constantly note how this deviates from the requirements of more formal style as well as of conservative normativism.

This brings us to another extra-linguistic factor motivating a work of the kind undertaken here: the puristic, normative tradition characteristic of much of Hebrew scholarship and the powerful impact of the usage-correctness controversy still raging strongly in Israeli scholarship and public life alike. The reasons for the puristic outlook are manifold, and they are bound up with the special history of Modern Hebrew. . . . Thus, there seems to be a special reverence accorded by "the people of the Book" to the written word; to this day the Bible and the rabbinical are not only the fountainheads of Israeli religious, historical, and literary heritage, they are the sources of its linguistic authoritarianism par excellence. Until quite recently, few of the leading figures in Israel's political and public life were native speakers of Hebrew, and it is only in the past decade or two that native speakers have become teachers of Hebrew language and literature in the schools and universities. Thus the "norms" have quite generally been set up by people who tended to rely heavily on the literary sources of the language.

All this has had rather far-reaching consequences for the study of Modern Hebrew. Firstly, it explains the highly prescriptive approach to the teaching of Hebrew in the Israeli school system. Hebrew textbooks currently in use typically illustrate rules by excerpts from the Bible and Mishnaic Hebrew, "modern" usage being illustrated—if at all—by literary language of several decades past. School Hebrew lessons are devoted in large part to two major areas, neither of which gives scholarly weight to the language actually used by students: i) the intricate system of *nikud* "(vowel) pointing", in the form of the Tiberian vocalization system added to the consonant alphabet approximately a thousand years ago—a system which bears a very indirect relation to the contemporary pronunciation of Hebrew; and ii) the area of *šibušey lašon* "language abuses" in the sense of solecisms drilled into students preparing for their school-leaving examinations with little heed as to how they themselves actually speak—except as a model for what is "wrong".

All this has had what seems to us an unfortunate effect on the attitudes of native Israelis to their language and their own usage thereof; while keeping the usage-correctness controversy noted earlier very much in the forefront of interest among educated speakers, it has created an atmosphere where Hebrew-users tend to be irrationally puristic or to feel quite insecure with respect to their own language.

This passage is followed by a note relating Berman's experience with the insecurity that native-speaker informants, who are linguistics majors, feel when making judgments about their own language despite the fact that they have been trained to avoid prescriptive kinds of judgments in general and in languages other than Hebrew in particular. I too can add a myriad of similar anecdotal accounts of native speakers with both a linguistic and a nonlinguistic professional background who seem to be irrationally influenced by the puristic attitudes prevalent in Israel (cf. Tobin 1991). This question of what to teach and what not to teach in Hebrew grammar as "wishful thinking" is discussed in Schwarzwald (1986).

3. This historical (panchronic) conflation of various (diachronic) sources shaping the (synchronic) structure of Hebrew has been discussed in Ben-Hayim (1953), Kaddari (1983), and Kutscher (1982). The effects that this may have on the creative use of the language and the problems that it may have for translation are discussed in Tobin (1981a, 1981b).

4. The issue of borrowing is also a subject of much controversy for language purists and members of the Hebrew Language Academy, who view the wholesale importation of foreign words (called *loazit*)—especially English words—as a threat to the language even today. The broader issue of relexification is discussed in Berman (1987), Fisherman (1985), Rosén (1953), Rubenshtein (1981), Sivan (1970), and Wexler (1990), among others.

5. Other than those immigrants speaking the various Indo-European and Finno-Ugric languages and the Holocaust survivors who came to Israel speaking Yiddish and Ladino, most of the Jews from the various Arabic- or Berber-speaking countries arrived in Israel in the early 1950s. There were also waves of immigration from India, Iran, Afghanistan, and other Asian countries that brought with them a wide assortment of tongues. It is estimated that over 120 languages are spoken by these various immigrant groups. Today, Israel has a large new population from the former Soviet Union that speaks Russian, Byelorussian, and Ukranian as well as the languages of the Asian republics such as Georgian and various other Caucasian and Turkish-based languages, not to mention the Amharic speaking Jews of Ethiopia who have recently been brought to Israel en masse.

6. Much of this complex linguistic, psycholinguistic, sociolinguistic, and anthropological linguistic situation is directly involved with the phonological problem at hand, particularly with regard to the issue of normative as opposed to current pronunciation. The literature on these matters may be found in Bachi (1957), Fellman (1973a), and Schmelz and Bachi (1973), among others.

7. I would like to thank Dorit Ravid for permitting me to use the proofs of her article prior to publication.

8. This kind of opaque rule is typical of early generative work in phonology. It must be remembered that Davis has contrasted how the notion of explanation differs in generative theory and the Columbia school, a point briefly mentioned before (see chap. 3, n. 1). However, given that Davis used Lightfoot (1982) as an example of generative grammar and that the issues employed in the latter's argument dealt with first language acquisition and deficiencies (such as opaque rules), it may be appropriate here to quote Davis's statements (1984: 92, n. 2) in full:

> Generative grammar does aim for "explanatory adequacy," but the problem to be solved is a different one from ours. As stated by Lightfoot [1982] (*The Language Lottery*), "The central problem is to characterize how children can master their native

languages. The problem is one of the deficiencies of the stimulus" (p. 15). "Whatever a grammar is going to look like, it is clear that grammars, representations of mature psychological states, are of primary interest; the notion of a language is not central. Unlike much earlier work, the focus here is not on the properties of a particular language or even of general properties of many or all languages. A language under this view is an epiphenomenon, a derivative concept, the output of certain people's grammars . . ." (p. 26). The deficiency of the stimulus takes three forms: imperfection, finiteness, and unavailability. The first assumes the concept "complete, well-formed sentences" (p. 16) as the body of good data, a notion that language itself does not support. The second appeals to creativity, a facility well-known in other human endeavors. The third, said to be the most important, depends crucially on the absence of certain negative data concerning "ungrammatical sentences" (sentences not generated by the grammar) that do not occur. The perils of analyzing what has not been observed are obvious. Generally, whatever is underdetermined by available data is said to be innate, provided it is also universal.

To take an example from phonology (p. 134), occurring and non-occurring consonant clusters can be specified by descriptive "rules" written in terms of "features" that bear some resemblance to phonetics but that in fact respond solely to the distribution of phones themselves ("distribution" in a special sense). Other rules map the generative equivalent of phonemes [see chap. 1, n. 6] into a phonetic representation (p. 138). No real motivation is given for these descriptive rules, and, again, the underdetermined rules are attributed to the genotype (p. 144).

9. It might be argued by those in the diachronic know, particularly those with a purist, prescriptive background, that the word *sapa,* "sofa," is not really Hebrew or Semitic but a borrowed word (although the *Random House Dictionary* lists its possible origins as Arabic *suffah,* "platform used as a seat," or Turkish *sofa*). Regardless of its origin, naive native speakers would not identify it as being foreign. Furthermore, most foreign words are integrated into the Hebrew system in a way that strongly supports the argument that the *BeGeDKeFeT* rule is not naturally acquired and that *b-v, k-x,* and *p-f* are perceived as phonemes.

10. Most minimal pairs are elicited in word-initial position because of the communication factor: i.e., that is where the burden of communication is at its highest and the most likely place where as many communicative oppositions as possible should appear (see chap. 1, n. 12, and chap. 2, n. 14 and passim). Borrowed phonemes, or phonemes that are derived from language change, often do not appear in initial position (e.g., English /ŋ/ vs. /n/ in *sin* vs. *sing,* or /ʒ/ vs. /z/ in *rouge* vs. *ruse*), as we have seen in the new minimal pairs in Hebrew.

11. The same holds true for the /k/ = /x/ alternation (e.g., *kolera/xolera,* "cholera"; *akaf/axaf,* "he upheld") as well.

12. In addition to the fact that people are strongly influenced by written language, Israeli children often confuse the letters *p* and *f* in the Latin alphabet because they are both represented by the same letter in the Hebrew alphabet.

13. In fact, people who want to be perceived as speaking properly often correct others' "mispronunciation" of native and foreign words to make them fit the *BeGeD-KeFeT* alternations (e.g., they will correct *likfots,* "to jump," with *likpots,* which sounds a bit affected, especially when used in certain idioms, or they will correct *tilfanti,* "I phoned," with *tilpanti* or pronounce the infinitive "to telephone" as *le-talpen* rather than the more common *le-talfen.* Radio news broadcasters are required to use the *BeGeDKeFeT* rule and are monitored by language "experts" so that they do not make "mistakes." Very often their pronunciation is ridiculed or made the subject of jokes because of unintended puns and possible misinterpretations of their affected speech. The force of prescriptivism is so strong that rulings made by the Language Academy have succeeded in banning popular songs containing "poor grammar and pronunciation" from the state-controlled television and radio stations (*Time,* 14 February 1994, 8).

14. In addition to the linguistically oriented grammar books about Hebrew mentioned in n. 1 this chapter, a contrastive analysis of English and Hebrew based on the sign-oriented theoretical concepts of invariance, markedness, and distinctive feature theory is found in Tobin (1994). An entire chapter there is devoted to the verb conjugation patterns (*binyanim*).

15. Ravid (in press) provides another example of verb tense: *safar/sofer,* "counted/is counting," where the fricative is in syllable-initial position but tested 100 percent as *sapar/sofer* for all children and uneducated adult speakers. For this case, she maintains that the infinitive—not the usual base form—was postulated as the base form. It might also be mentioned that there is a minimal pair *sapar,* "barber," vs. *safar,* "he counted," in the language. It might also be that a similar level of stricture, airflow, and turbulence between the two phonemes /s/ and /f/ (sibilant and fricative) may be easier to maintain here as well. Ravid also provides another example across parts of speech: *kafa/kafu/kipaon-kifaon,* "froze/is frozen/freeze," which also has /f/ in initial position. The influence of a low as opposed to a high vowel may also be playing a role here. However, it must be remembered that these phonotactic favorings are gradient and not absolute because of the complexity of the interaction of the communication and human factors.

16. In biblical Hebrew, this efficient stop/spirant phonemic distinction was maintained only for the laryngeal pair of the voiceless glottal stop /ʔ/ *aleph* and /h/. The glottal stop is no longer part of the phonemic inventory of Israeli Hebrew, and, if one judges by the speech of the past two generations of native speakers, /h/ is on the way out as well. The pair voiced/voiceless pharyngeal fricative /ʕ/ *ayin* and /ħ/ *Het* has also been eliminated in general Israeli speech—thus keeping all the active articulators in the oral cavity only. The other sounds that have been lost—the posterodorsal and labial /q/ and /w/ and the emphatic /T/—have merged with their simpler counterparts requiring one set of articulators only. The new phonological system of Israeli Hebrew therefore involves fewer active articulators that are easier to control and limited to the oral cavity only as well as a more efficient exploitation of different degrees of stricture and airflow.

17. It would be interesting to see whether children acquiring the sociolect where the normative plurals are used first use normative forms (which are acquired lexically) and then use naive forms for the same word while acquiring the grammar, before reverting to the normative lexical forms again in a way similar to English-speaking children who first acquire *feet* then use *foots* or *feets* before reverting again to *feet*. This could also be examined in the verb system as well as the plural system.
18. There is a whole area of what is considered to be irregular phonological form classes in Hebrew verb morphology and diachronic phonological rules that are no longer part and parcel of Israeli Hebrew but are taught in school as belonging to correct Hebrew that should be further researched. One such analysis is found in Tobin (1993a: 327–36) for the defective I-NUN class of Hebrew verbs. Some other diachronic phonological rules have been explained by the principles of the theory of phonology as human behavior as well (Arielli 1994). The phonological aspects of Israeli slang have been analyzed according to the theory of phonology as human behavior by Pitusi (1995).

6 Pedagogical and Textual Applications

1. Although I have been teaching phonetics and phonology for over twenty years, most of the time either implicitly or explicitly according to this linguistic orientation, I shall not present here a detailed outline or a minitext for teaching a course in phonetics as human behavior. (I do, however, reserve the right to do so in the future.) I shall merely be presenting some basic guidelines on how this might be done. The reader interested in the isomorphic implications of invariance, markedness, and distinctive feature theory and their application to problems in morphology, syntax, and semantics is urged to read Tobin (1990c, 1993a, 1994) and Andrews and Tobin (in press).
2. The data presented here represent a revised and expanded version of Kurtz (1992), an assignment done for a linguistics course entitled "Phonology as Human Behavior" in the Department of English Language and Literature at Haifa University. In app. 1, the instructions for the assignment are reproduced.
3. In the *Annotated Alice* version (Carroll 1965 [1871]: 191–97), the poem "Jabberwocky" is thoroughly discussed and explained word by word in great and most interesting detail. In addition, French and German versions of the poem are presented. These translations also appear in app. 2 for any interested reader.
4. This is not to say that languages that do not favor initial stress are inefficient. More detailed typological studies should be made of languages with fixed stress as opposed to languages with free stress. Among the languages with fixed stress, further studies should be made of languages with word-initial, word-medial, or word-final stress. There are many factors—such as syllable- vs. stress-timed languages; synthetic, analytic, agglutinative, or polysynthetic types of word formation; prosody; etc.—that may influence syllable stress.

5. The distribution of the number of sets of articulators in word-final position is fairly random as well, with a slight favoring of voiceless phonemes of constriction in the general corpus and a random distribution (50 percent–50 percent) for the neologisms. However, many of the voiced phonemes of constriction are devoiced in actual speech, as we have heard and seen in recordings and spectrograms.

7 Developmental Phonology and Functional Clinical Applications

1. Most if not all discussions of child phonology begin with Jakobson's seminal work, and he is referred to in every major book that I have consulted (e.g., Atkinson 1982; Bruner 1983; de Villiers and de Villiers 1978; Locke 1983b; Owens 1988; Weir 1962). Many books follow Jakobson's original approach and combine the areas of child phonology and language disorders (e.g., Bleile 1991; Hedrick, Prather, and Tobin 1984; Stoel-Gammon and Dunne (1985).
2. The following studies have either supported or supplied counterevidence to Jakobson's hypotheses and claims regarding Jakobson's view of babbling and its role in phonological development (e.g., Blount 1970; Irwin 1947; Oller et al. 1976; Vihman 1988; Vihman et al. 1985; Vihman, Ferguson, and Elbert 1986); the order of acquisition of phonemes (e.g., Braine 1971, 1974; Ferguson 1977b; Ferguson and Farwell 1975; Ferguson and Garnica 1975; Garnica 1973; Leopold 1947; Moskowitz 1973; Shvachkin 1973; Velten 1943); the order of acquisition of distinctive features (e.g., Burling 1959; Menyuk 1968; Olmstead 1971, 1974; Smith 1973); the need for the child to acquire a large productive vocabulary based on the adult model before a systematic phonological system is developed (e.g., Glucksberg and Danks 1975); the need for the child to reach the onset of symbolic representation in the late sensorimotor period of intellectual development (Ingram 1976a, based on Piaget 1970).
3. I will not enter here into discussions of the pros and cons of generative and post-generative, nonlinear phonologies and their role in phonological or developmental theories. I will concentrate only on the natural functional processes that will be relevant to the clinical discussions in this and subsequent chapters. Among the leading researchers in the field of natural phonological processes are Ingram (1974, 1976b, 1979, 1981), Khan (1982), Menn (1971), Moskowitz (1970), Smith (1973), Stampe (1969, 1979 [1972]), and Vihman (1976). It should be noted, however, that many of these natural processes were already discussed explicitly in Jakobson (1941/1968), while others were alluded to implicitly as well. The major clinical applications of these natural processes are discussed in Ingram (1976a, 1989) and Grunwell (1981, 1982, 1985, 1987). Readers interested in a historical account of the early generative contributions to child phonology should read Menn (1980).
4. The difference between production and perception is crucial particularly in the areas of child phonology and clinical phonology, as evinced by separate volumes devoted to production and perception for child phonology (Yeni-Komshian, Kavanagh, and Ferguson 1980). Crystal (1987 [1981]: 38–42), Grunwell (1987: 4, 10, n. 5,

29, and passim), and others discuss the difference between perception and production as well. Grunwell also clearly indicates that the phonological processes that she is discussing are based on children's speech production, most of which, for my money, at least, generally represents phonetic rather than phonological processes if no deviance from the adult phonological system has been found in perception or discrimination tests.

5. I have found this to be particularly true for children diagnosed with a voicing problem. Listening to recordings and viewing spectrograms have often revealed that such a child's production is different for voiced and voiceless phonemes, but both sounds fall into the acoustic range of what is normally perceived as being voiceless by the language community. This phenomenon has been reported for Hebrew in Ben-Dor (1990) and Shachar (1990). Spectrographic evidence of children producing phonemic differences that cannot readily be detected by adult perception has also been attested to in English by Macken and Barton (1979) and Smit and Bernthal (1983) and is discussed in Menyuk, Menn, and Silber (1986).

6. The question of phonological and phonetic processes and errors is discussed in Hewlitt (1985) in general and in Katz (1993: 2–4) from the point of view of phonology as human behavior as opposed to natural phonology. Other scholars advocating a similar stand as to the phonetic or phonological categorization of such errors include Bernthal and Bankson (1988), Locke (1983a, 1983b), McReynolds and Elbert (1981), Pollack and Rees (1975), and Winitz (1969). It should also be remembered that many of the most current theories of cognitive and nonlinear phonology do not necessarily recognize or have buried the phoneme as a unit of phonological analysis (see chap. 1, nn. 6, 7).

7. I will not enter here into a discussion comparing and contrasting the relatively simple approximately five-member Hebrew vowel system and the relatively complex approximately fourteen- to fifteen-member vowel-diphthong system of English. The interested reader should consult Levenston's (1970) contrastive analysis. Halpern (1991) discusses the identification and perception of vowels in adults as part of an experiment in cross-language (Hebrew-English) vowel perception and the influence of consonant-vowel transitions on vowel identifications. O. Amir (1995) discusses the acoustic measurements of the Israeli Hebrew vowel system in an attempt to establish norms that might be applied to the clinic according to the theory of phonology as human behavior.

8. The various arguments regarding the relation or lack thereof between the complete or incomplete perception and production of adult and child phonological systems, which form the central theoretical and methodological arguments in the field, are found in Berko and Brown (1960), Edwards (1974), Grunwell (1981, 1985, 1987), Ingram (1976b, 1981, 1989), Jespersen (1964), Peizer and Olmstead (1969), Shvachkin (1973), and Stoel-Gammon and Dunne (1985), among others. However, it should be noted that both views of developmental phonological systems—either as a simplification of adult systems or as independent systems that are, by definition, simpler than adult systems—are consonant with the human factor of the theory of

phonology as human behavior concerning children's more limited motor abilities (cf. Kent 1992).

9. The state of the art of speech pathology and audiology in Israel as it may be compared and contrasted with other countries (particularly the United States) is discussed in Schwartz, Harris, and Most (1993). The application of the theory of phonology as human behavior to the speech clinic has centered primarily around my work in the Department of Communication Disorders, Speech, Language and Hearing of the School of Health Professions in the Sackler Faculty of Medicine of Tel-Aviv University at Tel-Hashomer. Studies of similar populations and first language acquisition have also been done in a graduate seminar in the Department of Behavioral Sciences at the Ben-Gurion University of the Negev and will be included in the following list.

There have been more than one hundred individual applications of the theory to the clinic for specific problems representing a wide array of speech disorders of the following kinds: general functional disorders (Argov 1990; Ashkenazi 1993; Ben-David 1994; Ben-Said 1991; Ben-Tsvi 1990; Berlin 1989; Corona 1993; Jehudah 1990; Katz 1989; Kortser 1994; Levi 1992; Neumann 1992; Rapoport 1994; Schecht 1995; Segal 1995; Zilberstein 1994); such idiosyncratic, unusual, or relatively rare functional disorders as backing and unusual sound substitutions (Ben-David 1994; Bohanda 1994; Libo 1989; Mor 1992; Nakash 1991; Pel-Zalit 1993; Shinter 1993); delayed language development (Cohen-Mimran 1992; Feldman 1994; Fomgrin 1995; Hamburger 1992; Rich 1994; Shaulsky 1994), including poor motor control, short auditory memory, and lack of oral sensory sensitivity (Levi 1994; Koby 1995) and a hyperactive bilingual child with late development (Yosef-Barak 1995); stuttering (Amir 1993; Apter 1989; Bezalel-Goldblatt 1990; Gorodisky 1990; Himmel 1995a, 1995b; Isaacson 1995; Othman Gabara 1994; Platzky 1995; Taler 1995); organic disorders such as apraxia and dyspraxia (Doron 1995; Kopold 1991; Meckler 1995; Raz Harel 1988; Segev 1993; Segal Friedenreich 1992; Shamir 1994; Weinreb 1991); Down's syndrome (Hagoel 1993; Sharabi 1995); mental retardation (Ablas 1995; Segal 1992; Nir 1993; Eibschitz-Levine 1994); autism (Koren 1991; Kantz 1995); cerebral palsy, ataxia, and the speech of spastics (Eibschitz-Levine 1994, 1995; Isan [Weinreb] 1994); cleft palate (Yagev 1996); and esophageal and tracheoesophageal speech production (Cohen-Mimran 1995).

In addition, the theory has also been applied to first language acquisition for Hebrew and bilingual Hebrew-English-speaking children (Segal 1993; Haran 1989; Gan 1994, 1995; Cohen 1995; Hevron 1995; S. Amir 1995) and a Russian-speaking child (Tsatkin-Pessin 1994); second language learning (Mendolowici 1995); learning disabled children with minimal brain damage or attention deficit disorders (Faianas 1993; Galpaz 1995; Shaulsky 1994); and the problems of naming (Davidi 1991; Feldman 1994), language retrieval (Ris 1994), and slips of the tongue (Sadka 1995a, 1995b). In a larger study, Katz (1993) compares and contrasts the theory of natural phonology predominant in Israeli speech clinics with the theory of phonology as human behavior for over 250 utterances made by eight children between 4:6 and

5:6 years of age who presented with a wide variety of functional disorders.

10. I have presented here an oversimplified view of Katz's and the other studies applying the theory of phonology as human behavior to the clinic as an explanatory device. More detailed clinical studies applying the theory of phonology as human behavior and contrasting it with natural phonology have appeared in a special issue of *Dibur u-Shmiya* (Speech and hearing disorders) (vol. 18, 1995), the journal of the Israeli Speech, Hearing and Language Association (Tobin 1995c).

8 Clinical Applications to Organic Disorders

1. Applications of generative phonology and distinctive feature analysis to the clinic include Camarata and Gandour (1984) (who consider complementary distribution as part of generative phonology!), Compton (1976), Dinnsen et al. (1990) for phonotactic analysis, Edwards and Shriberg (1983), Elbert and Gierut (1986), Leonard and Brown (1984) for phonological categories, Lowe (1994), McReynolds and Engmann (1975) for distinctive feature analysis, McReynolds, Engmann, and Dimmitt (1974) for an analysis based on phonological markedness, Oller (1973), Pollack and Rees (1975), and Weiner (1981) for systematic sound preferences. Applications of such nonlinear phonological approaches as autosegmental phonology, metric phonology, lexical phonology, and feature geometry to language acquisition and disorders are found in Bernhardt (1990, 1992a, 1992b), Bernhardt and Gilbert (1992), Bernhardt and Stoel-Gammon (in press), Schwartz (1992a, 1992b, 1992c), and Bjorklund and Schwartz (in press). Not surprisingly, much of the clinical application of nonlinear phonology uses the syllable as the unit of analysis and concentrates on prosodic and segmental levels of speech as separate and autonomous tiers.

2. Apraxia or apraxias indicating the different kinds of developmental and adult apraxias and the differences between apraxia and dysarthria have been discussed in Carrell (1968: chap. 7), Darley (1964: 36–38), Darley, Aronson, and Brown (1975), Brain (1961: chap. 13), Lapointe and Wertz (1974), Weiss, Lillywhite, and Gordon (1980), and Wertz, Lapointe, and Rosenbek (1984), among others. The theory of phonology as human behavior has been used in a number of cases of apraxia and dysarthria, including Kopold (1991), Segev (1993), and Isan (Weinreb) (1991, 1994). Apraxia and dysarthria per se, and applying phonological theories to their analysis in general and the theory of phonology as human behavior in particular, are certainly topics worthy of additional research and study.

3. As was mentioned in chap. 4, n. 1, it should also be noted that I have viewed the historical (and Oriental or Sephardic) Hebrew /r/ phoneme as an apical trill, although in Israeli Hebrew it is pronounced as a voiced dorsal fricative /ɣ/. In this chapter, when I discuss the /r/ phoneme of Hebrew, the reader should assume that I mean /ɣ/ unless otherwise stated.

4. It is interesting to note that the early texts in speech pathology that I have con-

sulted (e.g., Carrell 1968: chap. 7; Darley 1964: 36–38; and Brain 1961: chap. 13) discuss apraxia at great length but do not mention dyspraxia. A recent resource manual for speech pathologists (Shipley and McAfee 1992) lists dyspraxia in the index with a note to see apraxia. The same basically holds true for dysphasia as well, which is defined only as a less severe form of aphasia in Darley (1964: 31). Ingram (1976b) does not deal with either apraxia, dyspraxia, or dysphasia. As was mentioned in the preceding chapter, in this volume I will maintain a very broad distinction between functional articulatory disorders (discussed in chap. 7) and organic ones (discussed in the present chapter). The reader should be aware that these classifications are being used in an informal way and are based on the original nomenclature, classifications, and diagnoses of the individual speech therapists who worked with each subject or client.

5. In this chapter, I have summarized only a small number of the so-called pathological or organic clinical problems that have been analyzed by the theory of phonology as human behavior. As was stated in chap. 7, n. 9, there are more than one hundred additional studies of this nature covering a wide range of topics, including delayed language development, stuttering, autism, cerebral palsy, and learning disabled children that are certainly worthy of further consideration. Future research should analyze these phenomena according to phonological theories in general and the theory of phonology as human behavior in particular. In a special issue of *Dibur u-Shmiya* (Speech and hearing disorders) (vol. 18, 1995), articles discuss the application of the theory to celebral palsy, stuttering, aphasia, the hearing impaired, and slips of the tongue.

9 Audiology, Hearing Impairment, and Cochlear Implants

1. These studies include those already cited in Ingram (1976b) as well as Levitt and Smith (1972), Ling (1976), McGarr and Whitehead (1992), Osberger and McFarr (1983), and Smith (1975), among others. The reader interested in a comprehensive and up-to-date reference for the physiology, acoustics, and perception of speech in general is advised to consult Borden, Harris, and Raphael (1993).

2. Some of the most interesting clinical work relates to the language of twins. Edwards and Bernhardt (1973b) discuss twin speech as the sharing of a phonological system. Von Bremen (1990) applies the theory of nonlinear phonology to the analysis of and clinical work with the severely disordered phonological systems of identical twins. Tromer Uziel (1992) applies the theory of phonology as human behavior to the disordered phonological systems of identical twins. Alfasa (1993) discusses the disordered system of a fraternal twin. Tobin and Segev (1992) analyze the identification of the voices of identical twins by trained and naive listeners, and Gal (1993) compares and contrasts the identification of the voices of identical twins by blind and hearing listeners. Weissfer (1994) analyzes the language of a triplet with language delay and fine and general motor control deficiency.

3. I have presented a very brief and oversimplified view of audiology and hearing impairment. For a more detailed view of the subject, the interested reader should consult Bess (1988), Bess and Humes (1990), Hannley (1986), Jerger and Jerger (1981), Katz (1978), Martin (1991), Northern (1984), Northern and Downs (1991), and Roeser (1986), among others.

4. These factors as well as others should also be further studied and researched. Other audiological analyses of the results of auditory discrimination tests for populations of normal and hearing-impaired children and adults based on the theory of phonology as human behavior include Fingleh (1995), Gabai (1993), Hurwitz (1993), and Sharoni (1992). The speech of hearing-impaired children and adults is analyzed according to the theory of phonology as human behavior in Halpern (1995).

5. I have presented a very brief and oversimplified view of cochlear implants. For a more detailed view of the subject, the interested reader should consult Aronson (1990), Cooper (1991), Dowell et al. (1982), and Owens and Kessler (1989), among others. Much interesting work and research in this field is being carried out under Professor Minka Hildesheimer (1989) and Dr. Hava Muchnik, the former and present chairs of the Department of Communication Disorders, Speech, Language and Hearing of the School of Health Professions in the Sackler Faculty of Medicine of Tel-Aviv University at Tel-Hashomer. Teitelbaum (1995) examined the segmental and prosodic differences in the speech of subjects before and after cochlear implants; this paper also includes a discussion of the human and communication factors in the light of these prosodic findings.

6. I have compared S.'s results with those of Rovel's (1990) subjects because both deal with the hearing impaired and/or those with normal hearing under adverse acoustic conditions, both tested for similar tasks under similar circumstances, and the kind of test (closed) and the stimuli (monosyllabic CVC words) were very similar as well. Further comparative and contrastive studies of the hearing impaired, those with normal hearing, and people who have had cochlear implants should be done under identical conditions.

7. *Degrees of stricture* and *types of airflow* are the terms in the theory of phonology as human behavior that replace the traditional concept of manner of articulation. Therefore, when I discuss the densalization of nasals and their substitutions by fricatives and stops, I will refer to changes in stricture and airflow in fricative and stop replacement (cf. chap. 3).

10 Aphasia

1. The literature on aphasia is vast and rapidly expanding. The bibliographies and lists of references in the works cited in the text should be consulted by the interested reader. The specific clinically oriented works used by Ani (1990) and Gvion (1989) that have applied phonological theory to aphasic patients include Albert et al. (1981), Benson (1979), Blumstein (1973, 1981), Friedrich et al. (1984), Gandour et al. (1982),

Keller (1978, 1981, 1984), Kohn (1984), Monoi et al. (1983), and Trost and Canter (1974), among others. Ani (1995, 1996) applies the theory of phonology as human behavior to a population of over thirty aphasics with different categories of aphasia: Broca's aphasia, conductive aphasia, and Wernicke's aphasia. A study of child aphasia applying the theory appears in Bar-Lev (1995a, 1995b). A further study of adult aphasia according to the theory of phonology as human behavior can be found in Levi and Kluck (1995).

2. I have not specifically dealt with functional load, frequency, and a connection to errors in the clinic in general and in aphasics in particular. Although, on the surface at least, the last principle makes sense, it—as well as all the other principles—should be examined and researched further. It should also be mentioned that frequency and markedness value are not necessarily connected with each other. A further area of research would be to classify so-called general and idiosyncratic processes according to distinctive features and markedness theory from the point of view of description and explanation in general and phonology as human behavior in particular.

Appendix 2

1. This translation, by Frank L. Warren, appeared in the *New Yorker* (10 January 1931).

2. This translation, by Robert Scott, appeared in "The Jabberwock Traced to Its True Source" *Macmillan's Magazine* (February 1872).

References

Ablas, Yifat. 1995. Applying the theory of phonology as human behavior to a mentally retarded child with anatomical problems of the speech mechanism (in Hebrew). Department of Communication Disorders, Speech, Language and Hearing, Sackler Faculty of Medicine, Tel-Aviv University. Typescript.

Akamatsu, Tsutomu. 1988. *The theory of neutralization and the archiphoneme in functional phonology.* Amsterdam and Philadelphia: John Benjamins.

Albert, M. L., H. Goodglass, N. A. Helm, A. I. Rubens, and M. P. Alexander. 1981. *Clinical aspects of dysphasia.* Berlin and New York: Springer.

Alcalay, Reuben. 1990. *Ha-Milon Ha-Ivri Ha-Shalem* [1975]. Ramat Gan and Jerusalem: Massada.

Alfasa, Anat. 1993. The theory of phonology as human behavior and its application to the disordered speech of a girl (5:3) (in Hebrew). Department of Communication Disorders, Speech, Language and Hearing, Sackler Faculty of Medicine, Tel-Aviv University. Typescript.

Ali, Latif H., Raymond G. Danilof, and Paul Hoffman. 1988. Acoustic properties of Arabic "ain." Paper presented at the Sixth International Phonology Meeting, Krems, Austria, 2 July.

Alster-Zini, Ruth. 1993. An analysis of the articulatory errors of a girl aged 4:5 according to the theory of phonology as human behavior (in Hebrew). Department of Communication Disorders, Speech, Language and Hearing, Sackler Faculty of Medicine, Tel-Aviv University. Typescript.

Altmann, Gabriel. 1978. Towards a theory of language. In *Glottometrika 1,* ed. G. Altmann. Bochum: Brockmeyer.

Altmann, G., and W. Lehfeldt. 1980. *Einführung in die quantitative Phonolgie.* Bochum: Brockmeyer.

Amir, Ofer. 1993. An analysis of stuttering based on the theory of phonology as human behavior (in Hebrew). Department of Communication Disorders, Speech, Language and Hearing, Sackler Faculty of Medicine, Tel-Aviv University. Typescript.

Amir, Ofer. 1995. Acoustic measurements of the modern Hebrew vowel system (in Hebrew). M.A. thesis, Department of Communication Disorders, Speech, Language and Hearing, Sackler Faculty of Medicine, Tel-Aviv University.

Amir, Sharon. 1995. Phonology as human behavior: First language acquisition (in Hebrew). *Dibur u-Shmiya* (Speech and hearing disorders) 18:37–50.

Andrews, Edna, and Yishai Tobin, eds. In press. *Invariance, markedness, distinctive feature theory and deixis: Towards a calculus of meaning.* Amsterdam and Philadelphia: John Benjamins.

Ani, Betty. 1990. An analysis of the phonological errors of a Broca's aphasia patient according to the theory of phonology as human behavior (in Hebrew). Department of Communication Disorders, Speech, Language and Hearing, Sackler Faculty of Medicine, Tel-Aviv University. Typescript.

Ani, Betty. 1995. Phonology as human behavior: Aphasia (in Hebrew). *Dibur u-Shmiya* (Speech and hearing disorders) 18:105–28.

Ani, Betty. 1996. Phonological errors in aphasic patients in light of the theory of phonology as human behavior (in Hebrew). M.A. thesis, Department of Communication Disorders, Speech, Language and Hearing, Sackler Faculty of Medicine, Tel-Aviv University.

Aphek, Edna, and Yishai Tobin. 1988. *Word systems in modern Hebrew: Implications and applications.* Leiden and New York: E. J. Brill.

Aphek, Edna, and Yishai Tobin. 1989. *The semiotics of fortune-telling.* Amsterdam and Philadelphia: John Benjamins.

Apter, Gili. 1989. Phonetics and phonology (in Hebrew). Department of Communication Disorders, Speech, Language and Hearing, Sackler Faculty of Medicine, Tel-Aviv University. Typescript.

Arce, Joaquín. 1962. Il numero dei fonemi in italiano in confronto con lo spagnolo. *Lingua Nostra* 23:48–52.

Argov, Anat. 1990. An analysis of the speech errors of a normal child (4:9) according to the theory of phonology as human behavior (in Hebrew). Department of Communication Disorders, Speech, Language and Hearing, Sackler Faculty of Medicine, Tel-Aviv University. Typescript.

Arielli, Zev. 1994. Some diachronic phonological rules of Hebrew in light of the theory of phonology as human behavior (in Hebrew). Department of Behavioral Sciences, Ben-Gurion University of the Negev. Typescript.

Armstrong, D., and C. H. van Schooneveld, eds. 1977. *Roman Jakobson: Echoes of his scholarship.* Lisse: Peter de Ridder.

Aronoff, Mark. 1976. *Word formation in generative grammar.* Cambridge, Mass.: MIT Press.

Aronson, L. 1990. Electronical parameters of cochlear prothesis adapted to deaf Hebrew speakers. Ph.D. diss., Technion-Israel Institute of Technology.

Ashkenazi, Orit. 1993. An analysis of a clinical case according to phonology as human behavior (in Hebrew). Department of Communication Disorders, Speech, Language and Hearing, Sackler Faculty of Medicine, Tel-Aviv University. Typescript.

Atkinson, Martin. 1982. *Explanations in the study of child language development.* Cambridge: Cambridge University Press.

Atkinson, Martin, David Kilby, and Iggy Roca. 1988. *Foundations of general linguistics.* London: Unwin Hyman.

Austerlitz, Robert. 1983. A curious surrogate for R in the English of New York City. In *From sounds to words,* Umea Studies in the Humanities no. 60. Umea.

Azim, Abdul. 1989. Some problems in the phonology of modern standard Urdu. Paper presented at the First International Columbia School Conference on Linguistics, 24 August.

Azim, Abdul. 1993. Problems of aspiration in modern standard Urdu. Paper presented at the Third International Columbia School Conference on Linguistics, 11 October.

Azim, Abdul. 1995. The phonology of the vocalic systems of modern standard Urdu. Paper presented at the Fourth International Columbia School Conference on Linguistics, 20 February.

Bachi, R. 1957. The revival of Hebrew in a statistical mirror (in Hebrew). *Leshonenu* 20:65–82, 21:41–68.

Bailey, Ch.-J. N. 1980. Über den gerechten Tod des Phonems. *Papiere zur Linguistik* 22:47–57.

Baltaxe, C. A. M. 1978. *Foundations of distinctive feature theory.* Baltimore: University Park Press.

Bangs, J. 1942. A clinical analysis of the articulatory defects of the feebleminded. *Journal of Speech and Hearing Disorders* 7:343–56.

Bar-Adon, Aaron. 1959. The spoken language of Israeli children (in Hebrew). Ph.D. diss., Hebrew University in Jerusalem.

Bar-Adon, Aaron. 1971. Primary syntactic structures in Hebrew child language. In *Child language: A book of readings,* ed. A. Bar-Adon and W. F. Leopold, 433–72. Englewood Cliffs, N.J.: Prentice-Hall.

Bar-Adon, Aaron. 1975. *The rise and decline of a dialect.* The Hague: Mouton.

Barkai, Malachi. 1972. Problems in the phonology of Hebrew. Ph.D. diss., University of Illinois at Urbana.

Bar-Lev, Ayala. 1995a. Applying the theory of phonology as human behavior to a child with aphasia (in Hebrew). Department of Communication Disorders, Speech, Language and Hearing, Sackler Faculty of Medicine, Tel-Aviv University. Typescript.

Bar-Lev, Ayala. 1995b. Phonology as human behavior: An analysis of the articulatory disorders of an aphasic hearing-disabled girl (in Hebrew). *Dibur u-Shmiya* (Speech and hearing disorders) 18:147–58.

Bates, E., and B. MacWhinney. 1982. Functionalist approaches to grammar. In *Language acquisition: The state of the art,* ed. E. Wanner and L. R. Gleitman. Cambridge: Cambridge University Press.

Battisti, Carlo, and Giovanno Alessio. 1950–57. *Dizionario etimologico italiano.* 5 vols. Florence: G. Barbera.

Ben-Asher, M. 1969. *The consolidation of normative grammar in modern Hebrew* (in Hebrew). Tel-Aviv: Hakibbutz Hameuchad.

Ben-David, Nofar. 1994. An analysis of the articulatory errors of a 5:6-year-old child according to the theory of phonology as human behavior (in Hebrew). Department of Communication Disorders, Speech, Language and Hearing, Sackler Faculty of Medicine, Tel-Aviv University. Typescript.

Ben-Dor (Tamir), Avivit. 1990. Auditory perception and speech production of (/d/, /g/, /t/, /k/) in 4–5-year-old speaking-impaired children (in Hebrew). M.A. thesis, Department of Communication Disorders, Speech, Language and Hearing, Sackler Faculty of Medicine, Tel-Aviv University.

Ben-Hayim, Z. 1953. An ancient language in a new reality (in Hebrew). *Leshonenu La'Am* 5:35–37.

Ben-Horin, Gadi, and Shmuel Bolozky. 1972. Hebrew *bkp*—rule opacity or data opacity? *Hebrew Computational Linguistics* 5:E24–E35.

Ben-Said, Limor. 1991. An analysis of speech errors according to the theory of phonology as human behavior (in Hebrew). Department of Communication Disorders, Speech, Language and Hearing, Sackler Faculty of Medicine, Tel-Aviv University. Typescript.

Benson, D. F. 1979. *Aphasia, alexia and agraphia.* London: Churchill Livingstone.

Ben-Tsvi, Tamar. 1990. An analysis of a case of a speech-impaired child according to a phonological theory (in Hebrew). Department of Communication Disorders, Speech, Language and Hearing, Sackler Faculty of Medicine, Tel-Aviv University. Typescript.

Berg, Thomas. 1993. The phoneme through a psycholinguist's looking-glass. *Theoretical Linguistics* 19, no. 1:39–76.

Berko, J., and R. Brown. 1960. Psycholinguistic research methods. In *Handbook of research methods in child development,* ed. P. Mussen, 517–77. New York: Wiley.

Berlin, Mira. 1989. Phonology and phonetics (in Hebrew). Department of Communication Disorders, Speech, Language and Hearing, Sackler Faculty of Medicine, Tel-Aviv University. Typescript.

Berman, Ruth A. 1977. Natural phonological processes at the one-word stage. *Lingua* 43:1–21.

Berman, Ruth A., ed. 1978. *Modern Hebrew structure.* Tel-Aviv: University Publishing Projects.

Berman, Ruth A. 1985. Acquisition of Hebrew. In *The crosslinguistic study of language acquisition,* ed. D. I. Slobin. Hillsdale, N.J.: Lawrence Erlbaum.

Berman, Ruth A. 1987. Productivity in the lexicon: New-word formation in modern Hebrew. *Folia Linguistica* 21:225–54.

Bernhardt, Barbara. 1990. Applications of nonlinear phonological theory to intervention with six phonologically disordered children. Ph.D. diss., University of British Columbia.

Bernhardt, Barbara. 1992a. The application of nonlinear phonological theory to intervention with one phonologically disordered child. *Clinical Linguistics and Phonetics* 6, no. 4:283–316.

Bernhardt, Barbara. 1992b. Developmental implications of nonlinear phonological theory. *Clinical Linguistics and Phonetics* 6, no. 4:259–81.

Bernhardt, Barbara, and John Gilbert. 1992. Applying linguistic theory to speech-language pathology: The case of non-linear phonology. *Clinical Linguistics and Phonetics* 6, nos. 1–2:123–45.

Bernhardt, Barbara, and Carol Stoel-Gammon. In press. Nonlinear phonology: Introduction and clinical application. *Journal of Speech and Hearing Research.*

Bernholtz-Priner, Ronit. 1993. The nonrandom distribution of initial consonant clusters in Yiddish according to the theory of phonology as human behavior (in Hebrew). Department of Communication Disorders, Speech, Language and Hearing, Sackler Faculty of Medicine, Tel-Aviv University. Typescript.

Bernstein, D. S., and E. Tigerman, eds. 1985. *Language and communication disorders in children.* Columbus, Ohio: Merrill.

Bernthal, J. E., and N. W. Bankson, eds. 1988. *Articulation and phonological disorders in children.* 2d ed. Englewood Cliffs, N.J.: Prentice-Hall.

Bess, F. H., ed. 1988. *Hearing impairment in children.* Parkton, Md.: York Press.

Bess, F. H., and L. E. Humes. 1990. *Audiology: The fundamentals.* Baltimore: Williams & Wilkins.

Bezalel-Goldblatt, Esther. 1990. Speech errors and fluency disturbances: Phonology as human behavior (in Hebrew). Department of Communication Disorders, Speech, Language and Hearing, Sackler Faculty of Medicine, Tel-Aviv University. Typescript.

Bierwisch, Manfred. 1971. *Modern linguistics.* The Hague: Mouton.

Bjorklund, David F., and Richard G. Schwartz. In press. The adaptive nature of developmental immaturity: Implications for language acquisition and language disabilities. In *Childhood language disorders,* ed. M. Smith and J. Damico. New York: Thieme Medical.

Bleile, Ken M. 1982. Consonant ordering in Down's syndrome phonology. *Journal of Communication Disorders* 15:275–85.

Bleile, Ken M. 1991. *Child phonology.* San Diego: Singular.

Bleile, Ken M., and Richard Schwartz. 1984. Three perspectives on the speech of children with Down's syndrome. *Journal of Communication Disorders* 17:87–94.

Bliss, S. L., D. V. Allen and G. Walker. 1978. Sentence structure of TMR and EMR subjects. *Journal of Speech and Hearing Research* 21:722–31.

Bloomfield, Leonard. 1933. *Language.* New York: Holt, Rinehart & Winston.

Blount, B. 1970. The pre-linguistic system of Luo children. *Anthropological Linguistics* 12:326–42.

Bluhme, Hermann. 1964. *Beitrag zur deutschen und zur polnischen Mundart im oberschlesischen Industriegebiet unter besonder Berücksichtigung phonometrischer Methoden.* The Hague: Martinus Nijhoff.

Blumstein, Sheila. 1973. *A phonological investigation of aphasic speech.* The Hague: Mouton.

Blumstein, S. 1981. Phonological aspects of aphasia. In *Acquired aphasia,* ed. M. Taylor-Sarno, 129–59. New York: Academic.

Blumstein, S., W. E. Cooper, H. Goodglass, S. Statlender, and J. Gottleib. 1980. Production deficits in aphasia: A voice-onset time analysis. *Brain and Language* 9: 153–70.

Blumstein, S., and P. Shinn. 1984. The spectral characteristics of stop consonants provide important cues to the nature of place of articulation production in Broca's aphasia: A reply to W. Ziegler. *Brain and Language* 23:171–74.

Bodine, A. 1974. A phonological analysis of the speech of two mongoloid (Down's syndrome) boys. *Anthropological Linguistics* 16:1–24.

Bohanda, Penina. 1994. Phonology as human behavior (in Hebrew). Department of Communication Disorders, Speech, Language and Hearing, Sackler Faculty of Medicine, Tel-Aviv University. Typescript.

Bolinger, Dwight, and Donald A. Sears. 1981. *Aspects of language.* New York: Harcourt Brace Jovanovich.

Bolozky, Shmuel. 1978. Some aspects of modern Hebrew phonology. In *Modern Hebrew structure,* ed. Ruth A. Berman. Tel-Aviv: University Publishing Projects.

Bolozky, Shmuel. 1982. Strategies of modern Hebrew word formation. *Hebrew Annual Review* 6:69–80.

Boone, D. R. 1987. *Human communication and its disorders.* Englewood Cliffs, N.J.: Prentice-Hall.

Borden, Gloria J., Katherine S. Harris, and Lawrence J. Raphael. 1993. *Speech science primer: Physiology, acoustics, and perception of speech.* 3d ed. Baltimore: Williams & Wilkins.

Brain, Russell Sir. 1961. *Speech disorders: Aphasia, apraxia, and agnosia.* Washington, D.C.: Butterworth.

Braine, M. D. S. 1971. The acquisition of language in infant and child. In *The learning of language,* ed. C. Reed. New York: Appleton-Century-Crofts.

Braine, M. D. S. 1974. On what might constitute learnable phonology. *Language* 50: 270–99.

Bronstein, Arthur J. 1960. *The pronunciation of American English: An introduction to phonetics.* New York: Appleton-Century-Crofts.

Bruner, J. 1983. *Child's talk: Learning how to use language.* New York: Norton.

Buck, C. D. 1933. *Comparative grammar of Greek and Latin.* Chicago: University of Chicago Press.

Buckley, S. 1985. Attaining basic educational skills: Reading, writing and numbers. In *Current approaches to Down's syndrome,* ed. D. Lane and B. Stratford. New York: Praeger.

Burling, R. 1959. Language development of a Garo and English-speaking child. *Word* 15:45–68.

Burt, C. 1937. *The backward child.* New York: Appleton-Century-Crofts.

Bybee, Joan. 1985. *Morphology: A study of the relationship between meaning and form.* Amsterdam and Philadelphia: John Benjamins.

Calvert, D. R. 1962. Speech sound duration and the surd-sonant error. *Volta Review* 64:101–2.

Camarata, Stephen, and Jack Gandour. 1984. On describing idiosyncratic phonological systems. *Journal of Speech and Hearing Disorders* 49:262–66.

Camilli, Amerindo. 1965. *Pronuncia e grafica dell'italiano.* Florence: Sansoni.

Caplan, David. 1987. Neurolinguistics and linguistic aphasiology. Cambridge: Cambridge University Press.

Carr, J. 1953. An investigation of the spontaneous speech sounds of five-year-old deaf-born children. *Journal of Speech and Hearing Disorders* 18:22–29.

Carrell, James A. 1968. *Disorders of articulation.* Englewood Cliffs, N.J.: Prentice-Hall.

Carroll, Lewis. 1961. *Alice in Wonderland* [1865]. London: Dent.

Carroll, Lewis. 1965. *Through the looking glass* [1871]. In *The Annotated Alice.* Harmondsworth: Penguin.

Castellani, A. 1956. Fonotipi e fonemi in italiano. *Studi di filologia italiana* 9:435–53.

Catford, J. C. 1977. *Fundamental problems in phonetics.* Bloomington: Indiana University Press.

Catford, J. C. 1988. Functional load and diachronical phonology. In *The Prague school and its legacy,* ed. Yishai Tobin, 3–20. Amsterdam and Philadelphia: John Benjamins.

Chomsky, Noam. 1951. Morphophonemics of modern Hebrew. M.A. thesis, University of Pennsylvania.

Chomsky, Noam. 1964. *Current issues in linguistic theory.* The Hague: Mouton.

Chomsky, Noam. 1966. Topics in the theory of generative grammar. In *Current trends in linguistics 3: Linguistic theory,* ed. T. Sebeok. Bloomington: Indiana University Press. Reprint, Janua Linguarum no. 56, The Hague: Mouton, 1968.

Chomsky, Noam, and Morris Halle. 1965. Some controversial questions in phonological theory. *Journal of Linguistics* 1, no. 2:97–138.

Chomsky, Noam, and Morris Halle. 1968. *The sound pattern of English.* New York: Harper & Row.

Clark, Eve. 1981. Lexical innovations: How children learn to create new words. In *The child's construction of language,* ed. W. Deutsch. New York: Academic.

Clark, Eve. 1982. The young wordmaker: A case study of innovation in the child's lexicon. In *Language acquisition,* ed. E. Wanner and L. R. Gleitman. Cambridge: Cambridge University Press.

Clark, Eve, and R. A. Berman. 1984. Structure and use in the acquisition of word formation. *Language* 60:542–90.

Clark, Herbert H., and Eve V. Clark. 1977. *Psychology and language.* New York: Harcourt Brace Jovanovich.

Cohen, A., and M. P. R. van der Broecke, eds. 1983. *Abstracts of the Tenth International Congress of Phonetic Sciences.* Dordrecht: Foris.

Cohen, Boaz. 1995. Phonology as human behavior: First language acquisition (in Hebrew). Department of Behavioral Sciences, Ben-Gurion University of the Negev. Typescript.

Cohen-Mimran, Ravit. 1992. The application of the theory of phonology as human behavior to phonological errors in Hebrew (in Hebrew). Department of Communication Disorders, Speech, Language and Hearing, Sackler Faculty of Medicine, Tel-Aviv University. Typescript.

Cohen-Mimran, Ravit. 1995. Acoustic and perceptual characteristics of esophageal and tracheoesophageal speech production (in Hebrew). M.A. thesis, Department of Communication Disorders, Speech, Language and Hearing, Sackler Faculty of Medicine, Tel-Aviv University.

Collins, Michael J. 1989. Differential diagnosis of aphasic syndromes and apraxia of speech. In *Acquired apraxia of speech in aphasic adults: Theoretical and clinical issues,* ed. Paula Square-Storer, 87–114. Hillsdale, N.J.: Erlbaum.

Compton, Arthur J. 1975. Generative studies of children's phonological disorders: A strategy for therapy. In *Measurement procedures for speech, hearing and language,* ed. S. Singh, 55–90. Baltimore: University Park Press.

Compton, Arthur J. 1976. Generative studies of children's phonological disorders: Clinical ramifications. In *Normal and deficient child language,* ed. Donald M. Morehead and Anne E. Morehead, 61–96. Baltimore: University Park Press.

Contini-Morava, Ellen. 1989. *Discourse pragmatics and semantic categorization: The case of negation and tense-aspect with special reference to Swahili.* Berlin and New York: Mouton de Gruyter.

Contini-Morava, Ellen, and Barbara Sussman Goldberg, eds. 1995. *Meaning as explanation: Advances in sign-based linguistics.* Berlin and New York: Mouton de Gruyter.

Cooper, H., ed. 1991. *A practical guide to cochlear implants.* London: Whurr.

Corona, Sharon. 1993. An analysis of a speech sample according to the theory of phonology as human behavior (in Hebrew). Department of Communication Disorders, Speech, Language and Hearing, Sackler Faculty of Medicine, Tel-Aviv University. Typescript.

Crary, M. A., and J. Fokes. 1980. Phonological processes in apraxia of speech: A systemic simplification of articulatory performance. *Aphasia, Apraxia, Agnosia* 4:1–13.

Crystal, David. 1980. *An introduction to language pathology.* London: Edward Arnold

Crystal, David. 1982. *Profiling language disability.* London: Edward Arnold.

Crystal, David. 1987. *Clinical linguistics* [1981]. 2d ed. London: Edward Arnold.

Culler, Jonathan. 1976. *Saussure.* London: Fontana.

Dale, P. S 1976. *Language development: Structure and function.* 2d ed. New York: Holt, Rinehart & Winston.

Daniloff, R. G., and J. R. Adams. 1985. Verbalizable knowledge of certain speech articulations. *Journal of Communication Disorders* 8:343–47.

Darley, Frederic L. 1964. *Diagnosis and appraisal of communication disorders.* Englewood Cliffs, N.J.: Prentice-Hall.

Darley, F. L. 1982. *Aphasia.* Philadelphia: W. B. Saunders.

Darley, F. L., A. E. Aronson, and J. R. Brown. 1975. *Motor speech disorders.* Philadelphia: W. B. Saunders.

Davidi, Shira. 1991. Naming problems from the point of view of the theory of phonology as human behavior (in Hebrew). Department of Communication Disorders, Speech, Language and Hearing, Sackler Faculty of Medicine, Tel-Aviv University. Typescript.

Davis, Joseph Clair, Jr. 1984. A combinatory phonology of Italian (Part I: Initial constriction to maximal aperture). M.A. thesis, Columbia University. Reprinted in *Columbia University Working Papers in Linguistics* 8 (1987): 3–100.

Davis, Joseph Clair, Jr. 1989. How a Columbia linguist does phonology. Paper presented at the First International Columbia School Conference on Linguistics, 24 August.

Délas, D. 1973. Phonétique, phonologie et poétique chez R. Jakobson. *Langue Française* 19:108–19.

Denes, Peter B., and Elliott N. Pinson. 1963. *The speech chain.* Bell Telephone Laboratories.

de Villiers, Jill G., and Peter A. de Villiers. 1978. *Language acquisition.* Cambridge, Mass.: Harvard University Press.

Devoto, Giacomo, and Gian Carlo Oli. 1967. *Vocabolario illustrato della lingua italiana.* 2 vols. New York: Funk & Wagnalls.

Diamant, Bilha. 1994. A phonological analysis of a hearing-impaired child according to the theory of phonology as human behavior of William Diver (in Hebrew). Department of Communication Disorders, Speech, Language and Hearing, Sackler Faculty of Medicine, Tel-Aviv University. Typescript.

Dinnsen, Daniel A., Steven B. Chin, Mary Elbert, and Thomas Powell. 1990. Some constraints of functionally disordered phonologies: Phonetic inventories and phonotactics. *Journal of Speech and Hearing Research* 33:28–37.

Diver, William. 1974. Substance and value in linguistic analysis. *Sémiotext(e)* 1, no. 2: 11–30.

Diver, William. 1975. Introduction. *Columbia University Working Papers in Linguistics* 2:1–20.

Diver, William. 1979. Phonology as human behavior. In *Psycholinguistic research: Implications and applications,* ed. D. Aaronson and J. Reiber, 161–98. Hillsdale, N.J.: Lawrence Erlbaum.

Diver, William. 1984. The grammars of Homeric Greek and classical Latin. Department of Linguistics, Columbia University. Typescript.

Diver, William. 1993. The phonology of the extremes: The correlation of initials and finals. Paper presented at the Third International Columbia School Conference on Linguistics, 11 October.

Diver, William. 1995. The theory. In *Meaning as explanation: Advances in linguistic sign theory,* ed. E. Contini-Morava and B. Sussman Goldberg, 43–114. Berlin: Mouton de Gruyter.

Dizionario Garzanti della lingu italiana. 1977. Rome: Aldo Garzanti.

Dodd, B. 1975. Recognition and reproductions of words by Down's syndrome and non-Down's retarded children. *American Journal of Mental Deficiency* 80:45–69.

Dorman, Michael, Lawrence Raphael, Frances Freeman, and Charles (Yishai) Tobin. 1974. Vowel and nasal duration as perceptual cues to voicing in word-final stop consonants. *Haskins Laboratories Status Report on Speech Research,* nos. 37/38: 263–70.

Doron, Dana. 1995. Applying the theory of phonology as human behavior to the speech of a dyspraxic child (in Hebrew). Department of Communication Disorders, Speech, Language and Hearing, Sackler Faculty of Medicine, Tel-Aviv University. Typescript.

Dowell, R. C., L. F. A. Martin, Y. C. Tong, and G. M. Clark. 1982. A-12 consonant confusion study on multiple channel cochlear implant patient. *Journal of Speech and Hearing Research* 25:509–16.

Dressler, Wolfgang. 1988. A linguistic classification of phonological paraphasias. In *Linguistic analyses of aphasic language,* ed. Wolfgang U. Dressler and Jacqueline A. Stark, 1–22. New York: Springer.

Dressler, Wolfgang U., W. Mayertaler, O. Panagl, and W. Wurzel, eds. 1987. *Leitmotifs in natural phonology.* Amsterdam and Philadelphia: John Benjamins.

Dressler, Wolfgang U., and Jacqueline A. Stark. 1988a. Introduction. In *Linguistic analyses of aphasic language,* ed. Wolfgang U. Dressler and Jacqueline A. Stark, xi–xiii. New York: Springer.

Dressler, Wolfgang U., and Jacqueline A. Stark, eds. 1988b. *Linguistic analyses of aphasic language.* New York, Berlin, and Heidelberg: Springer.

Durand, Jacques. 1990. *Generative and non-linear phonology.* London and New York: Longman.

Edwards, M. L. 1974. Perception and production in child phonology: The testing of four hypotheses. *Journal of Child Language* 1:205–19.

Edwards, M. L., and B. Bernhardt. 1973a. Phonological analyses of the speech of four children with language disorders. Stanford University. Typescript.

Edwards, M. L., and B. Bernhardt. 1973b. Twin speech as the sharing of a phonological system. Stanford University. Typescript.

Edwards, M. L., and L. D. Shriberg. 1983. *Phonology: Applications in communicative disorders.* San Diego: College Hill.

Eibschitz-Levine, Carmit. 1994. The theory of phonology as human behavior: The analysis of the articulatory errors of an ataxic girl with cerebral palsy (in Hebrew). Department of Communication Disorders, Speech, Language and Hearing, Sackler Faculty of Medicine, Tel-Aviv University. Typescript.

Eibschitz-Levine, Carmit. 1995. The speech of an ataxic cerebral palsy child: Phonology as human behavior (in Hebrew). *Dibur u-Shmiya* (Speech and hearing disorders) 18:79–96.

Eisenson, J. 1972. *Aphasia in children.* New York: Harper & Row.

Elbert, M., and J. Gierut. 1986. *Handbook of clinical phonology.* London: Taylor & Francis.

Eling, Paul, ed. 1991. *Reader in the history of aphasia from Franz Gall to Norman Geschwind.* Amsterdam and Philadelphia: John Benjamins.

Elman, J., and J. L. McClelland. 1986. Exploiting lawful variability in the speech wave. In *Intervariance and variability in speech processes,* ed. J. S. Perkell and D. H. Klatt, 360–80. Hillsdale, N.J.: Erlbaum.

Ephrat, M. 1980. Prenominal *bkp* after a preposition (in Hebrew). *Leshonenu* 45: 40–55.

Even Shoshan, A. 1978. *Milon Xadash.* Jerusalem: Kiryat Hasefer.

Even Shoshan, A. 1988. *Milon Ivri Merukaz.* Jerusalem: Kiryat Hasefer.

Faber, A. 1983. On the origin and development of Hebrew spirantization. *Mediterranean Language Review* 4:53–78.

Faianas, Rachel. 1993. Phonological processes in a learning-disabled child (in Hebrew). Department of Communication Disorders, Speech, Language and Hearing, Sackler Faculty of Medicine, Tel-Aviv University. Typescript.

Feldman, Irit. 1994. Articulatory disturbances as an expression of phonology as human behavior (in Hebrew). Department of Communication Disorders, Speech, Language and Hearing, Sackler Faculty of Medicine, Tel-Aviv University. Typescript.

Fellman, J. 1973a. Concerning the "revival" of the Hebrew language. *Anthropological Linguistics* 15 (May): 250–57.

Fellman, J. 1973b. *The revival of a classical tongue: Eliezer ben-Yehuda and the modern Hebrew language.* The Hague: Mouton.

Ferguson, C. A. 1964. Baby talk in six languages. *American Anthropologist* 66: 103–14.

Ferguson, C. A. 1977a. Baby talk as a simplified register. In *Talking to children: Language input and acquisition,* ed. Charles Ferguson and Catherine Snow. Cambridge: Cambridge University Press.

Ferguson, C. A. 1977b. Learning to pronounce: The earliest stages of phonological development in the child. In *Communication and cognitive abilities: Early behavioral assessment,* ed. F. D. Minifie and L. L. Lloyd. Baltimore: University Park Press.

Ferguson, C. A., and C. Farwell. 1975. Words and sounds in early language acquisition: English consonants in the first 50 words. *Language* 51:419–39.

Ferguson, C. A., and O. K. Garnica. 1975. Theories of phonological development. In *Foundations of language development: A multidisciplinary approach,* vol. 1, ed. E. H. Lennenberg and E. Lennenberg. New York: Academic.

Fingleh, Bili. 1995. Phonology as human behavior in a case of a severe hearing loss (in Hebrew). Department of Communication Disorders, Speech, Language and Hearing, Sackler Faculty of Medicine, Tel-Aviv University. Typescript.

Fischler, Ben-Ziyon. 1975. Unlicensed *bkp* in Israeli Hebrew (in Hebrew). In *A tribute to Kodesh,* ed. U. Ornan and B.-Z. Fischler. Jerusalem: Council on the Teaching of Hebrew.

Fisherman, A. 1985. Foreign words in Hebrew: A sociolinguistic description (in Hebrew). Ph.D. diss., Hebrew University in Jerusalem.

Fletcher, P., and M. Garman, eds. 1979. *Language acquisition: Studies in first language development.* Cambridge: Cambridge University Press.

Fomgrin, Vered. 1995. Phonology as human behavior: A case study of late language development (in Hebrew). Department of Communication Disorders, Speech, Language and Hearing, Sackler Faculty of Medicine, Tel-Aviv University. Typescript.

Fowles, John. 1984. *The ebony tower.* London: Jonathan Cape.

Fraser, W. I. 1978. Speech and language development of children with Down's syndrome. *Developmental Medicine and Child Neurology* 20:106–8.

Friedrich, F. J., et al. 1984. Interruption of phonological coding in conduction aphasia. *Brain and Language* 22:266–91.

Fry, D. B. 1966. The development of the phonological system in the normal and deaf child. In *The genesis of language,* ed. F. Smith and G. Miller, 187–206. Cambridge, Mass.: MIT Press.

Fujimara, O. 1962. Analysis of nasal consonants. *Journal of the Acoustic Society of America* 34:1865–75.

Gabai, Edna. 1993. Analyses of the speech errors made in audiological evaluations according to the theory of phonology as human behavior (in Hebrew). Department of Communication Disorders, Speech, Language and Hearing, Sackler Faculty of Medicine, Tel-Aviv University. Typescript.

Gal, Efrat. 1993. Identifying the voices of identical twins by blind and seeing listeners (in Hebrew). Department of Communication Disorders, Speech, Language and Hearing, Sackler Faculty of Medicine, Tel-Aviv University. Typescript.

Galpaz, Na'ama. 1995. A clinical discussion and application of the theory of phonology as human behavior (in Hebrew). Department of Communication Disorders, Speech, Language and Hearing, Sackler Faculty of Medicine, Tel-Aviv University. Typescript.

Gan, Romi. 1994. Phonological processes in bilingual children (in Hebrew). Department of Communication Disorders, Speech, Language and Hearing, Sackler Faculty of Medicine, Tel-Aviv University. Typescript.

Gan, Romi. 1995. Phonology as human behavior: The phonological development of bilingual children (in Hebrew). *Dibur u-Shmiya* (Speech and hearing disorders) 18:51–62.

Gan, Romi, Ruth Ezrati, and Yishai Tobin. 1995. The phonological acquisition of Hebrew-English bilingual children: Phonology as human behavior. Paper presented at the International Conference on Bilingualism, Haifa University, 14 July.

Gandour, A., et al. 1982. Case study of a Thai conduction aphasic. *Brain and Language* 17:327–58.

Gandour, A., and R. Dardarananda. 1984. Voice onset time in aphasia: Thai. II. Production. *Brain and Language* 23:177–205.

Garbell, I. 1959. The phonemic status of the schwa, the *Hatafim,* and *bkp* in Masoretic Hebrew (in Hebrew). *Leshonenu* 23:152–56.

García, Erica C. 1975. *The role of theory in linguistic analysis: The Spanish pronoun system.* Amsterdam: North-Holland.

Garfunkel, Shelli. 1989. Phonology as human behavior (in Hebrew). Department of Communication Disorders, Speech, Language and Hearing, Sackler Faculty of Medicine, Tel-Aviv University. Typescript.

Garfunkel-Aloufy, Shelli. 1992. Sex differences in lip-reading among native Hebrew and native English speakers (in Hebrew). M.A. thesis, Department of Communication Disorders, Speech, Language and Hearing, Sackler Faculty of Medicine, Tel-Aviv University.

Garnica, O. K. 1971. The development of the perception of phonemic differences in initial consonants in English speaking children. *Papers and Reports on Child Language Development* (Stanford University) 3:1–29.

Garnica, O. K. 1973. The development of phonemic speech perception. In *Cognition and the acquisition of language,* ed. T. E. Moore. New York: Academic.

Geschwind, N. 1965. Disconnection syndromes in animals and man. *Brain* 33:237–94.

Givón, Talmy, ed. 1979. *Syntax and semantics 12: Discourse and semantics.* New York: Academic.

Glinert, Lewis. 1989. *The grammar of modern Hebrew.* Cambridge: Cambridge University Press.

Glucksberg, S., and J. H. Danks. 1975. *Experimental psycholinguistics: An introduction.* Hillsdale, N.J.: Lawrence Erlbaum.

Goodglass, H., and E. Kaplan. 1983a. *The assessment of aphasia and related disorders.* Philadelphia: Lea & Febinger.

Goodglass, H., and E. Kaplan. 1983b. *Boston diagnostic aphasia examination.* Malvern, Pa.: Lea & Febinger.

Gorodisky, Orli. 1990. Phonology as human behavior (in Hebrew). Department of Communication Disorders, Speech, Language and Hearing, Sackler Faculty of Medicine, Tel-Aviv University. Typescript.

Gorup, R. J. 1987. *The semantic organization of the Serbo-Croatian verb.* Munich: Francke.

Greenberg, Joseph. 1950. The patterning of root morphology in Semitic. *Word* 6: 162–81.

Griffen, T. D. 1984. *Aspects of dynamic phonology.* Amsterdam and Philadelphia: John Benjamins.

Grossman, H. 1983. *Classification in mental retardation.* Washington, D.C.: American Association on Mental Deficiency.

Grunwell, Pamela. 1981. *The nature of phonological disability in children.* New York: Academic.

Grunwell, Pamela. 1982. *Clinical phonology.* 1st ed. London: Croom Helm.

Grunwell, Pamela. 1985. *Phonological assessment of child speech.* San Diego: College Hill.

Grunwell, Pamela. 1987. *Clinical phonology.* 2d ed. London: Croom Helm.

Grunwell, P., and S. Huskins. 1979. Intelligibility in acquired dysarthria: A neurophonetic approach. *Journal of Communication Disorders* 12:9–22.

Gunn, P. 1985. Speech and language. In *Current approaches to Down's syndrome,* ed. D. Lane and B. Stratford. New York: Praeger.

Gvion, Avia. 1989. An analysis of phonemic paraphasia in an aphasic patient (in Hebrew). Department of Communication Disorders, Speech, Language and Hearing, Sackler Faculty of Medicine, Tel-Aviv University. Typescript.

Hagège, Claude. 1993. *The language builder.* Amsterdam and Philadelphia: John Benjamins.

Hagoel, Yonit. 1993. Phonological aspects in the speech of a Down's syndrome child according to the theory of phonology as human behavior (in Hebrew). Department of Communication Disorders, Speech, Language and Hearing, Sackler Faculty of Medicine, Tel-Aviv University. Typescript.

Hall, Robert A., Jr. 1948. *Describing Italian grammar.* Ithaca, N.Y.: Cornell University Press/Linguistic Society of America.

Hall, Robert A., Jr. 1964. *Introductory linguistics.* Philadelphia and New York: Chilton.

Halle, Morris. 1959. *The sound pattern of Russian.* The Hague: Mouton.

Halle, Morris. 1977. Roman Jakobson's contribution to the modern study of speech sounds. In *Roman Jakobson: Echoes of his scholarship,* ed. D. Armstrong and C. H. van Schooneveld, 123–44. Lisse: Peter de Ridder.

Halperin, R. 1984. The phenomenon of phonological processes in the speech of Hebrew-speaking children from one and a half to three years of age (in Hebrew). Department of Communication Disorders, Speech, Language and Hearing, Sackler Faculty of Medicine, Tel-Aviv University. Typescript.

Halpern, Orly. 1991. Dynamic information in the identification and perception of vowels in adults: An experiment in cross-language (Hebrew-English) vowel perception influence on consonant-vowel transitions on vowel identifications (in Hebrew). M.A. thesis, Department of Communication Disorders, Speech, Language and Hearing, Sackler Faculty of Medicine, Tel-Aviv University.

Halpern, Orly. 1995. Phonology as human behavior: Hearing-impairment (in Hebrew). *Dibur u-Shmiya* (Speech and language disorders) 18:129–46.

Hamburger, Anat. 1992. An application of the theory of phonology as human behavior to the phonological system of a child with functional speech errors (in Hebrew). Department of Communication Disorders, Speech, Language and Hearing, Sackler Faculty of Medicine, Tel-Aviv University. Typescript.

Hannley, M. 1986. *Basic principles of audiological assessment.* Boston: Little, Brown.

Haran, Idit. 1989. A comparison of the speech of Hebrew and English in a bilingual child (in Hebrew). Department of Communication Disorders, Speech, Language and Hearing, Sackler Faculty of Medicine, Tel-Aviv University. Typescript.

Harkave, Alexander. 1988. *Yiddish-English-Hebrew dictionary* [1928, expanded 2d ed.]. With a new introduction by David Katz. New York: Yivo Institute for Jewish Research/Schocken.

Harmes, S. R., G. Daniloff, P. R. Hoffman, J. Lewis, M. B. Kramer, and R. Absher. 1984. Temporal and articulatory control of fricative articulation by speakers with Broca's aphasia. *Journal of Phonetics* 12:367–85.

Harshav, Benjamin. 1993. *Language in time of revolution.* Berkeley and Los Angeles: University of California Press.

Hebb, Donald O. 1966. *A textbook of psychology.* 2d ed. Philadelphia: Saunders.

Hedrick, D., E. Prather, and A. Tobin. 1984. *Sequenced inventory of communication development.* Seattle: University of Washington Press.

Hegde, M. N. 1991. *Introduction to communicative disorders.* Austin, Tex.: PRO-ED.

Herdan, Gustav. 1962. The patterning of Semitic verbal roots subjected to combinatory analysis. *Word* 18:262–68.

Herdan, Gustav. 1966. *The advanced theory of language as choice and chance.* New York, Heidelberg, and Berlin: Springer.

Heres, Nava. 1993. Phonology as human behavior: The theory and its application to a child with a severe hearing impairment (in Hebrew). Department of Communication Disorders, Speech, Language and Hearing, Sackler Faculty of Medicine, Tel-Aviv University. Typescript.

Hevron, Reut. 1995. Phonology as human behavior: First language acquisition (in Hebrew). Department of Behavioral Sciences, Ben-Gurion University of the Negev. Typescript.

Hewlitt, N. 1985. Phonological versus phonetic disorders: Some suggested modifications of the current use of the distinction. *British Journal of Disorders of Communication* 20:155–64.

Hildesheimer, Minka. 1989. Cochlear implants: Essence and application. Paper presented at the annual meeting of Israel Society of Speech Pathologists, Jerusalem, 12 February.

Himis, Rim. 1995. Comparing and contrasting two Palestinian Arab dialects: Phonology as human behavior (in Hebrew). Department of Communication Disorders, Speech, Language and Hearing, Sackler Faculty of Medicine, Tel-Aviv University. Typescript.

Himmel, Vardia. 1995a. The distribution of stuttering according to the theory of phonology as human behavior (in Hebrew). Department of Communication Disorders, Speech, Language and Hearing, Sackler Faculty of Medicine, Tel-Aviv University. Typescript.

Himmel, Vardia. 1995b. Phonology as human behavior: Stuttering (in Hebrew). *Dibur u-Shmiya* (Speech and hearing disorders) 18:97–104.

Himsworth, Harold. 1986. *Scientific knowledge and philosophic thought.* Baltimore: Johns Hopkins University Press.

Hodson, B. W., and E. P. Paden. 1981. Phonological processes which characterize unintelligible and intelligible speech in early childhood. *Journal of Speech and Hearing Disorders* 46:369–73.

Hodson, B. W., and E. P. Paden. 1983. *Targeting intelligible speech—a phonological approach to remediation.* San Diego: College Hill.

Hoffman, P. R., and G. H. Schuckers. 1984. Articulation remediation treatment models. In *Articulation assessment and treatment issues,* ed. R. G. Daniloff. San Diego: College Hill.

Hooper, Joan Bybee. 1979. Child morphology and morphophonemic change. *Linguistics* 17:21–50.

Hudgins, C. V. 1934. A comparative study of the speech coordination of deaf and normal subjects. *Pedagogical Seminary* 44:3–48.

Hudgins, C. V., and F. C. Numbers. 1942. An investigation of the intelligibility of the speech of the deaf. *Genetic Psychology Monographs* 25:289–392.

Hurwitz, Gila. 1993. An analysis of the errors in an audiological discrimination test of a subject with difficulties in speech perception (in Hebrew). Department of Communication Disorders, Speech, Language and Hearing, Sackler Faculty of Medicine, Tel-Aviv University. Typescript.

Hutt, M. L., and R. G. Gribby. 1973. *The mentally retarded child.* London: Allyn & Bacon.

Ingram, David. 1974. Phonological rules in young children. *Journal of Child Language* 1:49–64.

Ingram, David. 1976a. Current issues in child phonology. In *Normal and deficient child language,* ed. Donald M. Morehead and Anne E. Morehead, 3–27. Baltimore: University Park Press.

Ingram, David. 1976b. *Phonological disability in children.* London: Edward Arnold.

Ingram, David. 1979. Phonological patterns in the speech of young children. In *Language acquisition: Studies in first language development,* ed. P. Fletcher and M. Garman, 133–48. Cambridge: Cambridge University Press.

Ingram, David. 1981. *Procedures for the phonological analysis of children.* Baltimore: University Park Press.

Ingram, David. 1989. *Phonological disability in children: Studies in disorders of communication.* 2d ed. London: Cole & Whurr.

Irwin, O. 1942. The developmental status of speech sounds of ten feeble-minded children. *Child Development* 13:29–39.

Irwin, O. 1947. Infant speech: Consonantal sounds according to place of articulation. *Journal of Speech and Hearing Disorders* 12:397–401.

Isaacson, Ofra. 1995. Phonology as human behavior: Application to stuttering (in Hebrew). Department of Communication Disorders, Speech, Language and Hearing, Sackler Faculty of Medicine, Tel-Aviv University. Typescript.

Isan (Weinreb), Niva. 1991. An analysis of a cerebral palsy child according to the theory of phonology as human behavior (in Hebrew). Department of Communication Disorders, Speech, Language and Hearing, Sackler Faculty of Medicine, Tel-Aviv University. Typescript.

Isan (Weinreb), Niva. 1994. The phonetic characteristics in the speech of children with spastic cerebral palsy (in Hebrew). M.A. thesis. Department of Communication Disorders, Speech, Language and Hearing, Sackler Faculty of Medicine, Tel-Aviv University. Typescript.

Ivić, P. 1965. Roman Jakobson and the growth of phonology. *Linguistics* 18:35–78.

Izmailov, L. 1983. Phonological processes appearing in Hebrew-speaking children 3–4 years of age (in Hebrew). Department of Communication Disorders, Speech, Language and Hearing, Sackler Faculty of Medicine, Tel-Aviv University. Typescript.

Izre'el, S. 1986. Was the revival of Hebrew a miracle? or, The linguistic essence of the creation of modern Hebrew. Tel-Aviv University. Typescript.

Jabeen, Shazi Shah. 1993. Economy of articulation in the phonology of Bihar Urdu (as spoken in and around Gaya). Ph.D. diss., Aligarh Muslim University.

Jakobson, Roman. 1929. Remarques sur l'évolution phonologique de Russe. *Travaux du Cercle Linquistique de Prague* 2:161–83.

Jakobson, Roman. 1941. Kindersprache, Aphasie, une allgemeine Lautgesetze. *Uppsala Universiteits arsskift* 1:1–83. Translated as *Child language, aphasia and phonological universals.* The Hague and Paris: Mouton, 1968.

Jakobson, Roman. 1955. *Aphasia as a linguistic topic.* Monographs on Psychology and Related Disciplines. Worcester: Clarke University. Reprinted in *Selected writings,* 2:229–39 (The Hague: Mouton, 1971).

Jakobson, Roman. 1962a. *Selected writings,* vol. 1, *Phonological studies.* The Hague: Mouton.

Jakobson, Roman. 1962b. Why "mama" and "papa"? In *Selected writings,* vol. 1, *Phonological studies.* The Hague: Mouton.

Jakobson, Roman. 1971. *Studies on child language and aphasia.* The Hague and Paris: Mouton.

Jakobson, Roman. 1978. *Six lectures on sound and meaning.* Cambridge, Mass.: MIT Press.

Jakobson, R., G. Fant, and M. Halle. 1952. *Preliminaries to speech analysis.* Cambridge, Mass.: MIT Press.

Jakobson, R., and M. Halle. 1956. *Fundamentals of language.* The Hague: Mouton.

Jakobson, R., and M. Halle. 1962. Mufaxxama—the "emphatic" phonemes in Arabic. In *Selected writings,* vol. 1, *Phonological studies,* 510–52. The Hague: Mouton.

Jakobson, R., and M. Halle. 1968. Phonology in relation to phonetics. In *Manual of phonetics,* ed. B. Malmberg, 411–49. Amsterdam: North-Holland.

Jakobson, R., and L. Waugh. 1987. *The sound shape of language* [1979]. 2d ed. Berlin and New York: Mouton de Gruyter.

Jehudah, Na'ama. 1990. The theory of phonotactics in modern linguistics as it is expressed in the speech disorders of a child (4:6) (in Hebrew). Department of Communication Disorders, Speech, Language and Hearing, Sackler Faculty of Medicine, Tel-Aviv University. Typescript.

Jehudah, Na'ama. 1991. Vowel duration preceding stops as a cue to perception and production of voicing in word final position: A correlation between perception and production in Hebrew-speaking subjects (in Hebrew). M.A. thesis. Department of Communication Disorders, Speech, Language and Hearing, Sackler Faculty of Medicine, Tel-Aviv University.

Jerger, S., and J. Jerger. 1981. *Auditory disorders: A manual for clinical evaluation.* Boston: Little, Brown.

Jespersen, Otto. 1964. *Language: Its nature, development and origin.* New York: Norton.

John, J. E., and J. N. Howarth. 1965. The effect of time distortions on the intelligibility of deaf children's speech. *Language and Speech* 8:127–34.

Johns, D. A. 1969. Phonemics and generative phonology. In *Papers from the Fifth regional meeting of the Chicago Linguistic Society,* 374–81. Chicago: Chicago Linguistic Society.

Joos, Martin, ed. 1975. *Readings in linguistics.* Washington, D.C.: American Council of Learned Societies.

Kaddari, M. Z. 1983. Contemporary Hebrew: The state of the art (in Hebrew). In *Min Hasadna.* Jerusalem: Council on the Teaching of Hebrew.

Kantz, Helit. 1995. An attempt to apply the theory of phonology as human behavior to an autistic child (in Hebrew). Department of Behavioral Sciences, Ben-Gurion University of the Negev. Typescript.

Kaplan, Shirli. 1990. Phonology as human behavior and its application to the clinic (in Hebrew). Department of Communication Disorders, Speech, Language and Hearing, Sackler Faculty of Medicine, Tel-Aviv University. Typescript.

Karlin, I. W., and M. Strazulla. 1952. Speech and language problems of mentally deficient children. *Journal of Speech and Hearing Disorders* 17:286–94.

Katz, J. 1978. *Handbook of clinical audiology.* Baltimore: Williams & Wilkins.

Katz, Lilach. 1989. Phonology as human behavior: Functional disorders (in Hebrew). Department of Communication Disorders, Speech, Language and Hearing, Sackler Faculty of Medicine, Tel-Aviv University. Typescript.

Katz, Lilach. 1993. An analysis of the phonological errors of children according to the theory of phonology as human behavior (in Hebrew). M.A. thesis. Department of Communication Disorders, Speech, Language and Hearing, Sackler Faculty of Medicine, Tel-Aviv University.

Katz, Lilach. 1995. The theory of phonology as human behavior: a clinical application to functional articulatory problems (in Hebrew). *Dibur u-Shmiya* (Speech and language disorders) 18:63–78.

Kaye, Jonathan. 1989. *Phonology: A cognitive view.* Hillsdale, N.J.: Lawrence Erlbaum.

Keller, E. 1978. Parameters for vowel substitution in Broca's aphasia. *Brain and Language* 5:265–86.

Keller, E. 1981. Competence and performance in aphasia within a reference model of language. *Cortex* 17:349–56.

Keller, E. 1984. Simplification and gesture reduction in phonological disorders of apraxia and aphasia. In *Apraxia of speech,* ed. J. C. Rosenbek, M. R. McNeil, and A. E. Aaronson, 57–89. San Diego: College Hill.

Keller, Eric. 1988. The phonetic sciences as a pivotal science. *Phonetician* 47/48: 16–19.

Kent, Raymond D. 1990. *Intelligibility in speech disorders: Theory measurement and management.* Amsterdam and Philadelphia: John Benjamins.

Kent, Raymond D. 1992. Phonological development as biology and behavior. In *Processes in language acquisition and disorders,* ed. R. S. Chapman, 67–78. St. Louis: Mosby Yearbook.

Khan, L. M. L. 1982. A review of 16 major phonological processes. *Language, Speech and Hearing Services in Schools* 13, no. 2:77–85.

Kiparsky, Paul. 1982. *Explanation in phonology.* Dordrecht: Foris.

Kiparsky, Paul, and Lise Menn. 1977. On the acquisition of phonology. In *Language, learning and thought,* ed. J. McNamara. New York: Academic.

Kirsner, Robert S. 1979. *The problem of presentative sentences in modern standard Dutch.* Amsterdam: North-Holland.

Klein-Andreu, Flora, ed. 1983. *Discourse perspectives on syntax.* New York: Academic.

Koby, Edna. 1995. Final paper on late language development: Phonology as human behavior (in Hebrew). Department of Communication Disorders, Speech, Language and Hearing, Sackler Faculty of Medicine, Tel-Aviv University. Typescript.

Kohn, S. E. 1984. The nature of the phonological disorder in conduction aphasia. *Brain and Language* 23:97–115.

Kohn, S. E., P. Schoenle, and W. Hawkins. 1984. Identification of pictured homonyms: Latent phonological knowledge in Broca's aphasia. *Brain and Language* 22:160–66.

Kopold, Avigail. 1991. Phonology as human behavior: Apraxia (in Hebrew). Department of Communication Disorders, Speech, Language and Hearing, Sackler Faculty of Medicine, Tel-Aviv University. Typescript.

Koren, Ronit. 1991. Phonology as human behavior: Testing the theory on two autistic children (in Hebrew). Department of Communication Disorders, Speech, Language and Hearing, Sackler Faculty of Medicine, Tel-Aviv University. Typescript.

Kortser, Efrat. 1994. An analysis of articulatory errors in light of the theory of phonology as human behavior (in Hebrew). Department of Communication Disorders, Speech, Language and Hearing, Sackler Faculty of Medicine, Tel-Aviv University. Typescript.

Kotten, A. 1984. Phonematische und phonetische Probleme in Sprachproduktion und Rezeption für die Aphasietherapie. In *Sprachtherapie,* ed. V. M. Roth, 83–99. Tübingen: Gunter Narr.

Kurtz, Jael. 1992. Applying the theory of phonology as human behavior to two poems by Lewis Carroll. Department of English, Haifa University. Typescript.

Kutscher, E. Y. 1982. *A history of the Hebrew language.* Jerusalem: Magnes.

Lachner, R. J. 1968. A development study of language behavior in retarded children. *Neuropsychology* 6:59–73.

Ladefoged, Peter. 1982. *A course in phonetics.* 2d ed. New York: Harcourt Brace Jovanovich.

Lane, D., and B. Stratford, eds. 1985. *Current approaches to Down's syndrome.* New York: Praeger.

Lapointe, L. L., and R. T. Wertz. 1974. Oral-movement abilities and articulatory characteristics of brain-injured adults. *Perceptual and Motor Skills* 39:39–46.

Lavi, Shulamit. 1978. Norms in the development of Hebrew consonants for the ages of 3–5 years (in Hebrew). M.A. thesis. Department of Communication Disorders, Speech, Language and Hearing, Sackler Faculty of Medicine, Tel-Aviv University. Typescript.

Lebrun, Y. 1970. On the so-called phonemic pattern of language dissolution. *PICL* 10:703–7.

Lebrun, Y., L. Lenaerts, K. Goiris, and O. Demol. 1969. Aphasia and the concept of the phoneme. *Logopedie en foniatrie* 41:127–35.

Lecours, A. R., and F. Lhermitte. 1969. Phonemic paraphasias. *Cortex* 5:193–228.

Leonard, Laurence B., and Barbara L. Brown. 1984. Nature and boundaries of phonological categories: A case study of an unusual phonological pattern in a language-impaired child. *Journal of Speech and Hearing Disorders* 49:419–28.

Leopold, W. F. 1947. *Speech development of a bilingual child: A linguist's record.* Vol. 2, *Sound learning in the first two years.* Evanston, Ill.: Northwestern University Press.

Leopold, W. F. 1953. Patternings in children's language learning. *Language Learning* 5:1–14. Reprinted in *Child language: A book of readings,* ed. A. Bar-Adon and N. F. Leopold, 134–41. Englewood Cliffs, N.J.: Prentice-Hall.

Le Prevost, P. A. 1983. Using a Makoton vocabulary in early language training with Down's syndrome. *Mental Handicap* 2:28–39.

Lepschy, Giulio. 1970. *A survey of structural linguistics.* London: Faber & Faber.

Le Roy, Maurice. 1967. *The main trends in modern linguistics.* Translated by G. Price. Oxford: Basil Blackwell.

Lesser, Ruth. 1978. *Linguistic investigations of aphasia.* London: Edward Arnold.

Lesser, Ruth, and Lester Milroy. 1992. *Linguistics and aphasia: Psycholinguistic and pragmatic aspects of intervention.* London and New York: Longman.

Levenston, E. A. 1970. *English for Israelis.* Tel-Aviv: Israel Universities Press.

Levi, Oded, and Eti Kluck. 1995. Phonological aspects of aphasic patients (in

Hebrew). Department of Behavioral Sciences. Ben-Gurion University of the Negev. Typescript.

Levi, Ronit. 1992. Phonology as human behavior—an application of the theory to the errors of a child with a functional speech disorder (in Hebrew). Department of Communication Disorders, Speech, Language and Hearing, Sackler Faculty of Medicine, Tel-Aviv University. Typescript.

Levi, Sigalit. 1994. Phonology as human behavior: An analysis of the articulation of a child at the ages of 2:9 and 3:1 (in Hebrew). Department of Communication Disorders, Speech, Language and Hearing, Sackler Faculty of Medicine, Tel-Aviv University. Typescript.

Levinsky, Yom-Tov, ed. 1972. *A multilingual dictionary, Hebrew-Yiddish-English-French-Spanish-German-Russian.* Tel-Aviv: Adi.

Levitt, Harry. 1984. The phoneme: One of life's little uncertainties. In *Language and cognition: Essays in honor of Arthur J. Bronstein,* ed. Lawrence J. Raphael, Carolyn B. Raphael, and Miriam R. Valdovinos, 129–50. New York: Plenum.

Levitt, H., and R. Smith. 1972. Errors of articulation in the speech of profoundly hearing-impaired children. *Journal of the Acoustic Society of America* 51:102–3.

Liberman, Anatoly. 1988. Distinctive features in synchronic and diachronic phonology. In *The Prague school and its legacy,* ed. Yishai Tobin. Amsterdam and Philadelphia: John Benjamins.

Libo, Irit. 1989. Phonetics and phonology (in Hebrew). Department of Communication Disorders, Speech, Language and Hearing, Sackler Faculty of Medicine, Tel-Aviv University. Typescript.

Lightfoot, David. 1981. Explaining syntactic change. In *Explanation in lingusitics,* ed. N. K. Hornstein and D. W. Lightfoot. London: Longman.

Lightfoot, David. 1982. *The language of lottery: Towards a biology of grammars.* Cambridge, Mass.: MIT Press.

Lillywhite, H. S., and D. P. Bradley. 1969. *Communication problems in mental retardation: Diagnosis and management.* New York: Harper & Row.

Lindblom, B. 1986. On the origin and purpose of discreteness and invariance in sound patterns. In *Intervariance and variability in speech processes,* ed. J. S. Perkell and D. H. Klatt, 493–510. Hillsdale, N.J.: Lawrence Erlbaum.

Ling, D. 1976. *Speech and the hearing-impaired child: Theory and practice.* Washington, D.C.: Alexander Graham Bell Association for the Deaf.

Litowitz, Bonnie E., and Phillip S. Epstein. 1991. *Semiotic perspectives on clinical theory and practice.* Berlin and New York: Mouton de Gruyter.

Locke, L. J. 1983a. Clinical phonology: The explanation and treatment of speech sound disorders. *Journal of Speech and Hearing Disorders* 48:339–41.

Locke, L. J. 1983b. *Phonological acquisition and change.* New York: Academic.

Lowe, Robert. 1994. *Phonology: Applications to assessment and intervention.* Baltimore: Williams & Wilkins.

Mackay, L., and B. W. Hodson. 1982. Phonological process identification of misarticulations of mentally retarded children. *Journal of Communication Disorders* 15:243–50.

Macken, M. A., and D. Barton. 1979. The acquisition of the voicing contrasts in English: A study of voice onset time in word initial stop consonants. *Journal of Child Language* 7:41–74.

MacKenzie, C. 1982. Aphasic articulatory defects and aphasic phonological defect. *British Journal of Disorders of Communication* 17:27–46.

MacNeil, M. R. 1988. Aphasia in the adult. In *Handbook of speech-language pathology and audiology,* ed. N. J. Lass, L. V. McReynolds, J. L. Northern, and D. E. Yoder, 738–86. Toronto: B. C. Decker.

Magister, Sandro. 1984. Come si parla in Italia: La multilingua. *L'Espresso* (Rome) 30:36.

Manaster-Ramer, A. 1988. The phoneme in generative phonology and in phonological change. *Diachronica* 5:109–39.

Markides, A. 1970. The speech of deaf and partially-hearing children with special reference to factors affecting intelligibility. *British Journal of Disorders of Communication* 5:126–39.

Marquardth, T., and J. B. Reinhart. 1979. Markedness analysis of phonemic substitution errors in apraxia at speech. *Journal of Communication Disorders* 12, no. 6: 481–93.

Martin, F. N. 1990. Hearing and hearing disorders. In *Human communication and its disorders,* 3d ed., ed. G. H. Shames and E. H. Wiig, 350–93. Columbus, Ohio: Merrill.

Martin, F. N. 1991. *Introduction to audiology.* 4th ed. Englewood Cliffs, N.J.: Prentice-Hall.

Martinet, André. 1949. *Phonology as functional phonetics.* London: Oxford University Press.

Martinet, André. 1955. *Économie des changements phonétiques: Traité de phonologie diachronique.* Berne: A. Francke.

Martinet, André. 1960. *Elements of general linguistics.* Translated by A. Palmer. Chicago: University of Chicago Press.

McGarr, H. S., and R. Whitehead. 1992. Contemporary issues in phoneme production in hearing-impaired children and youth: Theory and practice. *Volta Review* 94, no. 5:26–59.

McNeill, D. 1970. The development of language. In *Carmichael's manual of child phonology,* vol. 1, ed. P. Mussen. New York: Wiley.

McReynolds, L. V., and M. Elbert. 1981. Criteria for phonological process analysis. *Journal of Hearing and Speech Disorders* 46:197–204.

McReynolds, L. V., and D. Engmann. 1975. *Distinctive feature analysis of misarticulations.* Baltimore: University Park Press.

McReynolds, L. V., D. Engmann, and K. Dimmitt. 1974. Markedness theory and articulation errors. *Journal of Speech and Hearing Disorders* 39:93–103.

Meckler, Tamar. 1995. Phonology as human behavior: Functional speech errors (in Hebrew). Department of Communication Disorders, Speech, Language and Hearing, Sackler Faculty of Medicine, Tel-Aviv University. Typescript.

Mendolowici, Anat. 1995. Applying the theory of phonology as human behavior to second language learning (Spanish/Hebrew) (in Hebrew). Department of Behavioral Sciences, Ben-Gurion University of the Negev. Typescript.

Menn, Lise. 1971. Phonotactic rules in beginning speech. *Lingua* 26:225–51.

Menn, Lise. 1976. On the origin and function of rules of child phonology: Interactionist-discovery theory and new evidence for it. Paper presented at the Child Language Research Forum, Stanford University.

Menn, Lise. 1980. Phonological theory and child phonology. In *Child phonology,* vol. 1, *Production,* ed. Grace Yeni-Komshian, James F. Kavanagh, and Charles A. Ferguson, 32–41. New York: Academic.

Menn, Lise, and Lorraine K. Obler, eds. 1989. *Agrammatic aphasia: A cross-language narrative source book.* Amsterdam and Philadelphia: John Benjamins.

Menyuk, Paula. 1968. The role of distinctive features in children's acquisition of phonology. *Journal of Speech and Hearing Research* 7:138–46.

Menyuk, P., and L. Menn. 1979. Early strategies for the perception and production of words and sounds. In *Language acquisition: Studies in first language development,* ed. P. Fletcher and M. Garman, 49–70. Cambridge: Cambridge University Press.

Menyuk, P., L. Menn, and R. Silber. 1986. Early strategies for the perception and production of words and sounds. In *Language acquisition,* 2d ed., ed. P. Fletcher and M. Garman, 198–222. Cambridge: Cambridge University Press.

Mierzejewska, H. 1977. *Afatyczna dezintegracja fonetycznej postaci wyrazów.* Wrocław: Ossolineum.

Migliorini, Bruno. 1966. *The Italian language.* Abridged and recast by T. Gwynfor Griffith. New York: Barnes & Noble.

Milgram, N. H. 1973. Cognition and language in mental retardation. In *The experimental psychology of mental retardation,* ed. D. E. Routh. New York: American Publishing Co.

Miron, Nitsan. 1990. The principles of phonology as human behavior in monosyllabic words in Hebrew (in Hebrew). Department of Communication Disorders, Speech, Language and Hearing, Sackler Faculty of Medicine, Tel-Aviv University. Typescript.

Mohr, J., M. Pessin, S. Finkelstein, H. Funkenstein, G. Duncan, and K. Davis. 1978. Broca's aphasia: Pathological and clinical aspects. *Neurology* 28:311–24.

Monoi, M., et al. 1983. Speech sound errors in patients with conduction and Broca's aphasia. *Brain and Language* 20:175–94.

Mor, Michal. 1992. The analysis of the speech errors of two five-year-old children according to the theory of phonology as human behavior (in Hebrew). Department of Communication Disorders, Speech, Language and Hearing, Sackler Faculty of Medicine, Tel-Aviv University. Typescript.

Morag, Shlomo. 1960. *beged kefet* times seven (in Hebrew). In *The Tur-Sinai book.* Jerusalem: Council on the Teaching of Hebrew.

Moran, J. M. 1986. Identification of Down's syndrome adults from prolonged vowel samples. *Journal of Communication Disorders* 19:387–94.

Morehead, Donald M., and Anne E. Morehead. 1976. *Normal and deficient child language.* Baltimore: University Park Press.

Morgenbrod, H., and E. Serifi. 1981. The sound structure of verb roots in modern Hebrew. *Journal of Linguistics* 17:11–16.

Moskowitz, A. I. 1970. The two-year-old stage in the acquisition of English phonology. *Language* 46:426–41.

Moskowitz, A. I. 1973. Acquisition of phonology and syntax: A preliminary study. In *Approaches to natural language,* ed. I. Hintikka et al. Dordrecht: Reidel.

Muljačič, Zarko. 1969. *Fonologia generale e fonologia della lingua italiana.* Bologna: Societa editrice il Mulino.

Muljačič, Zarko. 1970. Phonologie théoretique et phonétique. In *Roman Jakobson: Echoes of his scholarship,* ed. D. Armstrong and C. H. van Schooneveld, 309–20. Lisse: Peter de Ridder.

Muraoka, Takamitsu. 1992. Much ado about nothing? A sore point or two of Hebrew grammarians. *Journal of the Ancient Near Eastern Society "Ex Oriente Lux"* 32: 131–40.

Nakash, Nava. 1991. The speech errors of a girl (4:5) (in Hebrew). Department of Communication Disorders, Speech, Language and Hearing, Sackler Faculty of Medicine, Tel-Aviv University. Typescript.

Naro, A. J. 1978. A study in the origins of pidgination. *Language* 54:314–447.

Nelson, K. 1973. Structure and strategy in learning to talk. *Monographs of the Society for Research in Child Development,* vol. 38, nos. 1–2.

Neumann, Einat. 1992. An analysis of speech errors using the theory of phonology as human behavior (in Hebrew). Department of Communication Disorders, Speech, Language and Hearing, Sackler Faculty of Medicine, Tel-Aviv University. Typescript.

Norris, M., and J. Harden. 1981. Natural processes in the phonologies of four error-rate groups. *Journal of Communication Disorders* 14:194–213.

Northern, J. L., ed. 1984. *Hearing disorders.* 2d ed. Boston: Little, Brown.

Northern, J. L., and M. Downs. 1991. *Hearing in children.* 4th ed. Baltimore: Williams & Wilkins.

Nuyts, Jan. 1982. Een psycholinguistische benadering van de fonologische aspekten van afasie. *Antwerp Papers in Linguistics* 26:45–73.

O'Connor, J. D. 1973. *Phonetics.* Harmondsworth: Penguin.

Ohala, John J. 1981. Discussion. In *The cognitive representation of speech,* ed. T. Meyers, J. Laver, and J. Anderson, 373. Amsterdam: North-Holland.

Ohala, John J. 1983a. The direction of sound change. In *Abstracts of the Tenth International Congress of Phonetic Sciences,* ed. A. Cohen and M. P. R. van der Broecke, 253–58. Dordrecht: Foris.

Ohala, John J. 1983b. The origin of sound patterns in vocal tract constraints. In *The production of speech,* ed. Peter F. MacNeilage, 189–216. New York, Heidelberg, and Berlin: Springer.

Ohala, John J. 1983c. The phonological end justifies any means. In *Proceedings of the XIIIth International Congress of Linguists, August 29–September 4, 1982,* ed. S. Hattori and K. Inoue, 232–43. Tokyo: Sanseido Shoten.

Ohala, John J. 1984. Prosodic phonology and phonetics. *Phonology Yearbook* 1: 113–27.

Ohala, John J. 1985. Linguistics and the automatic processing of speech. In *New systems and architectures for automatic speech recognition and synthesis,* ed. R. De Mori and C. Y. Suen, 447–75. New York, Berlin, and Heidelberg: Springer.

Ohala, John J. 1986. Consumer's guide to evidence in phonology. *Phonology Yearbook* 3:3–26.

Ohala, John J. 1987. Experimental phonology. *Proceedings of the Annual Meeting of the Berkeley Linguistic Society* 13:207–22.

Ohala, John J. 1988. *The cognitive test of phonological analysis.* Berkeley Cognitive Science Report no. 53. Berkeley: Institute of Cognitive Studies, University of California, Berkeley.

Ohala, John J. 1990. There is no interface between phonology and phonetics: A personal view. *Journal of Phonetics* 18:152–72.

Ohala, John J., and Jeri J. Jaeger, eds. 1986a. *Experimental phonology.* Orlando, Fla.: Academic.

Ohala, John J., and J. J. Jaeger. 1986b. Introduction. In *Experimental phonology,* ed. J. J. Ohala and J. J. Jaeger, 1–12. Orlando, Fla.: Academic.

Ohala, John J., and James Lorentz. 1977. The story of [w]: An exercise in the phonetic explanation for sound patterns. *Proceedings of the 3rd Annual Meeting of the Berkeley Linguistics Society* 3:577–99.

Ohala, John J., and Manjari Ohala. 1986. Testing hypotheses regarding the psychological manifestation of morpheme structure units. In *Experimental phonology,* ed. J. J. Ohala and J. J. Jaeger, 239–52. Orlando, Fla.: Academic.

Oller, D. K. 1973. Regularities in abnormal child phonology. *Journal of Speech and Hearing Disorders* 38:35–46.

Oller, D. K., and R. Eilers. 1975. Phonetic expectation and transcription validity. *Phonetica* 3:13–29.

Oller, D. K., and C. A. Kelly. 1974. Phonological processes of a hard-of-hearing child. *Journal of Speech and Hearing Disorders* 39:65–74.

Oller, D. K., L. A. Wieman, W. J. Doyle, and C. Ross. 1976. Infant babbling and speech. *Journal of Child Language* 3:1–11.

Olmstead, D. K. 1974. Review of *The acquisition of phonology: A case study,* by Neil V. Smith. *Journal of Child Language* 1:133–38.

Olmstead, D. L. 1971. *Out of the mouths of babes.* The Hague: Mouton.

Ornan, Uzi. 1973. Regular rules and *bkp* phonemization. In *Readings in phonology,* ed. U. Ornan. Jerusalem: Hebrew University.

Osberger, M. S., and N. S. McFarr. 1983. Speech production of the hearing impaired. *Speech and Language* 8:221–83.

Othman Gabara, Rema. 1994. Phonology as human behavior: A case of stuttering in Arabic. Department of Communication Disorders, Speech, Language and Hearing, Sackler Faculty of Medicine, Tel-Aviv University. Typescript.

Owens, E., and D. K. Kessler, eds. 1989. *Cochlear implants in young deaf children.* Boston: College Hill.

Owens, Robert E., Jr. 1988. *Language development.* 2d ed. Columbus, Ohio: Merrill.

Peizer, D., and D. Olmstead. 1969. Modules of grammar acquisition. *Language* 45: 60–96.

Pel-Zalit, Tsafra. 1993. The analysis of the speech of a four-year-old girl according to the theory of phonology as human behavior (in Hebrew). Department of Communication Disorders, Speech, Language and Hearing, Sackler Faculty of Medicine, Tel-Aviv University. Typescript.

Penrose, L. S., and G. E. Smith. 1975. *Down's anomality.* London: J. & A. Churchill.

Perkell, J. S., and D. H. Klatt, eds. *Intervariance and variability in speech processes.* Hillsdale, N.J.: Lawrence Erlbaum.

Piaget, J. 1950. *The language and thought of the child.* Cleveland: World.

Piaget, J. 1970. Piaget's theory. In *Carmichael's manual of child psychology,* 3d ed., vol. 1, ed. P. H. Mussen. New York: Wiley.

Pickett, J. M. 1988. Some thoughts about the state of phonetics. *Phonetician* 47/48: 5–7.

Pilch, H., and R. Hemmer. 1970. Phonematische Aphasie. *Phonetica* 22:231–39.

Pitusi, Dani. 1995. A phonological analysis of Israeli slang (in Hebrew). Department of Behavioral Sciences, Ben-Gurion University of the Negev. Typescript.

Platzky, Rozanne. 1995. Applying Diver's theory to developmental phonology and stuttering. Department of Communication Disorders, Speech, Language and Hearing, Sackler Faculty of Medicine, Tel-Aviv University. Typescript.

Pollack, E., and N. S. Rees. 1975. Disorders of articulation: Some applications of distinctive feature theory. *Journal of Speech and Hearing Disorders* 35:451–61.

Pomorska, Krystyna, E. Chodakowska, H. McLean, and B. Vine, eds. 1987. *Language, poetry and poetics: The generation of the 1890s: Jakobson, Trubetzkoy, Majakovskij.* Berlin, Amsterdam, and New York: Mouton de Gruyter.

Postal, Paul. 1962. Some syntactic rules in Mohawk. Ph.D. diss., Yale University.

Postal, Paul. 1968. *Aspects of phonological theory.* New York: Harper & Row.

Powers, M. H. 1959. Functional disorders of articulation. In *Handbook of speech pathology,* ed. L. E. Travis, 837–75. New York: Appleton Century Crofts.

Prater, R. J. 1982. Functions of consonant assimilation and reduplication in the early words of mentally retarded children. *American Journal of Mental Deficiency* 86: 399–404.

Priestley, T. M. S. 1977. One idiosyncratic strategy in the acquisition of phonology. *Journal of Child Language* 4:45–66.

Propp, Vladimir. 1984. *Theory and history of folklore.* Translated by A. Y. and R. P.

Martin et al. Edited, with an introduction and notes, by A. Liberman. Minneapolis: University of Minnesota Press.

Rabin, C. 1974. *A short history of the Hebrew language.* Jerusalem: Jewish Agency.

Rabin, C. 1977. Acceptability in a revived language. In *Acceptability in language,* ed. S. Greenbaum. The Hague: Mouton.

Raphael, Lawrence, Michael Dorman, Frances Freeman, and Charles (Yishai) Tobin. 1975. Vowel and nasal duration as cues to voicing in word-final stop consonants: Spectrographic and perceptual studies. *Journal of Speech and Hearing Research* 18, no. 3:389–400.

Raphael, Lawrence, Michael Dorman, Charles (Yishai) Tobin, and Frances Freeman. 1974. Vowel and nasal duration in vowel-nasal consonant sequences in American English: Spectrographic studies. *Haskins Laboratories Status Report on Speech Research* SR 37/38:252–62.

Raphael, Lawrence, and Yishai Tobin. 1983. Perception and acoustic studies of voice onset time in Hebrew. In *Abstracts of the Tenth International Congress of Phonetic Sciences,* ed. A. Cohen and M. P. R. van der Broecke, 516. Dordrecht: Foris.

Raphael, Lawrence J., Yishai Tobin, Alice Faber, Tova Most, H. Betty Kollia, and Doron Milstein. 1995. Intermediate values of voice onset time. In *Producing speech: Contemporary issues: For Katherine Safford Harris,* ed. F. Bell-Berti and L. J. Raphael. Woodbury, N.Y.: American Institute of Physics.

Raphael, Lawrence, Yishai Tobin, and Tova Most. 1983. Atypical categories in Hebrew and Spanish. *Journal of the Acoustic Society of America,* suppl. 1, 74:89.

Rapoport, Sharon. 1994. An analysis of the articulatory errors of a 3:7-year-old boy according to the theory of phonology as human behavior (in Hebrew). Department of Communication Disorders, Speech, Language and Hearing, Sackler Faculty of Medicine, Tel-Aviv University. Typescript.

Ravid, Dorit. 1978. Word formation processes in modern Hebrew nouns and adjectives. M.A. thesis, Tel-Aviv University.

Ravid, Dorit. 1988. Transient and fossilized phenomena in inflectional morphology: Varieties in spoken Hebrew. Ph.D. diss., Tel-Aviv University.

Ravid, Dorit. 1991. Internal structure constraints on new-word formation devices in modern Hebrew. *Folia Linguistica* 24:289–347.

Ravid, Dorit. In press. Modern Hebrew spirantization and language change. *Mediterranean Language Review.*

Raz Harel, A. 1988. The articulation behavior of an apraxic child in light of the theory of phonology as human behavior (in Hebrew). Department of Communication Disorders, Speech, Language and Hearing, Sackler Faculty of Medicine, Tel-Aviv University. Typescript.

Recasens, Daniel. 1984. V-to-C coarticulation in Catalan VCV sequences: An articulatory and acoustical study. *Journal of Phonetics* 12:61–73.

Reid, Wallis. 1991. *Verb and noun number in English.* London and New York: Longman.

Rees, Ilanit. 1994. An analysis of articulatory errors according to the theory of phonology as human behavior (in Hebrew). Department of Communication Disorders, Speech, Language and Hearing, Sackler Faculty of Medicine, Tel-Aviv University. Typescript.

Rich, Shanit. 1994. An analysis of the articulatory errors of a 2:10-year-old girl based on the theory of phonology as human behavior (in Hebrew). Department of Communication Disorders, Speech, Language and Hearing, Sackler Faculty of Medicine, Tel-Aviv University. Typescript.

Ris, M. 1994. Phonology as human behavior: Language retrieval (in Hebrew). Department of Communication Disorders, Speech, Language and Hearing, Sackler Faculty of Medicine, Tel-Aviv University. Typescript.

Roach, Peter. 1983. *English phonetics and phonology: A practical course.* Cambridge: Cambridge University Press.

Roeser, R. J. 1986. *Diagnostic audiology: The PRO-ED studies in communicative disorders.* Austin, Tex.: PRO-ED.

Rosén, Haiim. 1953. Spoken Hebrew phenomena (in Hebrew). *Leshonenu La'Am* 3: 3–32.

Rosén, Haiim. 1977. *Contemporary Hebrew.* The Hague: Mouton.

Rosenthal, Naomi. 1995. Analyzing the dialect of Rio de Janeiro according to the theory of phonology as human behavior (in Hebrew). Department of Communication Disorders, Speech, Language and Hearing, Sackler Faculty of Medicine, Tel-Aviv University. Typescript.

Rothschild, Zviya. 1992. Phonology as human behavior—theory and application (in Hebrew). Department of Communication Disorders, Speech, Language and Hearing, Sackler Faculty of Medicine, Tel-Aviv University. Typescript.

Rovel, Jehudit. 1990. An analysis of the errors in a speech discrimination test (in Hebrew). Department of Communication Disorders, Speech, Language and Hearing, Sackler Faculty of Medicine, Tel-Aviv University. Typescript.

Rubinshtein, Eliezer. 1981. *Modern Hebrew and ancient Hebrew.* Tel-Aviv: Israel Ministry of Defense Publishing House.

Sadka, Yair. 1995a. An analysis of slips of the tongue according to the theory of phonology as human behavior (in Hebrew). Department of Behavioral Sciences, Ben-Gurion University of the Negev. Typescript.

Sadka, Yair. 1995b. Porno . . . : Phonology as human behavior and sri . . . slips of the tongue (in Hebrew). *Dibur u-Shmiya* (Speech and hearing disorders) 18:159–73.

Salus, P. H., and M. W. Salus. 1974. Developmental neurophysiology and phonological acquisition order. *Language* 50:151–60.

Samet, Mirit. 1993. An analysis of the speech of a hearing child (2:8) of deaf parents according to the theory of phonology as human behavior (in Hebrew). Department of Communication Disorders, Speech, Language and Hearing, Sackler Faculty of Medicine, Tel-Aviv University. Typescript.

Sampson, Geoffrey. 1980. *Schools of linguistics.* Stanford, Calif.: Stanford University Press.

Sander, E. K. 1961. When are speech sounds learned? *Journal of Speech and Hearing Disorders* 37:55–63.

Sangster, R. B. 1982. *Roman Jakobson and beyond.* The Hague: Mouton.

Sapir, Edward. 1921. *Language.* New York: Harcourt, Brace & World.

Sapir, Edward. 1933. La realité psychologique des phonèmes. *Journal de psychologie normale et pathologique* 30:247–65.

Saussure, Ferdinand de. 1966. *Course in general linguistics* [1916]. Edited by C. Bally and A. Sechehaye, in collaboration with A. Riedlinger. Translated by W. Baskin. New York: Philosophical Library/McGraw-Hill.

Saussure, Ferdinand de. 1983. *Course in general linguistics* [1916]. Edited by C. Bally and A. Sechehaye, in collaboration with A. Riedlinger. Translated and annotated by Roy Harris. London: Duckworth.

Schane, Sanford A. 1971. The phoneme revisited. *Language* 47, no. 3:503–21.

Schecht, Tamar. 1995. Phonology as human behavior: Theory and application (in Hebrew). Department of Communication Disorders, Speech, Language and Hearing, Sackler Faculty of Medicine, Tel-Aviv University. Typescript.

Schlanger, B. 1953a. Speech examination of a group of institutionalized mentally handicapped children. *Journal of Speech and Hearing Disorders* 18:339–49.

Schlanger, B. 1953b. Speech measurements of institutionalized mentally handicapped children. *American Journal of Mental Deficiency* 58:114–22.

Schlanger, B. 1973. *Mental retardation.* Indianapolis: Merrill.

Schmelz, U., and R. Bachi. 1973. Hebrew as the daily spoken language of Jews in Israel (in Hebrew). *Leshonenu* 37:50–68, 187–201.

Schwartz, Richard. 1992a. Clinical applications of advances in phonological theory. Paper presented at the Department of Communication Disorders, Speech, Language and Hearing, Sackler Faculty of Medicine, Tel-Aviv University.

Schwartz, Richard. 1992b. Nonlinear phonology as a framework for phonological acquisition. In *Child talk: Processes in language acquisition and disorders,* ed. R. Chapman, 108–24. Chicago: Mosby Yearbook.

Schwartz, Richard. 1992c. Recent advances in phonological theory: Clinical applications. Paper presented at the meeting of the American Speech and Hearing Association, 13 October. Atlanta.

Schwartz, Richard, Katherine S. Harris, and Tova M. Most. 1993. Speech, language, and hearing in Israel. American Journal of Speech and Language Pathology. (September): 5–7.

Schwarzwald, Ora Rodrigue. 1976. Theoretical and concrete methods in the analysis of *beged kefet* in Hebrew (in Hebrew). *Leshonenu* 40:211–32.

Schwarzwald, Ora Rodrigue. 1980. Normativity and naturalness in a morphophonemic rule in modern Hebrew. In *Bar-Ilan University yearbook.* Ramat-Gan: Bar-Ilan University Press.

Schwarzwald, Ora Rodrigue. 1981. *Grammar and reality in the Hebrew verb* (in Hebrew). Ramat-Gan: Bar-Ilan University Press.

Schwarzwald, Ora Rodrigue. 1986. Hebrew grammar: Wishful thinking. Bulletin of Hebrew and Hebrew Education 1, no. 2:7–14.

Segal, Elna. 1995. Phonology as human behavior: The theory and its application (in Hebrew). Department of Communication Disorders, Speech, Language and Hearing, Sackler Faculty of Medicine, Tel-Aviv University. Typescript.

Segal, Haviva. 1990. Phonology as human behavior (in Hebrew). Department of Communication Disorders, Speech, Language and Hearing, Sackler Faculty of Medicine, Tel-Aviv University. Typescript.

Segal, Iris. 1992. An analysis of the language of a mentally retarded girl according to the principles of the theory of phonology as human behavior (in Hebrew). Department of Communication Disorders, Speech, Language and Hearing, Sackler Faculty of Medicine, Tel-Aviv University. Typescript.

Segal, Orna. 1993. An analysis of language development in the preverbal phase according to the theory of phonology as human behavior (in Hebrew). Department of Communication Disorders, Speech, Language and Hearing, Sackler Faculty of Medicine, Tel-Aviv University. Typescript.

Segal Friedenreich, Asnat. 1992. An analysis of the errors of a child suffering from developmental dyspraxia according to the theory of phonology as human behavior (in Hebrew). Department of Communication Disorders, Speech, Language and Hearing, Sackler Faculty of Medicine, Tel-Aviv University. Typescript.

Segev, Einat. 1993. An analysis of the speech patterns of an apraxic child according to the principles of the theory of phonology as human behavior (in Hebrew). Department of Communication Disorders, Speech, Language and Hearing, Sackler Faculty of Medicine, Tel-Aviv University. Typescript.

Seltzer, Nitsa. 1992. Phonological aspects in the speech of a child suffering from developmental dysphasia according to the theory of phonology as human behavior (in Hebrew). Department of Communication Disorders, Speech, Language and Hearing, Sackler Faculty of Medicine, Tel-Aviv University. Typescript.

Shachar, Na'ama. 1990. The sensorimotor ability of children unable to produce voiced stops in word-initial position. M.A. thesis, Department of Communication Disorders, Speech, Language and Hearing, Sackler Faculty of Medicine, Tel-Aviv University. Typescript.

Shaked, Galia. 1990. Early phonological development: Phonological processes in children 1:7–2:7-years-old (in Hebrew). M.A. thesis, Department of Communication Disorders, Speech, Language and Hearing, Sackler Faculty of Medicine, Tel-Aviv University. Typescript.

Shamir, Rachel. 1994. Phonology as human behavior: A case of developmental oral dyspraxia (in Hebrew). Department of Communication Disorders, Speech, Language and Hearing, Sackler Faculty of Medicine, Tel-Aviv University. Typescript.

Shannon, C. E., and W. Weaver. 1949. *The mathematical theory of communication.* Urbana: University of Illinois Press.

Shapiro, Michael, and Marianne Shapiro. 1988. *Figuration in verbal art.* Princeton, N.J.: Princeton University Press.

Sharabi, Gil. 1995. Phonology as human behavior: An application to Down's syndrome (in Hebrew). Department of Behavioral Sciences, Ben-Gurion University of the Negev. Typescript.

Sharoni, Rakefet. 1992. The theory viewing phonology as human behavior and its clinical application (in Hebrew). Department of Communication Disorders, Speech, Language and Hearing, Sackler Faculty of Medicine, Tel-Aviv University. Typescript.

Sharoni, Zohara. 1992. Phonology as human behavior (in Hebrew). Department of Communication Disorders, Speech, Language and Hearing, Sackler Faculty of Medicine, Tel-Aviv University. Typescript.

Shaulsky, Limor. 1994. Phonology as human behavior: The theory and its application (in Hebrew). Department of Communication Disorders, Speech, Language and Hearing, Sackler Faculty of Medicine, Tel-Aviv University. Typescript.

Shibamoto, J. S., and D. L. Olmstead. 1978. Lexical and syllabic patterns in phonological acquisition. *Journal of Child Language* 5:417–56.

Shinn, P., and S. Blumstein. 1983. Phonetic disintegration in aphasia: Acoustic analysis of spectral characteristics for place of articulation. *Brain and Language* 20: 90–114.

Shinter, N. 1993. Phonology as human behavior: Backing (in Hebrew). Department of Communication Disorders, Speech, Language and Hearing, Sackler Faculty of Medicine, Tel-Aviv University. Typescript.

Shipley, Kenneth G., and Julie G. McAfee. 1992. *Assessment in speech-language pathology.* San Diego: Singular.

Shvachkin, N. Kh. 1973. The development of phonemic speech perception in early childhood. In *Studies of child language development,* ed. C. A. Ferguson and D. Slobin. New York: Holt, Rinehart & Winston.

Sivan, Reuven. 1970. 80 years, 1890–1970 (in Hebrew). *Leshonenu La'am* 20:10–60.

Slobin, D. I. 1977. Language change in childhood and in history. In *Language learning and thought,* ed. J. MacNamara. New York: Academic.

Slobin, D. I. 1985a. Crosslinguistic evidence for the language-making capacity. In *The crosslinguistic study of language acquisition,* ed. D. I. Slobin. Hillsdale, N.J.: Lawrence Erlbaum.

Slobin, D. I., ed. 1985b. *The crosslinguistic study of language acquisition.* Hillsdale, N.J.: Lawrence Erlbaum.

Smit, A. B., and J. E. Bernthal. 1983. Voicing contrasts and their phonological implications in the speech of articulation disordered children. *Journal of Speech and Hearing Disorders* 48:114–18.

Smith, B. L. 1981. Explaining the development of speech production skills in young children. *Journal of the National Student Speech-Language-Hearing Association* 9:9–19.

Smith, B. L., and C. Stoel-Gammon. 1983. A longitudinal study of stop consonant production in normal and Down's syndrome children. *Journal of Speech and Hearing Disorders* 48:114–18.

Smith, C. R. 1975. Residual hearing and speech production in deaf children. *Journal of Speech and Hearing Research* 18:795–811.

Smith, Neil V. 1973. *The acquisition of phonology: A case study.* Cambridge: Cambridge University Press.

Smith, N. V. 1974. The acquisition of phonological skills in children. *British Journal of Disorders of Communication* 9:17–23.

Spradlin, Joseph E. 1963. Language and communication of mental defectives. In N. R. Ellis (ed.), *Handbook of mental deficiency.* New York: McGraw-Hill.

Spreen, O. 1965. Language function in mental retardation: A review. *American Journal of Mental Deficiency* 69:45–68.

Square-Storer, Paula, ed. *Acquired apraxia of speech in aphasic adults: Theoretical and clinical issues.* Hillsdale, N.J.: Lawrence Erlbaum.

Stampe, David. 1969. The acquisition of phonetic representation. In *Papers from the Fifth Regional Meeting of the Chicago Linguistic Society,* 443–54. Chicago: Chicago Linguistic Society.

Stampe, David. 1979. *A dissertation on natural phonology* [1972]. New York: Garland.

Steiner, Smadar. 1993. Final paper: Phonetics and phonology (in Hebrew). Department of Communication Disorders, Speech, Language and Hearing, Sackler Faculty of Medicine, Tel-Aviv University. Typescript.

Stoel-Gammon, C. 1980. Phonological analysis of four Down's syndrome children. *Journal of Applied Psycholinguistics* 1:31–45.

Stoel-Gammon, C., and C. Dunne. 1985. *Normal and disordered phonology in children.* Baltimore: University Park Press.

Strazulla, M. 1953. Speech problems of the Mongoloid child. *Quarterly Review of Pediatrics* 8:268–73.

Studdert-Kennedy, M. 1987. The phoneme as a perceptuomotor structure. In *Language perception and production,* ed. A. Allport, D. G. Mackay, W. Prinz, and E. Scheerer, 67–84. London: Academic.

Sturtevant, Edgar H. 1949. *The pronunciation of Greek and Latin.* 2d ed. Philadelphia: Linguistic Society of America/University of Pennsylvania.

Szende, T. 1976. Intra- and interlingual specifics in distributional phenomena. *Acta Linguistica Acadamiae Scientiarum Hungaricae* 26, nos. 1–2:67–76.

Szende, T. 1980. Defining the phoneme: Phenomenological aspects. *Acta Linguistica Acadamiae Scientiarum Hungaricae* 30, nos. 1–2:63–66.

Taler, Inbal. 1995. Stuttering—according to the theory of phonology as human behavior (in Hebrew). Department of Behavioral Sciences, Ben-Gurion University of the Negev. Typescript.

Teitelbaum, Riki. 1990. Phonology as human behavior applied to cochlear implants (in Hebrew). Department of Communication Disorders, Speech, Language and Hearing, Sackler Faculty of Medicine, Tel-Aviv University. Typescript.

Teitelbaum, Riki. 1995. An evaluation of the speech of deaf post-cochlear implant patients. M.A. thesis, Department of Communication Disorders, Speech, Language and Hearing, Sackler Faculty of Medicine, Tel-Aviv University. Typescript.

Templin, M. 1957. *Certain language skills in children: Their development and interrelationships.* Institute for Child Welfare Monograph no. 26. Minneapolis: University of Minnesota Press.

Téné, David. 1985. The historical unity of Hebrew (in Hebrew). In *Language Studies I,* ed. M. Asher. Jerusalem: Jewish Studies Institute/Hebrew University in Jerusalem.

Thass-Thinemann, T. 1973. *The interpretation of language.* Vol. 1, *Understanding the symbolic meaning of language.* New York: Jason Aronson.

Tobin, Yishai. 1981a. The biblical connection: Sociolinguistic problem of modern Hebrew to English translation. *Jewish Education* 49:40–44.

Tobin, Yishai. 1981b. Introduction. In *Little Tel-Aviv,* by Nathan Alterman, trans. Yishai Tobin. Tel-Aviv: Hakibbutz Hameuchad.

Tobin, Yishai. 1983. The role of morphology and morphophonemics in the development of transformational generative grammar from *Syntactic structures* to *Aspects of the theory of syntax. Language Forum* 9:117–38.

Tobin, Yishai. 1985. Two aspects of sign theory. *Bulletin CILA* 41:120–41.

Tobin, Yishai. 1986. Review of *Schools of linguistics,* by Geoffrey Sampson. *Lingua* 68:141–50.

Tobin, Yishai. 1988a. Phonetics versus phonology: The Prague school and beyond. In *The Prague school and its legacy,* ed. Yishai Tobin, 49–70. Amsterdam and Philadelphia: John Benjamins.

Tobin, Yishai, ed. 1988b. *The Prague school and its legacy.* Amsterdam and Philadelphia: John Benjamins.

Tobin, Yishai. 1988c. Review of *Language, poetry and poetics,* ed. Krystyna Pomorska et al. *Lingua* 75, no. 4:373–79.

Tobin, Yishai. 1988d. Two quantitative approaches to phonology: A contrastive analysis. In *Descriptio linguistica,* ed. H. Bluhme, 51–75. Tübingen: Gunter Narr.

Tobin, Yishai, ed. 1989. *From sign to text: A semiotic view of communication.* Amsterdam and Philadelphia: John Benjamins.

Tobin, Yishai. 1990a. A combinatory phonology of the Hebrew triconsonantal (CCC) root system. *La linguistique* 26:100–114.

Tobin, Yishai. 1990b. Principles for contrastive phonotactics: The Hebrew triconsonantal root (CCC) system a case in point. *Papers and Studies in Contrastive Linguistics* 26:137–53.

Tobin, Yishai. 1990c. *Semiotics and linguistics.* London and New York: Longman.

Tobin, Yishai. 1991. Review article: Comparing and contrasting grammars. *Studies in Language* 15, no. 2:423–52.

Tobin, Yishai. 1993a. *Aspect in the English verb: Process and result in language.* London and New York: Longman.

Tobin, Yishai. 1993b. Phonology as human behavior: Theoretical implications and clinical applications. Paper presented at the Third International Columbia School Conference on Linguistics, 11 October.

Tobin, Yishai. 1994. *Invariance, markedness and distinctive feature theory: A contrastive study of sign systems in English and Hebrew.* Amsterdam and Philadelphia: John Benjamins.

Tobin, Yishai. 1995a. Phonology as human behavior: Further applications. Paper presented at the Fourth International Columbia School Conference on Linguistics, 18 February.

Tobin, Yishai. 1995b. Introduction to special issue on phonology (in Hebrew). *Dibur u-Shmiya* (Speech and hearing disorders) 18:1–18.

Tobin, Yishai, ed. 1995c. Phonology as human behavior: Theoretical implications and cognitive and clinical applications (Special issue on phonology). *Dibur u-Shmiya* (Speech and hearing disorders) 18.

Tobin, Yishai, and Sima Segev. 1983a. The functional load of phonemes in modern Hebrew as cues for speaker identification: A pilot study of acoustic phonetic parameters. Research Report no. CID 83-11. Jerusalem: Department of Research and Development, Israel Ministry of Police.

Tobin, Yishai, and Sima Segev. 1983b. The functional load of phonemes in modern Hebrew as cues for speaker identification: A pilot study of articulatory phonetic parameters. Research Report no. CID 83-10. Jerusalem: Department of Research and Development, Israel Ministry of Police.

Tobin, Yishai, and Sima Segev. 1983c. The spectrographic method of voice identification: Theoretical and practical aspects. Research Report no. CID 83-9. Jerusalem: Department of Research and Development, Israel Ministry of Police.

Tobin, Yishai, and Sima Segev. 1984a. The Chomsky-Halle phonological feature system as potential parameters for spectrographic speaker identification: A pilot study. Research Report no. CID 84-02. Jerusalem: Department of Research and Development, Israel Ministry of Police.

Tobin, Yishai, and Sima Segev. 1984b. Roman Jakobson's distinctive phonological features as potential parameters for spectrographic speaker identification: A pilot study. Research Report no. CID 84-01. Jerusalem: Department of Research and Development, Israel Ministry of Police.

Tobin, Yishai, and Sima Segev. 1992. Identifying the voices of identical twins: An empirical forensic study using the spectrographic method of voice identification. In *Forensic sciences,* ed. C. Wecht, 20–35. New York: Matthew Bender.

Tobin, Yishai, and Norman Simms. 1988. Seeds of the pomegranate: A dual evaluation of Vladimir Propp (Review essay of Vladimir Propp's *Theory and history of folklore*). *Mentalities/Mentalités* 5, no. 1:4–13.

Tromer Uziel, Vered. 1992. The analysis of the phonological systems of twins aged 5:6 (in Hebrew). Department of Communication Disorders, Speech, Language and Hearing, Sackler Faculty of Medicine, Tel-Aviv University. Typescript.

Trost, J., and G. J. Canter. 1974. Apraxia of speech in patients with Broca's aphasia. *Brain and Language* 1:63–80.

Trubetzkoy, N. S. 1931. Die phonologischen System. *Travaux du Cercle Linguistique de Prague* 4:96–116.

Trubetzkoy, N. S. 1939. Grundzüge der Phonologie. *Travaux du Cercle Linguistique de Prague,* vol. 7.

Trubetzkoy, N. S. 1949. *Principes de phonologie.* Paris: C. Klincksieck.

Trubetzkoy, N. S. 1969. *Principles of phonology.* Translated by C. A. M. Baltaxe. Berkeley: University of California Press.

Tsatkin-Pessin, Helen. 1994. Phonology as human behavior: Phonological acquisition in Russian. Department of Foreign Literatures and Linguistics, Ben-Gurion University of the Negev. Typescript.

Tsuf-Mosisko, Racheli. 1993. An analysis of the speech errors of a hearing-impaired child (in Hebrew). Department of Communication Disorders, Speech, Language and Hearing, Sackler Faculty of Medicine, Tel-Aviv University. Typescript.

Tur-Sinai, N. H. 1954. The pronunciation of *beged kefet* in the history of Hebrew. In *The language and the book.* Jerusalem: Bialik Institute.

van Schooneveld, C. H. In press. Phoneme and morpheme and the sign nature of language. In *Invariance, markedness, distinctive feature theory and deixis: Toward a calculus of meaning,* in Edna Andrews and Yishai Tobin. Amsterdam and Philadelphia: John Benjamins.

Velten, H. V. 1943. The growth of phonemic and lexical patterns in infant language. *Language* 19:281–92.

Vihman, Marilyn May. 1976. From pre-speech to speech: On early phonology. *Papers and Reports on Child Language Development* 3:51–94.

Vihman, M. M. 1988. Later phonological development in articulation and phonological disorders. In *Articulation and phonological disorders in children,* 2d ed., ed. J. E. Bernthal and W. W. Bankson. Englewood Cliffs, N.J.: Prentice-Hall.

Vihman, M. M., C. A. Ferguson, and M. Elbert. 1986. Phonological development from babbling to speech: Common tendencies and individual differences. *Applied Psycholinguistics* 7:3–4.

Vihman, M. M., M. A. Macken, R. Miller, H. Simmons, and J. Miller. 1985. From babbling to speech: A reassessment of the continuity issue. *Language* 61:395–443.

Voiers, W. 1977. Diagnostic evaluation of speech intelligibility. In *Speech intelligibility and recognition,* ed. M. E. Hawley. Stroudsburg, Pa.: Dowden, Hutchinson & Ross.

von Bremen, V. 1990. A nonlinear phonological approach to intervention with severely phonologically disordered twins. M.A. thesis, University of British Columbia.

Walden (Peres), Z. 1982. The root of roots: Children's construction of word formation processes in Hebrew. Ph.D. diss., Harvard University.

Walgren, Ronit. 1989. The human and communication aspects in the speech of a hearing disabled child (in Hebrew). Department of Communication Disorders,

Speech, Language and Hearing, Sackler Faculty of Medicine, Tel-Aviv University. Typescript.

Wang, William. 1968. Vowel features, paired variables, and the English vowel shift. *Language* 44:695–708.

Waterson, N. 1971. Child phonology: A prosodic view. *Journal of Linguistics* 7: 170–221.

Weber, J. 1970. Patterning of deviant articulation behavior. *Journal of Speech and Hearing Disorders* 35:135–41.

Weiner, Frederick F. 1981. Systematic sound preference as a characteristic of phonological disability. *Journal of Speech and Hearing Disorders* 46:281–86.

Weir, Ruth. 1962. *Language in the crib.* The Hague: Mouton.

Weiss, C. E., H. S. Lillywhite, and M. E. Gordon. 1980. *Clinical management of articulation disorders,* 2d ed. St. Louis: C. V. Mosby.

Weissfer, Sarah. 1994. An analysis of the articulatory errors of a 3:6-year-old boy based on the theory of Diver: Phonology as human behavior (in Hebrew). Department of Communication Disorders, Speech, Language and Hearing, Sackler Faculty of Medicine, Tel-Aviv University. Typescript.

Weissman-Gordon, A. 1978. The patterning of root morphemes in biblical Hebrew. Department of Linguistics, Tel-Aviv University. Typescript.

Wertz, R. T., L. L. Lapointe, and J. C. Rosenbek. 1984. *Apraxia of speech in adults: The disorder and its management.* Orlando, Fla.: Grune & Stratton.

West, J. J., and J. L. Weber. 1973. A phonological analysis of the spontaneous language of a four-year-old hard-of-hearing child. *Journal of Speech and Hearing Disorders* 38:25–35.

Wetherby, A. M., D. A. Yonclas, and A. A. Bryan. 1989. Communication profiles of preschool children with handicaps. *Journal of Speech and Hearing Disorders* 54, no. 2:148–58.

Wexler, Paul. 1990. *The schizoid nature of modern Hebrew: A Slavic language in search of a Semitic past.* Wiesbaden: Otto Harrassowitz.

Wilde, Oscar. 1965. *The picture of Dorian Gray* [1891]. New York: Harper & Row.

Wilson, F. 1966. Efficacy of speech therapy with educable mentally retarded children. *Journal of Speech and Hearing Research* 9:423–33.

Winitz, Harry. 1969. *Articulatory acquisition and behavior.* Englewood Cliffs, N.J.: Prentice-Hall.

Winitz, H. 1975. *From syllable to conversation.* Baltimore: University Park Press.

Winitz, H. 1978. *Human communication and its disorders.* Norwood, N.J.: Ablex.

Yagev, Irit. 1996. Phonology as human behavior: Cleft palates (in Hebrew). Department of Communication Disorders, Speech, Language and Hearing, Sackler Faculty of Medicine, Tel-Aviv University. Typescript.

Yaves, Mehmet S. 1991. *Phonological disorders in children.* London: Routledge.

Yehene, Vered. 1994. Phonology as human behavior from an evolutionary point of view (in Hebrew). Department of Behavioral Sciences, Ben-Gurion University of the Negev. Typescript.

Yehene, Vered. 1995. Phonology as human behavior: An analysis of the development of memory systems from an evolutionary point of view (in Hebrew). *Dibur u-Shmiya* (Speech and hearing disorders) 18:19–36.

Yeni-Komshian, Grace, James F. Kavanagh, and Charles A. Ferguson, eds. 1980. *Child phonology.* Vol. 1, *Production.* Vol. 2, *Perception.* New York: Academic.

Yosef-Barak, Ofra. 1995. An analysis of the speech of a hyperactive, bilingual child with a language delay (in Hebrew). Department of Communication Disorders, Speech, Language and Hearing, Sackler Faculty of Medicine, Tel-Aviv University. Typescript.

Zeitchik, Ariella. 1992. The perception of auditory, visual and audio-visual sensitivity in the hearing impaired (in Hebrew). M.A. thesis, Department of Communication Disorders, Speech, Language and Hearing, Sackler Faculty of Medicine, Tel-Aviv University.

Zilberstein, Iris. 1994. Phonological aspects of the slurred speech of a child with a motor-tactile deficiency according to the theory of phonology as human behavior (in Hebrew). Department of Communication Disorders, Speech, Language and Hearing, Sackler Faculty of Medicine, Tel-Aviv University. Typescript.

Zipf, G. K. 1949. *Human behavior and the principle of least effort.* Cambridge, Mass.: Addison-Wesley.

Zonshain, Y. 1974. One-word utterances of Hebrew-speaking children aged 12 to 18 months (in Hebrew). M.A. thesis, Department of Communication Disorders, Speech, Language and Hearing, Sackler Faculty of Medicine, Tel-Aviv University. Typescript.

Zwirner, E. 1938a. Langue et parole en phonométrie. *Annu. Inst. Philol. et Hist. Orient et Slav.* 6:135–44.

Zwirner, E. 1938b. L'opposition phonologique et la variation des phonèmes. *Archiv für vergleichende Phonetik* 2:391–94.

Zwirner, E. 1963. New trends in linguistic research. In *Education in Europe Section IV—General—No. 2,* 47–98. Strasbourg: Council for Cultural Cooperation of the Council of Europe.

Zwirner, E., and Zwirner, K. 1970. *Principles of phonometrics.* Translated by H. Bluhme. Alabama Linguistic and Philological Series no. 1. University: University of Alabama Press.

Index

Aaronson, A. E., 333 n.2
Adams, J. R., 316 n.6
Afrikaans, 49, 118
Akamatsu, Tsutomu, 314 n.10
Albert, M. L., 298, 335 n.1
Alcalay, Reuben, 105, 110
Alfasa, Anat, 334 n.2
Ali, Latif H., 323 n.6
Allen, D. V., 239
Altmann, Gabriel, 89, 314 n.11
Amharic, 326 n.5
Amir, Ofer, 331 n.7
Andrews, Edna, 311 n.1, 315 n.1, 329 n.1
Ani, Betty, 285, 293–97, 335–36 n.1
Aphasia: apraxia and, 286, 290–92, 332 n.9, 333 n.2, 334 n.4; Broca's, 285, 286, 289–90, 292–97, 298–99, 303; conduction, 286, 291, 297–303; definition and classification, 284–85; linguistics, phonology, and, 285–87; paraphasia, 286–87, 288, 289, 298; phonetics vs. phonology, 287–90, 299, perseverations, 293, 295–96, 302
Aphek, Edna, 311 n.1
Arabic, 49, 118, 326 n.5, 327 n.9
Aramaic, 49, 110, 118, 127
Arce, Joaquin, 319 n.4
Arielli, Zev, 329 n.18
Aronoff, Mark, 137
Aronson, L., 335 n.5
Articulators: active articulators vs. passive receptors, xviii, 37–38, 59–85, 90–91, 97–106, 108–12, 178–79, 180–82, 190–94, 213–14, 316 n.6, 328 n.16; number of, xviii, 38–40, 63–66, 92–95, 108–9, 113–15, 183–84, 190–94, 213–14, 316 n.7, 317 nn.8; visible, 44–46, 66–68, 105–6, 117–18, 121, 214, 218
Atkinson, Martin, 176–79, 330 n.1
Audiology, 251–52, 270–79, 303, 332 n.9, 335 n.3
Azim, Abdul, 142, 321 n.18

Bachi, R., 326 n.6
Bailey, Ch.-J. N., 313 n.7
Bally, Charles, 313 n.8
Baltaxe, C. A. M., 14, 312 n.4, 314 n.10
Bangs, J., 240–42, 261
Bankson, N. W., 206–8, 217–18, 331 n.6
Bar-Adon, Aaron, 129, 192, 324 n.1
Bar-Lev, Ayala, 336 n.1
Barkai, Malachi, 130, 138
Barton, D., 331 n.5
Bates, E., 138
Beckett, Samuel, 210
BeGeDKeFeT, 113, 121, 125–44, 320–21 n.12, 321 n.1, 328 n.13
Ben Horin, Gadi, 130
Ben Yehuda, Eliezer, 324 n.1
Ben-Asher, Moshe, 130
Ben-Dor (Tamir), Avivit, 317 n.7, 331 n.5
Ben-Hayim, Z., 326 n.3
Benson, D. F., 298, 335 n.1
Berber, 326 n.5

Berg, Thomas, 313 n.7
Berko, Jean, 331 n.8
Berman, Ruth A., 125, 137, 138, 139, 192, 324–25 nn.1, 2, 32
Bernhardt, Barbara, 263–64, 333 n.1, 334 n.2
Bernholtz-Priner, Ronit, 24, 88, 112–18, 323–24 n.11
Bernthal, J. E., 207–8, 217–18, 331 nn.5, 6
Bess, F. H., 279, 335 n.3
Bierwisch, Manfred, 311 n.1
Bjorklund, David F., 333 n.1
Bleile, Ken, 231, 330 n.1
Bliss, S. L., 239
Bloomfield, Leonard, 55, 63, 312 nn.4, 6
Blount, B., 330 n.2
Blumstein, Sheila, 289–90, 291–92, 299, 335 n.1
Bodine, A., 231, 233, 236
Bolozky, Shmuel, 130, 137
Boone, D. R., 285
Borden, Gloria J., 334 n.1
Brain, Russel Sir, 333 n.2, 334 n.4
Braine, Martin D. S., 330 n.2
Bremen, V. von, 334 n.2
Bronstein, Arthur, 159
Brown, Barbara L., 333 n.1
Brown, J. R., 333 n.2
Brown, R., 331 n.8
Bruner, J., 330 n.1
Bryan, A. A., 231
Buck, C. D., 73, 78
Buckley, S., 232
Bukharian (Judaeo-Persian), 49, 118
Bulgarian, 49, 118
Burling, R., 330 n.2
Burt, C., 237
Byelorussian, 326 n.5

Calvert, D. R., 261
Camarata, Stephen, 333 n.1
Camili, Amerindo, 319 n.4
Canter, G. J., 336 n.1
Carr, J., 261
Carrell, James A., 216–17, 237–38, 258–60, 333 n.2, 334 n.4
Carroll, Lewis, xviii, 1, 123, 151–52, 329 n.3
Castellani, A., 319 n.4
Catalan, 49, 118
Catford, J. C., 59–60, 141–42, 313 n.9, 314 n.11, 319 n.1
Child phonology. *See* Developmental phonology
Chomsky, Noam, 48, 129, 304, 311 n.2, 312 n.6, 313 n.7
Clark, Eve, 138, 139, 175
Clark, Herbert, 175
Clinical organic disorders, 210–51, 263, 291, 303, 334 n.4; apraxia, 212, 215–21, 222–23, 249, 332 n.9, 333 n.2; ataxia, 332 n.9; autism, 332 n.9, 334 n.5; cerebral palsy, 332 n.9, 334 n.5; cleft palate, 332 n.9; Down's syndrome, 212, 230–37, 249; dysarthria, 216–17, 220, 249, 333 n.2; dysphasia, 221–22, 227–29, 334 n.4; dyspraxia, 212, 221–30, 332 n.9, 334 n.4; learning disabled, 332 n.9, 334 n.5; mental retardation, 216, 237–50, 332 n.9; tracheo/esophageal speech, 332 n.9
Clinical phonology, 173–74, 303–4; functional, 195–209, 215, 291, 303, 332 n.9, 334 n.4; naming (lexical retrieval), 220, 228, 332 n.9; stuttering, 332 n.9, 334 n.5
Cochlear implants, 251, 257, 279–83, 303, 335 n.5
Collins, Michael, 286, 292–93, 297–99
Columbia School, xvii, 3, 10, 25–28, 312 n.5, 315 nn.1, 2
Combinatory phonology. *See* Phonotactics
Competence vs. performance, 290–92, 311 n.2

Compton, Arthur J., 141, 199–200, 333 n.1
Consonant clusters, 34–42, 81–84, 106–18, 168–69, 227, 291, 327 n.8
Consonants emphatic, 108–9, 111–12, 131, 322 n.1
Contini-Morava, Ellen, 315 n.1
Cooper, H., 335 n.5
Crary, M. A., 211
Crystal, David, 141, 182, 185–86, 198–99, 200–1, 216, 222
Culler, Jonathan, 5
Czech, 49, 118

Dale, P. S., 175
Daniloff, Raymond G., 316 n.6, 323 n.6
Danish, 49, 118
Danks, J. H., 330 n.2
Dardarananda, R., 290
Darley, Fredric L., 217, 292, 333 n.2, 334 n.4
Davis, Joseph Clair Jr., 53–87, 88, 105, 112, 115, 133, 140–42, 183, 319 nn.1, 2, 4, 321 nn.15, 16, 18, 322 n.2
de Courtenay, Baudoin, 288
de Saussure, Ferdinand, vii, 3, 4, 6, 8–11, 23–24, 25–26, 55, 311
de Villiers, Jill G., 176–78, 182–83, 184–85, 330 n.1
de Villiers, Peter A., 176–78, 182–83, 184–85, 330 n.1
Délas, D., 312 n.4
Demol, O., 288
Denes, Peter, 147, 256
Descartes, René, 304
Description vs. explanation, 129–33, 206–9, 312–13 n.6, 319 n.1, 326–27
Developmental phonology, 173–94, 211, 215, 250, 303–4, 318 n.12; babbling vs. speech, 176–78, 256, 330 n.2, bilingual language acquisition, 192–93, 332 n.9; delayed language development, 194, 218, 223, 224, 230, 236, 239, 243; twins, language acquisition of, 334 n.2
Devoto, Giacomo, 321 n.13
Diamant, Bilha, 270
Dimmitt, K., 333 n.1
Dinnsen, Daniel, 333 n.1
Distinctive features, xviii, 9, 13–15, 33–46, 176–78, 184–85, 314 n.10, 329 n.1, 330 n.2, 333 n.1
Diver, William, xvii, xviii, 8, 10, 24, 25–48, 53–56, 69, 156, 162, 166–67, 193, 283, 308, 312 n.4, 316 nn.5, 6, 318 nn.11, 13, 321 n.18, 322
Dodd, B., 233
Dorman, Michael, 317 n.9
Dowell, R. C., 335 n.5
Downs, M., 335 n.2
Dressler, Wolfgang, 186, 284, 288–89
Dufriche-Desegenettes A., 313 n.7
Dunne, C., 330 n.1, 331 n.8
Dutch, 49, 118, 315 n.1

Economy of effort, 15–23
Edwards, M. L., 185, 263–64, 331 n.8, 333 n.1, 334 n.2
Eilers, R., 261, 263
Eisenson, J., 224
Elbert, M., 330 n.2, 331 n.6, 333 n.1
Elman, J., 313 n.7
Encoder and decoder, 21–23, 147–48, 169–70, 208–9, 290
English, xviii, 24, 33–46, 74, 80, 88–89, 93, 95, 142, 143, 152–69, 182, 192–93, 297, 303, 318 nn.10, 15, 326 n.4, 327 n.10, 328 n.14
Engmann, D., 333 n.1
Ephrat, Michael, 130
Esperanto, 49, 118
Estonian, 49, 118
Even Shoshan, Abraham, 90, 105
Ezrati, Ruth, 193

Faber, Alice, 128, 130

Fant, Gunnar, 13, 174
Farwell, C., 183, 199, 330 n.2
Fellman, Jack, 324 n.1, 326 n.6
Ferguson, Charles A., 183, 184, 199, 330 nn.2, 4
Fingleh, Bill, 335 n.4
Finnish, 49, 118
Fischler, Ben-Ziyon, 130, 138
Fisherman, A., 326 n.4
Fokes, J., 211
Fowles, John, 1
Frank, Yael, xx
Fraser, W. I., 231
Frei, Henri, 313 n.8
French, 49, 74, 118
Friedrich, F. J., 298, 335 n.1
Fry, D. B., 261
Fujimara, O., 323 n.8
Functional load, 313 n.9, 314 nn.10, 11, 319 n.1, 336 n.2

Gabai, Edna, 335 n.4
Gal (Korster), Efrat, 334 n.2
Gan, Romi, 192–93
Gandour, A., 290, 298, 335 n.1
Garbell, I., 128, 130
García, Erica C., 315 n.1
Garfunkel-Aloufi, Shelli, 44
Garnica, O. K., 177, 185, 330 n.2
Generative and postgenerative phonological theories, 173, 177–78, 184, 195, 210–11, 249, 311 n.3, 320 n.8, 326–27 n.8, 330 n.3, 331 n.6, 333
Geneva School, 313 n.8
Georgian (Grusinski), 49, 118, 326 n.5
German, 49, 61, 113, 288, 316 n.4
Gierut, J., 333 n.1
Gilbert, John, 333 n.1
Givón, T., 315 n.1
Glinert, Lewis, 125, 324 nn.1, 2
Glucksberg, S., 330 n.2
Godel, Robert, 313 n.8
Goiris, K., 288
Goodglass, H., 285, 286–87, 292–93, 297–98
Gordon, M. E., 333 n.2
Gorup, R. J., 315 n.1
Greek, 49, 74, 118, 318 n.13
Greenberg, Joseph, 90
Griffen, T. D., 313 n.7
Grunwell, Pamela, 187, 190–91, 195–200, 211, 217, 221–22, 287–88, 330–31 nn.3, 4, 8
Guillaume, Gustave, 315 n.1
Gunn, P., 231
Gvion, Avia, 285, 299–303, 335 n.1

Hagège, Claude, 304
Hagoel, Yonit, 233–36
Hall, Robert A. Jr., 49, 51, 315 n.10, 319 n.4
Halle, Morris, 13, 174, 180, 312 nn.4, 6, 314 n.10, 323 n.6
Halperin, R., 192
Halpern, Orli, 318 n.10, 331 n.7, 335 n.4
Hannley, M., 335 n.3
Haran, Idit, 193
Harden, J., 229
Harkave, Alexander, 112
Harmes, S. R., 289
Harris, Katherine S., 332 n.9, 334 n.1
Harshav, Benjamim, 324 n.1
Hawkins, W., 186, 289
Hearing impairment, 194–95, 251, 255–83, 303, 334 n.5, 335 n.3
Hebb, Donald O., 237–38
Hebrew, xviii, 24, 49, 87, 88–112, 116–21, 125–44, 299–303, 315 n.1, 317 nn.7, 8, 321 n.18, 328 nn.14, 15, 16, 330 n.5
Hedge, M. N., 298–99
Hedrick, D., 330 n.1
Hemmer, R., 289
Herdan, Gustav, 89, 90, 186
Heres, Nava, 270
Hewlitt, N., 331 n.6

Hildesheimer, Minka, 335 n.5
Himis, Rim, 49
Himsworth, Sir Harold, 304–5
Hodson, B. W., 211, 230, 231
Hoffman, Paul R., 207, 323 n.6
Hooper, Joan Bybee, 138, 142
Howarth, J. N., 261, 262
Hudgins, C. V., 261–62
Humes, L. E., 279, 335 n.3
Hungarian, 49, 118
Hurwitz, Gila, 335 n.4
Huskins, S., 217

Indo-European, 78, 126
Ingram, David, 175, 180–81, 182, 187, 195, 197, 202, 210–12, 330 nn.2, 3, 331 n.8, 334 n.1
Irwin, O., 240, 330 n.2
Isan (Weinreb), Niva, 221, 332 n.9, 333 n.2
Italian, viii, 24, 49, 53–87, 88–89, 93, 95, 98, 168, 303, 315 n.10, 318 nn.14, 15
Ivić, P., 312 n.4
Izmailov, L., 192
Izre'el, S., 129

Jabeen, Shazi Shah, 142, 321 n.18
Jaeger, J. J., 88, 123
Jakobson, Roman, xviii, xx, 9–14, 171, 173–84, 192, 195, 312 nn.4, 5, 313 n.6, 314 n.10, 315 n.1, 323 n.6, 330 nn.1, 2, 3
Jehudah, Na'ama, 317 n.7
Jerger, J., 335 n.3
Jerger, S., 335 n.3
Jespersen, Otto, 331 n.8
John, J. E., 261, 262
Johns, D. A., 313 n.7
Johnson, Samuel Dr., 1

Kaddari, M. Z., 326 n.3
Kalama Sutta, 305
Kaplan, E., 285, 286–87, 292–93, 297–98
Kaplan, Shirli, 270
Karcevskij, Serge, 10
Karlin, I. W., 239, 240, 242
Katz, J., 335 n.3
Katz, Lilach, 201–9, 214, 250, 331 n.6, 332 n.9, 333 n.1
Kavanagh, James F., 330 n.3
Kaye, Jonathan, 312 n.6, 313 n.7
Keller, E., 291, 336 n.1
Kelly, C. A., 261, 263
Kent, Raymond D., 173, 184, 313 n.7, 318 n.12, 332 n.8
Kessler, D. K., 279, 335 n.5
Khan, L. M. L., 330 n.3
Kilby, David, 176–79
Kiparsky, Paul, 129–31, 178
Kirsner, Robert S., 315 n.1
Klein-Andreu, Flora, 315 n.1
Klingon, 49, 118
Kluck, Esti, 336 n.1
Kohn, S. E., 186, 289, 298, 299, 336 n.1
Kopold, Avigail, 220, 332 n.9, 333 n.2
Kotten, A., 288
Kurtz, Yael, 165, 329 n.2
Kutscher, E. Y., 326 n.3

Lachner, R. J., 239
Ladefoged, Peter, 159, 319 n.5
Langue vs. *parole,* 4–6, 9–11, 19, 24, 311 n.2, 313 n.9
Lapointe, L. L., 333 n.2
Latin, xviii, 24, 49, 61–62, 72–75, 118, 133, 142
Lavi, Shulamit, 192
Le Roy, Maurice, 10, 16, 17, 18, 311 n.1, 312 n.4
Lebrun, Y., 288
Lecours, A. R., 289
Lehfeldt, W., 89, 314 n.11
Lenaerts, L., 288
Leonard, Laurence B., 333 n.1

Leopold, W. F., 175, 180, 183, 330 n.2
Lepschy, Giulio, 16–17, 311 n.1
Levenston, E. A., 331 n.7
Levi, Oded, 336 n.1
Levinsky, Yom-Tov, 112
Levitt, Harry, 85, 261, 313 n.7, 334 n.1
Lhermitte, F., 289
Liberman, Anatoly, xx, 4, 314 n.10
Lightfoot, David, 66–67, 129, 130, 138, 319 n.1, 326–27 n.8
Likes favored and differents disfavored, 36–37, 81–83, 107–9, 112–13, 168–69
Lillywhite, H. S., 333 n.2
Lindblom, B., 313 n.7
Ling, D., 334 n.1
Linguistic sign, 24–26, 311 n.3, 314 n.12, 315 nn.1, 2
Linguistic theories: cognitive, xviii; functional, xviii, 10–18, 177; structural, xviii, 4–18, 54–55, 175, 288–89, 311 n.1. *See also* Generative and post-generative phonological theories; Natural phonology; Sign-oriented linguistic theories
Lithuanian, 49, 118
Locke, L. J., 330 n.1, 331 n.6
Lorentz, James, 319 n.4
Lowe, Robert, 333 n.1

MacKay, L., 231
Macken, M. A., 331 n.5
MacKenzie, C., 287–88
MacNeil, M. R., 285
MacWhinney, B., 138
Magister, Sandro, 319 n.4
Manaster-Ramer, Alexis, 313 n.7
Manner of articulation. *See* Stricture and airflow; Stable vs. mobile
Markedness theory, 289–90, 291, 314 n.10, 329 n.1, 333 n.1
Markides, A., 261, 264
Marquardth, T., 218
Martin, F. N., 257, 279, 335 n.3
Martinet, André, xvii, xx, 3, 8, 15–18, 312 n.4, 314 nn.10, 11
Matthews, H., 123
McAfee, Julie G., 216, 220, 231, 256–57, 270–72, 279, 285
McClelland, J. L., 313 n.7
McFarr, N. S., 334 n.1
McGarr, H. S., 334 n.1
McNeill, David, 175
McReynolds, L. V., 331 n.6, 333 n.1
Menn, Lise, 174–76, 178, 180, 183, 199, 330 n.3, 331 n.5
Menyuk, Paula L., 199, 330 n.2, 331 n.5
Mierzejewska, H., 289
Migliorini, Bruno, 319 n.4
Milgram, N. H., 240
Miron, Nitsan, 24, 88, 106–12
Mohr, J. M., 293
Monoi, M., 299, 336 n.1
Morag, Shelomo, 130
Morgenbrod, H., 90, 318 n.13
Morphology, 136–39, 140–42, 312 n.6, 315–16 n.15
Moskowitz, Arlene, 330 nn.2, 3
Most, Tova, 317 n.8, 332 n.9
Muchnik, Hava, 335 n.5
Muljačič, Zarko, 312 n.4, 319 n.4
Muraoka, Takamitsu, 323 n.9
Mussen, P., 175

Naro, A. J., 138
Native speaker intuitions, 142–45, 311 n.1, 313–14 n.9, 314 n.13
Natural phonology, 184–95, 201–9, 211, 289–90, 330 n.3, 331 n.5
Natural processes: active articulators (apicalization, labialization), 188, 204–5, 214, 219–21, 229–30, 233–36, 273–79, 280–83, 295–96, 300–1; airflow (stopping, deaffrication, gliding, glottalization), 189–91, 205, 214, 224–26, 228–30, 233–36, 273–79, 295–96, 300–1; assimilation (velar, nasal,

labial), 188, 203, 214, 221, 230, 263, 264–65, 273–79); deletion (stressed syllable, cluster reduction), 187, 190–91, 194, 202–5, 219–21, 224–26, 228–30, 267–70, 273–79, 273–79, 281–83, 294–97; idiosyncratic, 189, 190, 196, 198–200, 205–6, 212, 229–30; metathesis, 191, 227, 278, 281, 293, 299, 303–4; number of articulators (devoicing, denasalization), 190, 202–5, 219–21, 229, 233–36, 262–63, 294–97; substitution (fronting, backing), 188–89, 204–5, 214, 218, 224–26, 230, 233–36, 281–83, 291, 294–97, 298, 299–302; syllable structure (reduplication, epenthesis), 187–88, 191, 202–3, 214, 224–26, 230, 248, 299, 302; vocalization, 188, 189–90, 205, 234, 242, 262–63, 265–66

Nelson, K., 180

Neologisms, 150–68, 195, 287, 298

Norris, M., 229

Northern, J. L., 335 n.3

Norwegian, 49, 118

Numbers, F. C., 261–62

Nuyts, Jan, 289

O'Connor, J. D., 51

Ohala, John J., vii, xvii, 3, 88, 123, 125, 143–44, 145, 173

Ohala, Manjari, 3

Oli, Gian Carlo, 321 n.13

Oller, D. K., 261, 263, 330 n.2, 333 n.1

Olmstead, D. K., 182, 331 n.8

Olmstead, D. L., 199, 330 n.2

Ornan, Uzi, 130

Osberger, M. S., 334 n.1

Owens, E., 279, 335 n.5

Owens, Robert E., 330 n.1

Paden, E. P., 211, 230

Peizer, D., 331 n.8

Penrose, L. S., 232

Phoneme vs. allophone, vxii–xviii, 6–8, 19–20, 100–5, 108–12, 128, 184–85, 206–7, 218, 223, 272, 288–90, 291–94, 314 nn.9, 10, 13, 314–15 n.14, 315 n.3, 331 n.6, 333 n.1

Phonetics vs. phonology, xviii, 1–24, 27–30, 66–86, 146–50, 184–87, 287–90, 299, 312 n.4, 313–14 n.9, 330–31 n.4

Phonotactics, viii, 33–47, 53–85, 91–118, 177–78, 185–95

Piaget, Jean, 210, 318 n.12, 330 n.2

Pickett, J. M., 255

Pilch, Herbert, 289

Pinson, Elliott, 147, 256

Pitusi, Dani, 329 n.18

Place of articulation. *See* Articulators: active articulators vs. passive receptors

Polish, 49, 118

Pollack, E., 331 n.6, 333 n.1

Pomorska, Krystyna, 311 n.1

Portuguese, 49, 118

Postal, Paul, 312 n.6

Powers, M. H., 197

Prague School, xviii, 8, 9–15, 16, 134, 177, 313 nn.7, 8

Prater, R. J., 231

Prather, E., 330 n.1

Prescriptivism, 126–27, 128, 324–26 n.2, 326 nn.4, 6, 327 n.9

Priestley, T. M., 198, 199

Provençal, 74

Rabin, Chaim, 129

Raphael, Lawrence J., xix, 317 nn.8, 9, 334 n.1

Ravid, Dorit, 128–44, 326 n.7, 328 n.15

Recasens, Daniel, 320 n.10

Rees, Norma S., 331 n.6, 333 n.1

Reid, Wallis H., 315 n.1

Reinhart, J. B., 218

Roca, Iggy, 176–79

Roeser, R. J., 335 n.3
Romanian, 49, 118
Romansch, 49, 118
Rosén, Haiim, 125, 129, 130, 324 n.1, 326 n.4
Rosenbek, J. C., 333 n.2
Rosenthal, Naomi, 49
Rothschild, Zviya, 270
Rovel, Jehudit, 272–79, 281–82, 335 n.6
Rubenshtein, Eliezer, 326 n.4
Rule opacity, 129–33, 319 n.1
Russian, 49, 118, 193, 326 n.5, 332 n.9

Samet, Mirit, 194–95
Sampson, Geoffrey, 48, 311 n.1, 313 n.7
Sander, E. K., 182
Sangster, Rodney, 315 n.3
Sapir, Edward, 55, 313 n.7
Sardinian, 49, 118
Schane, Sanford, 312 n.6, 313 n.7
Schlanger, B., 240
Schmelz, U., 326 n.6
Schoenle, P., 186, 289
Schooneveld, Cornelis H. van, xvii, xx, 313 n.6, 315 n.1
Schuckers, G. H., 207
Schwartz, Richard, 231, 332 n.9, 333 n.1
Schwarzwald, Ora Rodrigue, 128–30, 136–37, 322 n.4, 326 n.2
Sechehaye, Albert, 313 n.8
Segal, Haviva, 270
Segal, Iris, 243–50
Segal, Orna, 193
Segal-Friedenreich, Asnat, 224–26
Segev, Einat, 218–21, 332 n.9, 333 n.2
Segev, Sima, 314 n.10, 334 n.2
Seltzer, Nitsa, 227–29
Semiotics. *See* Sign-oriented linguistics
Serbo-Croatian, 49, 118, 315 n.1
Serifi, E., 90, 318 n.13
Shachar, Na'ama, 317 n.7, 331 n.5
Shaked, Galia, 191–92, 194
Shannon, C. E., 89
Shapiro, Marianne, 150
Shapiro, Michael, 150
Sharoni, Zohara, 270, 335 n.4
Shibamato, J. S., 199
Shinn, P., 289–90
Shipley, Kenneth G., 216, 220, 231, 256–57, 270–72, 279, 285
Shriberg, D., 333 n.1
Shvachkin, N. Kh., 177, 330 n.2, 331 n.8
Sign-oriented linguistics, 4–6, 311 nn.1, 3, 319 n.1
Silber, R., 331 n.5
Simms, Norman, 4
Sivan, Reuven, 129, 326 n.4
Slips of the tongue, 332 n.9, 334 n.5
Slobin, Dan, 138
Slovak, 49, 118
Smit, A. B., 331 n.5
Smith, B. L., 231, 233
Smith, C. R., 264, 334 n.1
Smith, G. E., 232
Smith, Neil, 185, 195, 199, 330 nn.2, 3
Smith, R., 261, 334 n.1
Spanish, 49, 74, 118, 315 n.1
Spradlin, Joseph E., 240
Spreen, O., 239
Stable vs. mobile, 34–36, 81–83, 107–10, 112–13, 141–43, 168–69, 280–83, 291, 320 n.6, 322 n.2, 323 n.10
Stampe, David, 190–91, 201, 211, 330 n.3
Stark, Jacqueline A., 284
Stoel-Gammon, C., 231, 233, 330 n.1, 331 n.8, 333 n.1
Strazulla, M., 231, 239, 240, 242
Stricture and airflow, 59–62, 90–91, 94–98, 117–18, 179–80, 183–88, 322 nn.1, 4, 323 n.10, 328 n.15, 335 n.7
Studdert-Kennedy, M., 313 n.7
Sussman Goldberg, Barbara, 315 n.1
Swahili, 315 n.1
Swedish, 49, 118
Syllables: number and stress, 152–55, 180–81, 182–84, 206, 213–14, 223–22;

syllable structure, 187–88, 206, 214, 223, 263, 293, 294–95
Synchrony vs. diachrony, xviii, 15–18, 23, 61–62, 90, 108–12, 251, 321 n.1, 326 n.3, 327 n.9, 329 n.17
Synergesis, xviii, 18–23, 119–20, 145–46, 150, 208–9
Szende, T., 312 n.6

Teitelbaum, Riki, 279–83, 335 n.5
Templin, M., 182
Téné, David, 129
Thass-Thinemann, T., 25
Tobin, A., 330 n.1
Tobin, Yishai, 4, 49, 89, 126, 193, 311 nn.1, 3, 312 n.5, 315 nn.1, 2, 317 n.8, 318 nn.11, 14, 15, 326 nn.2, 3, 328 n.14, 329 n.1, 334 n.2
Tromer Uziel, Vered, 334 n.2
Trost, J., 336 n.1
Trubetzkoy, Nikolai Count, xviii, xx, 10–14, 312 n.4, 314 n.10, 316 n.4
Tsatkin-Pessin, Helen, 193, 332 n.9
Tsuf-Mosisko, Racheli, 267–70
Tur-Sinai, N. H., 128, 131
Turkish, 326 n.5, 327 n.9

Ukrainian, 49, 118, 326 n.5
Universals (language, phonological), 178–82, 191, 319 n.1
Urdu, 142, 321 n.18

Velten, H. V., 175, 177, 180, 330 n.2
Vihman, M. M., 183, 330 nn.2, 3
Voice onset time (VOT), 39–40, 289–90, 317 n.8
Voiced and voiceless. *See* Articulators, number of

Walden, (Peres) Z., 192
Walgren, Ronit, 270
Walker, G., 239
Wang, William, 312 n.6
Waugh, Linda, 312 n.5, 313 n.6, 315
Weaver, W., 89
Weber, J. L., 241, 261
Weiner, Frederick, F., 333 n.1
Weir, Ruth, 330 n.1
Weiss, C. E., 333 n.2
Weissfer, Sara, 334 n.2
Weissman-Gordon, A., 90
Wertz, R. T., 333 n.2
West, J. J., 261
Wetherby, A. M., 231
Wexler, Paul, 326 n.4
Whitehead, R., 334 n.1
Wilde, Oscar, 150
Wilson, F., 240
Winitz, Harry, 331 n.6

Yehene, Vered, 313 n.7
Yeni-Komshian, Grace, 330 n.4
Yiddish, xviii, 24, 49, 112–20, 142, 168, 303, 321
Yonclas, D. A., 231

Zeitchik, Ariella, 44
Zipf, G. K., 20–21
Zonshain, Y., 192
Zwirner, Eberhard, 89, 312 n.4, 314 n.11
Zwirner, Karl, 89, 312 n.4, 314 n.11

Yishai Tobin is Professor of Linguistics
at Ben-Gurion University of the Negev, Israel.

Library of Congress Cataloging-in-Publication Data

Tobin, Yishai
Phonology as human behavior : theoretical implications and
clinical applications / Yishai Tobin.
p. cm.—(Sound and meaning)
Includes bibliographical references and indexes.
ISBN 0-8223-1808-3. — ISBN 0-8223-1822-9 (pbk.)
1. Grammar, Comparative and general—Phonology. 2. Phonetics.
3. Contrastive linguistics. 4. Language acquisition. 5. Speech
disorders—Diagnosis. 6. Language disorders—Diagnosis. I. Title. II. Series.
P217.T6 1997
414—dc20 96-13941
CIP